BONE

Volume 2 : The Osteoclast

BONE

Volume 2 : The Osteoclast

Brian K. Hall
Department of Biology
Dalhousie University
Halifax, Nova Scotia
Canada

CRC Press
Boca Raton   Ann Arbor   Boston

Library of Congress Cataloging-in-Publication Data
(Revised for volume 2)

Bone.

    Includes bibliographical references.
    Contents: v. 1. The Osteoblast and osteocyte -- v. 2. The osteoclast.
    1. Bones. I. Hall, Brian Keith, 1941- .
[DNLM: 1. Bone and Bones.   WE 200 B7113]
QP88.2.B58 1989 599'.01852   89-20391
ISBN 0-936923-24-5 (v. 1)
ISBN 0-8493-8822-8 (v. 2)

Developer: Telford Press

This book represents information obtained from authentic and highly regarded sources. Reprinted material is quoted with permission, and sources are indicated. A wide variety of references are listed. Every reasonable effort has been made to give reliable data and information, but the authors and the publisher cannot assume responsibility for the validity of all materials or for the consequences of their use.

International Standard Book Number 0-8493-8822-8

Library of Congress Card Number 89-20391

Printed in the United States

Contents

Preface

This is the second of seven volumes devoted to the biology of bone.The rational for the series was laid out in the preface to Volume 1, the volume that dealt with osteoblasts and osteocytes, the bone-forming cells. The present volume, which treats the bone-resorbing cell, the osteoclast, parallels Volume 1, in that structural, functional, biochemical, metabolic, molecular and clinical aspects of the osteoclast are integrated, and in that the organization of the chapters mirrors that of Volume 1.

As in Volume 1, a chapter by Marijke Holtrop begins the present volume, summarizing and analyzing the ultrastructural evidence both for the identification of osteoclasts as a separate cell type and for their bone-resorbing ability. Marijke particularly discusses the nature of the "ruffled border" which is so characteristic of osteoclasts and emphasizes interactions between osteoclasts and other cell types (chiefly osteoblasts) and between osteoclasts and their immediate environment. It is clear that we can no longer regard the osteoclast as a cell acting independently and/or in isolation.

The origin of the osteoclast remains enigmatic and our knowledge rudimentary in comparison with knowledge of the origin of the osteoblast. Elizabeth Burger and Peter Nijweide discuss theories of the cellular origins of the osteoclast in chapter 2. The importance for osteoclast function of the immediate microenvironment, a concept introduced in chapter 1 on the basis of structural analysis, is reinforced from *in vivo* and *in vitro* experimental analyses in chapter 2.

The very recent development of techniques to isolate osteoclasts for *in vitro* analysis, and the knowledge gained from such analyses, is the subject of chapters 4 and 6 by Alberta Zambonin Zallone, Anna Teti and Tim Chambers, authors whose pioneering work has enormously increased our knowledge of osteoclast behaviour and metabolism. The importance of osteoclast-osteoblast interactions in regulating osteoclastic bone resorption and a detailed evaluation of osteoclasts isolated from various sources and species are emphasized in these two chapters.

In chapter 5, Arnie Kahn and Nicola Partridge present a novel mechanism, the Mechanostat Hypothesis, for bone resorption *in vivo*.

Clinical application of knowledge of osteoclast biology is especially emphasized in chapters 7 and 8, in which Barbara Mills provides an in-depth synthesis of human clinical conditions that involve bone-resorbing cells (the partner to Michael Parfitt's chapter on clinical conditions and bone-forming cells in Volume 1), and Sandy Marks examines mutations, especially osteopetrosis, that act by modification of osteoclast function (the partner to David Cole and Michael Cohen's chapter on mutations and osteoblasts in Volume 1). Eighty six separate elements that affect osteoclasts in clinical conditions are identified by Barbara Mills. These range from elements such as calcium and phosphorus, through nutrition, hormonal status, metabolic instability, organ failure (chiefly the kidneys and gastrointestinal tract), drugs and neoplasms. Microenvironmental factors are emphasized by Sandy Marks in his analysis of osteopetrotic mutants in mice and man, bringing us full circle to chapter 1 and Marijke Holtrop's discussion of osteoclasts in relation to their environment. In concert, Volumes 1 and 2 provide current, authoritative reviews of the biology of bone-forming and bone-forming cells and of the interactions between these two cell lineages.

In preparing the subject index for this volume I have attempted to adhere to the format developed for volume 1 in the hope that this common approach will facilitate cross referencing between the two volumes.

Brian K. Hall
Halifax
August, 1990

1

Light and Electronmicroscopic Structure of Osteoclasts

MARIJKE E. HOLTROP
Vitamin D, Skin & Bone Research Laboratory
Boston University, School of Medicine
Boston, Massachusetts

Introduction
Morphology of the osteoclast
Relationship of the osteoclast to its environment
Morphological expression of the functional state of activity of the
    osteoclast
Osteoclastic and other cells
References

Introduction

"The purpose of exploring morphology is to learn about function, since the morphological image represents the visual expression of functional activity." These words, written in the introduction to chapter 1, volume 1 of this series, apply equally to this chapter. Morphology is expressed in images obtained by light- and by electronmicroscopy. Lightmicroscopy has limitations with respect to resolution, which is defined as the shortest distance between two points that can be seen separately. Resolution depends on the wavelength of the "light" sent through the tissue. Using electrons instead of light, resolution is greatly improved; emitted electrons have a much shorter wavelength than light. Hence, much greater detail can be obtained in electronmicroscopy, which becomes visible at much higher magnifications than in lightmicroscopy.

Tissue has to be prepared in certain ways for light or electrons to penetrate and form images. After fixation to prevent disintegration, the tissue is embedded in a fluid plastic that hardens during "curing". With high precision microtomes, and skill and patience on the part of the operator, thin slices of the tissue are cut for lightmicroscopy at 3-5μm thickness using a steel knife;

and for electronmicroscopy at 60 nm, using a diamond knife. Enhancement of the final image is obtained by staining: for lightmicroscopy colorful dyes are used that adhere to specific compounds; for electronmicroscopy heavy metals are used that attach in different degrees to tissue components and decrease or prevent electrons going through the tissue. The final image after magnification can be seen in lightmicroscopy by the eye of the observer or recorded on a photographic plate, or is made visible in electronmicroscopy after the electrons hit a fluorescent screen or photographic plate.

A special development of electronmicroscopy makes it possible to look at surfaces of tissue, for instance the surface of bone or the surface of a cell. These images, formed by scanning electronmicroscopy (SEM) as opposed to transmission electronmicroscopy (EM), show shadows indirectly caused by the electron beam, resulting in a 3-dimensional impression much like light photography of 3-dimensional forms.

These techniques are written about in greater detail in the introduction to the first chapter of volume 1 of this series.

The images obtained by lightmicroscopy or electronmicroscopy are 2-dimensional representations of 3-dimensional structures. It is a challenge for the mind to try to make the conversion in dimensions: to come closer to the structural reality of the tissue by imagining what was present in the tissue before the section we are looking at, and what was present beyond that section. Especially in electronmicroscopy, serious mistakes in interpretation of images have been made; the interested reader may refer to the article: *Three-Dimensional Structure Identified from Single Sections - Misinterpretation of Flat Images Can Lead To Perpetuated Errors* (Elias, 1971). Serial sections are helpful in forming a complete 3-dimensional image but are technically extremely difficult to obtain. An example of interval serial sections through one osteoblast is given in Chapter 1, volume 1 of this series.

Morphology of the Osteoclast

When looking at bone tissue through a light microscope, some cells stand out clearly by their size and shape, even though they are not frequent (Fig. 1). It is therefore not surprising that these cells were recognized and described as early as 1873 and attributed the important function of resorbing bone, which gave them the name of osteoclast (Kolliker, 1873). These cells are usually several times the size of osteoblasts (Fig. 1), are usually found on the bone surface and take many shapes: sometimes curling around a bony spicule or lamella, other times lined up along the bone surface. The diversity in shape

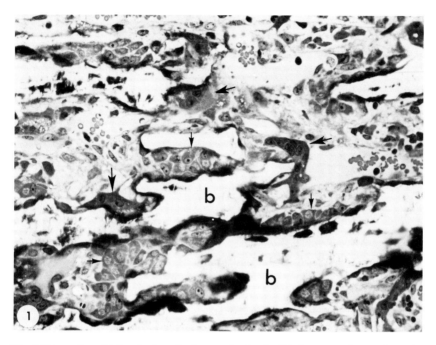

Fig. 1 This section of trabecular bone in the metaphysis of a tibia from a rat shows at least three osteoclasts (large arrows). They are large cells compared to osteoblasts (small arrows), and contain many nuclei with prominent nucleoli. Mineralized bone (b) is not stained. Between the trabecula are marrow cells and red blood cells. Toluidine blue, × 315

suggests cell movement and indeed, in cinematography of cultured osteoclasts, it was clearly shown that these cells not only wander from site to site, but also move while on the bone surface (Gaillard, 1961; Goldhaber, 1961; Hancox and Boothroyd, 1961). SEM of osteoclasts on bone also shows a great variety in cell shapes and cytoplasmic projections and makes clear that they "walk" along the surface of the bone, leaving a trail where the bone has just been resorbed (Fig. 2) (Jones and Boyde, 1977; Kanehisa and Heersche, 1988).

The osteoclast contains many nuclei that result from fusion of a number of mononuclear cells. Nucleoli can be so prominent that they are visible even at the lightmicroscopic level (Fig. 1). The cell stains less darkly than osteoblasts in routine staining with toluidine blue, suggesting less RER and hence less production of proteins for secretion. The cytoplasm can even look

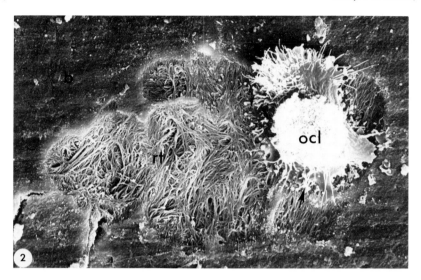

Fig. 2 Scanning electronmicrograph of a resorption trail (rt) made by an osteoclast (ocl) cultured on a slice of bone for 48 h. The surface of the resorbed area has a course fibrillar appearance and is clearly distinguishable from non resorbed bone surfaces (b). The osteoclast is dome-shaped in the center and has many peripheral cytoplasmic processes (arrows). × 1200 (Courtesy of Heersche and Kanehisa, University of Toronto).

vacuolated and has been described as "foamy", representing many vacuoles belonging to the lysosomal system.

At the electronmicroscopic level the osteoclast also stands out as very different from other cells in bone tissue, in particular osteoblasts (Fig. 3). The cytoplasm is so characteristic that it can easily be recognized even when other specific features of the osteoclast are not present in the plane of section (Fig. 4). Most striking is the abundance of mitochondria. They outnumber, per unit volume of cytoplasm, those in any other bone cell and indeed in any other cell type in the body (Figs 3,4). Because they are rather evenly distributed through the cytoplasm, their abundance is obvious regardless of the plane of section through the osteoclast (Fig. 4). Occasionally electrondense granules, similar to the ones observed at times in osteoblasts (Volume 1, chapter 1) have been seen in these mitochondria. The granules consist of clusters of finer particles and have been found using conventional fixation techniques (Gonzales and Karnovsky, 1961; Anderson and Parker, 1966; Cooper *et al.* 1966; Lucht and Maunsbach, 1973) and also after fixation in anhydrous organic solvents (Landis *et al.*, 1977). By means of X-ray analysis these granules proved to

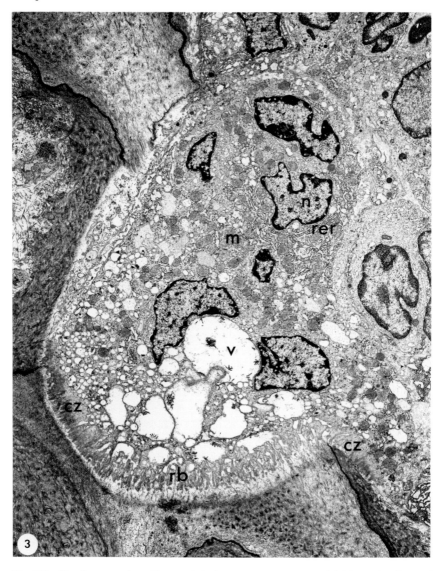

Fig. 3 Profile of an osteoclast. Characteristic features are numerous nuclei (n), an abundance of mitochondria (m), sparse rough endoplasmic reticulum (rer), many free ribosomes or clusters of ribosomes distributed throughout the cytoplasm, vacuoles (v), ruffled border (rb) and clear zone (cz) (Holtrop and King, 1977). × 8,600

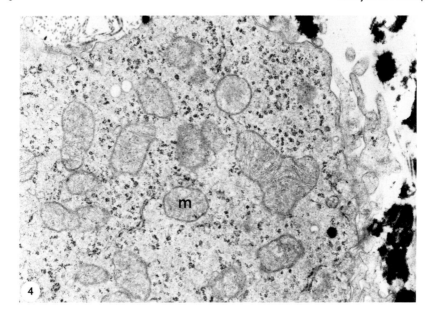

Fig. 4 Part of an osteoclast profile showing typical features of osteoclast cytoplasm as can be found throughout the cell: numerous mitochondria (m) and clusters of ribosomes. x 16,800

contain calcium (Lucht and Maunsbach, 1973), which led to the concept that mitochondria can function as site of storage of calcium on the pathway of transport from bone surface to cell uptake to extracellular fluid (Lehninger, 1970).

In the cytoplasm many free ribosomes are present, either singly or in clusters (Fig. 4), suggesting synthesis of proteins for use within the cell. Rough endoplasmic reticulum is present but in small quantity (Fig. 3). A Golgi area can also be found, but again is small. It is usually located adjacent to the nucleus (Fig. 5).

The most characteristic feature of an osteoclast is an area that is present when the cell is resorbing bone, as is evident by the frayed appearance of the bone surface under this specific area in undecalcified sections (Fig. 6). Over time a number of names have been given to this area, such as "brush border" or "striated border" (Kolliker, 1873), but since the first ultrastructural description (Scott and Pease, 1956), the name "ruffled border" has been most commonly used, a name which best describes the structure of the membrane in this area. The ruffled border can be opposed to a straight surface of bone (Fig. 7),

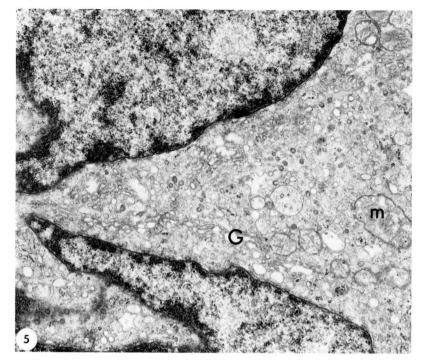

Fig. 5 Golgi area (G) alongside nuclei in an osteoclast profile; m: mitochondrion. × 16,000

or wrap around a spicule or lamella of bone (Fig. 6). A great number of "ruffles" or deep infoldings of the plasma membrane result in a complex system of what appears in a section as finger-like projections of the cytoplasm, separated by spaces (Fig. 6). The usual images of these projections could however also be plate-like and a rare section through a ruffled border roughly perpendicular to the usual ruffled border image shows that can indeed be the case (Fig. 8). There is a great variability in the length, width and shape of these projections (Lucht, 1972a; Holtrop, 1977) and also in the amount of space between the projections, from narrow channels (Fig. 6) to more bulbous areas (Gonzales and Karnovsky, 1961; Lucht, 1972a), that seem to be connected with large vacuoles in the cytoplasm adjacent to the ruffled border (Figs 3,7). No matter what the structure is, the ruffled border always represents an enormously extended area of interface between cell and extracellular environment, providing the potential for extensive exchange between cell and extracellular space. The extent to which the cell membrane can increase in

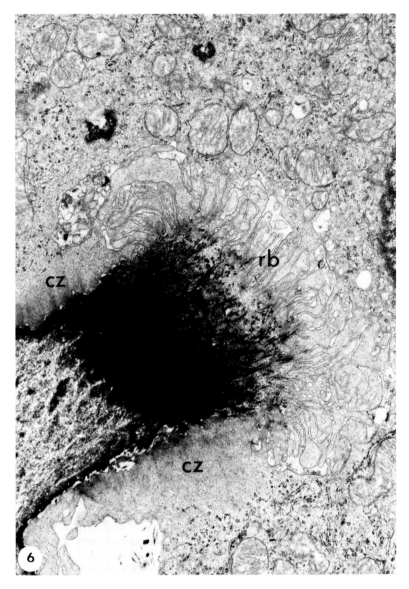

Fig. 6 Ruffled border (rb) and adjacent clear zone (cz) cover a bony spicule or lamella. The bone under the ruffled border looks disrupted, but not so under the clear zone. (Holtrop *et al.* 1974) × 12,700

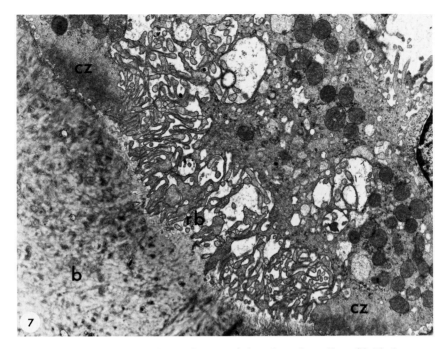

Fig. 7 Ruffled border (rb) and adjacent clear zone (cz) on the surface of bone (b). The bone was demineralized during processing. (Holtrop and King, 1977) × 6,800

length in these infoldings is well demonstrated in Fig. 8, an unusual section through a ruffled border. One can imagine that the bone surface is below the represented section at a plane roughly parallel to the plane of section. The cytoplasmic projections are hit in cross section and are very narrow.

The structure of the cell membrane in the ruffled border is somewhat different from the rest of the plasma membrane: the membrane is coated with fine bristle-like structures evenly spaced 20-25 nm apart and projecting perpendicularly into the cytoplasm (Kallio *et al.*, 1971). It was speculated that these might represent sites of enzymatic activity related to bone resorption (Kallio *et al.*, 1971).

Ruffled borders are not always present in sections of osteoclasts. In cultures of fetal rat bones only 11% of the osteoclast profiles showed ruffled borders (Holtrop *et al.*, 1974). The main reason for this is the limited area of the osteoclast represented in one section. A section is only a slice of 60 nm, hence 500 sections can be cut from a cell with a diameter of 30μm. Thus it

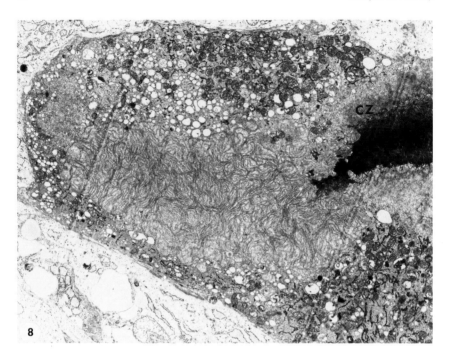

Fig. 8 Cross section through a ruffled border in a plane roughly parallel to the bone surface, showing an enormous increase in membrane surface in this area. Some clear zone (cz) can be seen along the bone surface. The straight parallel lines are caused by defects in the knife edge. Compare with Fig. 13. (Holtrop and King, 1977) × 4,700

depends greatly on the extent to which the ruffled border is part of the osteoclast whether it is included in any one section through the cell, or not. In unstimulated osteoclasts sampled from the metaphysis of rat long bones the average area of ruffled borders occupied only 3.4% of the area of cytoplasm in random sections through these cells (King *et al.*, 1976). Hence it is clear that ruffled borders can be easily missed in osteoclast sections. It is also possible that osteoclasts do not have ruffled borders, like osteoclasts that are not on the surface of the bone. Lucht (1972a) collected thin sections at an interval of 2.5μm and found that indeed some osteoclasts do not have a ruffled border. Sometimes two ruffled borders can be seen in one osteoclast profile, far enough apart from each other to assume that these are indeed two different ruffled borders in one cell. This usually happens only in very large osteoclasts. In cultures of osteoclasts on devitalized bone slices, observed by phase-contrast time-lapse cinemicrography and SEM, it was indeed evident that the

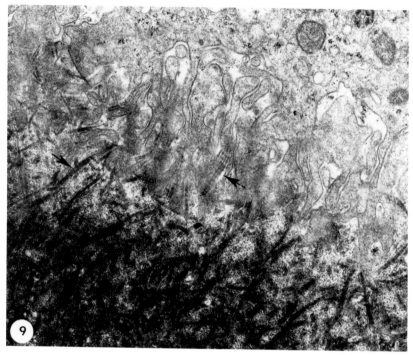

Fig. 9 Detail of bone - ruffled border interface. Some collagen fibers are partly demineralized (arrows). (Holtrop and King, 1977) × 22,100

same osteoclast can simultaneously resorb two lacunae, even at different rates (Kanehisa and Heersche, 1988).

The mechanism of resorption of bone at the site of the ruffled border will be discussed in Chapters 5 and 6 of this volume. A detail of the morphology of this process is presented in Figs 9 and 10. Fig. 9 represents an undemineralized section showing the frayed appearance of the surface of the bone during bone resorption and some collagen fibers more or less demineralized as part of the resorption process. Collagen fibers are usually not seen in this area between cell and bone, probably because the degradation of the collagen is so fast. In Fig. 10 many bone particles can be seen between the infoldings of the cell membrane at the ruffled border. Whether these particles are taken up by the cell or not is still a matter of debate and will be discussed in Chapter 5. Apart from resorbing bone matrix, the osteoclast is also capable of absorbing the cells in the bone matrix, the osteocytes. Soskolne (1978) demonstrated

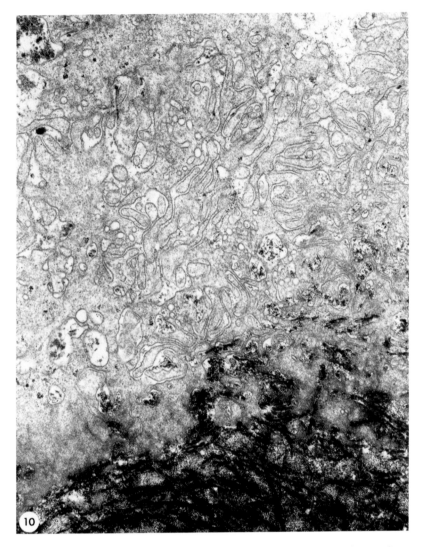

Fig. 10 Detail of bone - ruffled border interface. Bone mineral crystals can be seen between cytoplasmic processes of the ruffled border. × 17,100.

different stages of the phagocytosis of osteocytes by osteoclasts. Serial LM sections and multiple EM sections showed that osteocytes were completely engulfed by osteoclasts.

Always accompanying the ruffled border is a specific area along the cell membrane at the periphery of the ruffled border (Figs 6,7). Many names have been given to this area over time, such as transitional zone, (Lucht, 1972a,b; Scott and Pease, 1956); ectoplasmic layer (Gothlin and Ericson, 1972; Scott, 1967) granular zone (Schenk et al., 1967) contact zone (Malkani et al., 1973) and sealing zone (TranVan et al., 1982; Zambonin-Zallone et al., 1988). Of all these, the neutral name *clear zone* seems the most appropriate and is the most widely used. At low magnification the clear zone does indeed look clear, *i.e.* devoid of any specific cell organelles such as mitochondria, ribosomes or endoplasmic reticulum. Occasionally, a few small vesicles can be found. With optimal preservation of the cell, and at higher magnifications, more detailed structure can be recognized: parallel dark bands or electrondense material in a loose network (Malkani et al., 1973) turn out, when cut in a favorable plane, to consist of numerous thin filaments (Fig. 11). When these bundles are cut in cross section they show up as round accumulations of dots and short lines within an amorphous substance (Fig. 12) (Lucht 1972a; King et al., 1975). These filaments have a diameter of 5-7 nm and their property to bind specifically to heavy meromyosin makes them fall into the category of actin filaments (King et al., 1975). The filament bundles often extend into small protrusions that seem to fit into small indentations of the bone surface (King et al., 1975). Similar protrusions have been seen in isolated osteoclasts cultured *in vitro* on a bone slice (Zambonin-Zallone, 1988). They were shown by immunofluorescence of specific antibodies to contain F-actin and a group of cytoskeletal proteins involved in linking microfilaments to the points of adhesion of the osteoclast to the substratum, and they were named podosomes (Marchisio et al., 1984; Zambonin-Zallone et al., 1988). Between the bundles of filaments is a fine granular material that is morphologically very similar to the material in the cytoplasmic extensions of the ruffled border.

The clear zone is always present in an osteoclast profile that includes the ruffled border and is always at the edge of the ruffled border, where the cell membrane ceases to ruffle and starts to follow the contour of the cell smoothly. Imagining the consequence of this 3-dimensionally, one can infer that the clear zone encircles the ruffled border completely, as clarified in Fig. 13. Clear zones do also exist, although seldomly, in osteoclast profiles without a ruffled border. From Fig. 13 it is apparent that the clear zone may be included

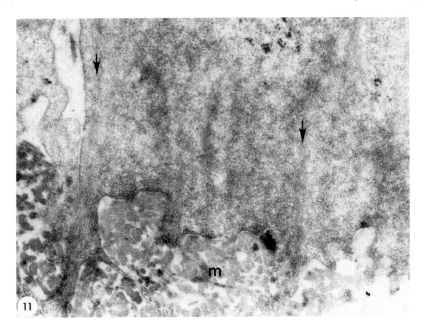

Fig. 11 Detail of a clear zone. Dark bands consisting of a bundle of filaments run through the clear zone perpendicular to the bone surface and end in short processes into irregularities of the bone matrix. The tissue has been demineralized during processing, leaving other matrix components (m). (King and Holtrop, 1975) × 39,000

in the section, but not the ruffled border. It is also possible that clear zones exist without ruffled border, if ruffled borders form after clear zones. From microcinematography of cultured bone it is known that osteoclasts move around and that once an osteoclast is adhered to bone, the ruffled border is highly motile. It is most likely from the structure and contents of the clear zone that this area attaches the cell to the bone surface, thereby giving support and stability to the motile ruffled border. Osteoclasts in cultured bones exposed to biophysical forces remained on the bone surface, whereas osteoblasts did not, thus providing evidence for the adherence of osteoclasts to bony surfaces (Ryder *et al.*, 1981). Some investigators have proposed that the attachment of the clear zone to the bone would be so tight that it would seal off the area under the ruffled border from the extracellular space, thus providing a contained space to maintain the acid environment necessary for the removal of mineral from the bone matrix and for lysosomal enzymes, secreted by the osteoclast, to degrade the bone matrix (Schenk *et al.*, 1967; Zambonin-

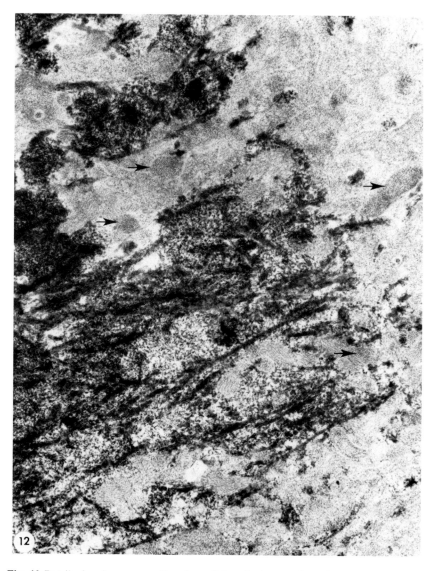

Fig. 12 Detail of a clear zone sectioned parallel to the bone surface close to the bone - cell interface. Bundles of filaments (arrows) appear as discrete, roughly circular, areas surrounded by amorphous material. Individual filaments are represented as dots when sectioned truly perpendicular, and as short lines when sectioned tangentially. (King and Holtrop, 1975) × 35,800

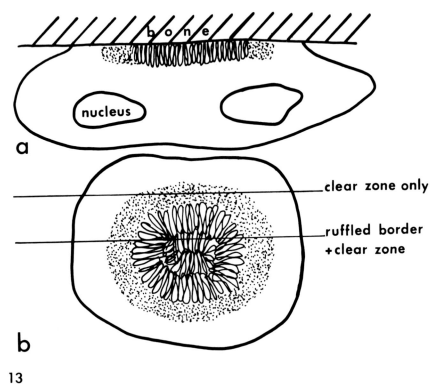

13

Fig. 13 Diagrammatic representations of an osteoclast; a: as usually seen in sections; b: surface of the cell opposed to the bone surface (compare with Fig. 8). Since a ruffled border in a section always shows adjacent clear zones (a), the clear zone must be surrounding the ruffled border completely (b) (Holtrop *et al.*, 1974).

Zallone, 1988). Although spaces can always be seen between clear zone and bone surface, even with the best tissue preservation, it is possible that the cell has retracted somewhat at the moment of submersion in fixative. However, the extracellular, electrondense, marker peroxide was seen in the channels of the ruffled border as early as 5 minutes after injection (Lucht, 1972c), thus questioning the theory of a seal.

Ruffled borders and clear zones are never seen in osteoclasts away from the bone surface. It is not known what happens to these areas when the osteoclast stops resorbing and starts moving away to another site on the bone. The disarrangement of the ruffled border and the clear zone may be too fast to see in an electronmicrograph. Laying hens go through cyclic changes in bone resorption in accordance with their egg-laying cycle. A study of Japanese quail showed that the numbers of osteoclasts and their nuclei remained unchanged during the egg cycle, implying that changes in bone resorption involved changes in individual cell activity. Indeed, during egg shell calcification ruffled borders were abundant. After completion of egg shell calcification osteoclasts remained attached to the bone surface, ruffled borders disappeared and extensive, interdigitated, cell processes appeared along the peripheral surface of the osteoclast away from the bone. These unusual structures were considered to serve as a reservoir of membrane (Miller, 1977). They have however not been observed in other species.

Another characteristic of osteoclast cytoplasm is the presence of vacuoles. These can be so numerous that, at the lightmicroscopic level, they give the appearance of a foamy cytoplasm. At the electronmicroscopic level there appears to be a great variety in the presence and size of vacuoles, probably dependent on the stage of activity of the cell (Scott, 1967). Most, and the largest, vacuoles are found next to the ruffled border, where it is sometimes difficult to determine where the ruffled border ends and the vacuoles begin (Figs 3,7). Actually, many structures may seem to be vacuoles, but may have a connection with the extracellular space between the ruffles, outside the plane of section, and therefore not be true vacuoles. The term vacuole is usually reserved for the larger membrane-bounded bodies that appear to be largely empty (Scott, 1967; Lucht, 1972b), which is probably an artifact. Their profiles in a section measure between 0.03 μm and 5 μm (Lucht, 1972b). Their membrane has the same diameter as the ruffled border membrane, roughly 9 nm (Lucht, 1972b; Thyberg et al., 1975), and is also coated (Kallio, 1971; Doty and Schofield, 1972; Lucht, 1972b; Thyberg, 1975; Thyberg et al., 1975). This morphological similarity of the membrane of vacuoles and ruffled border brings up the possibility of a functional relationship. Coated vesicles are generally believed to be specialized for the cellular uptake of extracellular material, in particular proteins. They can then fuse to form larger vacuoles, usually referred to as phagosomes (Daems et al., 1969). Pierce and Lindskog (1988) pointed out that the coating of the ruffled border membrane is different from the coating of coated pits and vesicles in osteoclasts and based this statement on a difference in reaction with clathrin. These pits and vesicles were easily detected on the dorsal (away from the bone surface) and lateral membrane areas, just peripheral to the clear zone, and not in the clear zone or ruffled border. Interestingly, pits and vesicles were seen on the cell membrane facing, or immediately associated with, the osteoblast plasma membrane that in turn also showed these structures along the membrane facing the osteoclast. The authors conclude that the osteoclast appears to exhibit morphological evidence for two distinctly different membrane structures for endocytosis (Pierce and Lindskog, 1988). How much of the degraded bone matrix is then taken up by the osteoclast during resorption is still unknown. Morphologically it seems that crystals from the bone matrix are taken up by the cell (Fig. 10) (Scott, 1967; Fetter and Capen, 1971; Kallio, 1971), but vacuoles or vesicles containing crystals may have been invaginations instead of true vacuoles. Also, relocation of calcium could have occurred during fixation in aqueous solutions. Details about the issue of uptake of components of the bone matrix by the osteoclast and degradation within the cell will be discussed in Chapter 5.

Vacuoles and vesicles may also be involved in the secretion of material, such as enzymes for the degradation of bone matrix. Lucht (1972b) distinguished vacuoles with a coating and vacuoles without, the coated vacuoles probably functioning in endocytosis and the non-coated vacuoles functioning in exocytosis.

A variety of smaller membrane bound bodies, measuring 0.02-3 μm in diameter, with an internal structure or a stainable constituent of varying density can be present in osteoclasts (Lucht, 1972b). It is not always possible to distinguish these from vacuoles because of intermediate forms (Scott, 1967; Lucht, 1972b). Their many different appearances and the lack of insight into their function are reflected in the many names given to these structures, such as: vesicles containing electron opaque material (Schenk *et al.* 1967), specific granules (Scott, 1967), dense bodies (Freilich, 1971), dense granules (Fetter and Capen, 1971), cytoplasmic dense bodies (Gothlin and Ericson, 1972; Thyberg, 1975), cytoplasmic bodies (Lucht, 1972b), and lysosomes (Yaeger and Kraucunas, 1969). Lucht (1972b) made the most distinct characterization and described: a) light cytoplasmic bodies, b) dense cytoplasmic bodies, c) coated cytoplasmic bodies and d) cytoplasmic bodies with inclusions. Some bodies and small, uncoated, vacuoles may be associated with the Golgi apparatus and may be lysosomes (Schenk *et al.*, 1967; Scott, 1967; Lucht, 1972b). Residual bodies that are membrane bound, acid phosphatase-negative, and contain electron dense material of various shapes, probably representing indigestible products, are also present in the osteoclast.

Giving names to structures without knowledge of their function seems rather academic, but is a first step towards understanding mechanisms within the cell. Histochemical studies have further advanced our knowledge of the role of the osteoclast in bone resorption and these will be discussed in Chapter 3.

There are some organelles in the osteoclast that are not easily seen or are rare.

Microtubules are present, with no apparent preferential orientation as seen in EM (Lucht, 1973; Holtrop *et al.*, 1974), although Lucht (1973) noticed that they can be especially numerous in regions close to centrioles. However, the distribution of microtubules in cultured osteoclasts, as observed by indirect immunofluorescence microscopy, showed a complex array of fibers extending towards the cell margin, or in very large cells extending from different origins in the cell (Zambonin-Zallone, *et al.*, 1983). Microtubules do seem to play a role in the activity of the osteoclasts, because when microtubules are disintegrated by colchicine in osteoclasts stimulated to resorb by parathyroid hormone in bone cultures, bone resorption is inhibited (Raisz *et al.*, 1973; Holtrop *et al.*,1974). They may play a role in the secretion of lysosomal enzymes, as has been suggested in human leukocytes (Zurier *et al.*, 1973). However, in cultured bones in which the stimulation of bone resorption by parathyroid hormone was inhibited by colchicine, the frequency of ruffled borders in osteoclast profiles decreased from 68% in controls to 19% in treated bones, an effect very similar to that of calcitonin (Holtrop *et al.*, 1974). This may mean that microtubules play a role in the formation of ruffled borders. This effect may be primary or secondary and is not understood.

Centrioles are rarely seen, usually in a cluster close to the Golgi area (Matthews *et al.*, 1967; Cameron, 1968; Lucht, 1973; Sapp, 1976). They have the same structure as those in other cell types (Fig. 14). Because osteoclasts are post-mitotic cells, these centrioles are thought to have come from fusion with mononuclear mitotic precursors (Sapp, 1976).

Relationship of the Osteoclast to the Environment

Very little attention has been given to the direct environment of the osteoclast, in particular the relationship of this cell to other cells. Since osteoclasts move around, the assumption probably has been that no relationships exist with neighboring cells. However, Soskolne (1979) looked carefully at the osteoclast-endothelium interface in the femurs of young rabbits and noted in lightmicroscopy that 85% of the osteoclasts made direct contact with

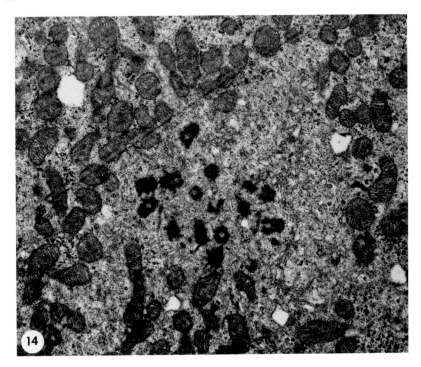

Fig. 14 Centrosphere consisting of centrioles in an osteoclast. × 13,500

the endothelial cells. Electronmicroscopy revealed that small processes reached out from the osteoclast towards the endothelial cells with, on rare occasions, the presence of specialized junctions (Soskolne, 1979). This finding was recently confirmed in rats, mice and humans (Cox *et al.*, 1988). Osteoclasts made contact not only with endothelial cells, but also with pericytes. Contact was made by touching with no clear indications of any specialization of the cell membrane. Sometimes the contact was made by two small cell processes hooking into each other (Cox *et al.*, 1988). The significance of these observations is not known.

Arising from an interest in the role of mononuclear cells in bone resorption (see below), it was noted that large numbers of mononuclear cells were present in close proximity to, and often lined up along the surface of, osteoclasts on the periosteal alveolar bone surface during active bone resorption in adult monkeys (Rifkin and Heijl, 1979) and during the bone remodeling sequence in rats (Tran Van *et al.*, 1982). They were recognized in EM as presumably fibroblasts and macrophages (Rifkin and Heijl, 1979), and mononuclear phagocytes (Tran Van et al., 1982). It may seem odd that such proximity had never been noticed before. However, EM images contain so much information in such a limited area that the mind must select and focus on a particular topic. Moreover, it is known that mononuclear cells fuse with osteoclasts and then become an intricate part of the osteoclast. Ascribing a specific function to mononuclear cells in bone resorption is a more recent concept.

Morphological Expression of the Functional State of Activity of the Osteoclast

If morphology is the visual expression of functional activity, a change in function would be expected to be accompanied by a change in morphology. Indeed, changes have been recorded, both in light- and in electronmicroscopy, concurrent with changes in cell activity.

The only morphological features that can be distinguished and quantitated at the lightmicroscopic level are the number of cell profiles per area of tissue in a section, and the number of nuclei in cell profiles. Parathyroid hormone has been the first and most tested hormone on cell changes. In organ cultures in which the rate of bone resorption is increased, as monitored by release of previously incorporated ^{45}Ca from the bone into the culture medium, parathyroid hormone increased the number of osteoclasts (Holtrop et al., 1974; Rowe and Hausmann, 1977; King et al., 1978; Holtrop and Raisz, 1979; Wezeman et al., 1979). This effect can also be seen in vivo directly (Bingham et al., 1969; Tatevossian, 1973; Vignery and Baron, 1978; VanderWiel and Talmage, 1979; Holtrop et al., 1979) or indirectly by calcium and phosphorus deficiency (Thompson et al., 1975). The number of nuclei per cell also increases after exposure to parathyroid hormone (Wezeman et al., 1979; Addison, 1980). Stimulation of bone resorption in cultures by PTH can be reversed by calcitonin and this is accompanied by a decrease in the number of osteoclasts to control (resting) values (Holtrop et al., 1974). This also occurred in patients with Paget's disease after administration of calcitonin (Singer et al., 1976). There are other hormones and compounds that affect osteoclast activity and morphology: the number of osteoclasts in vivo also increased after exposure to 1,25(OH)2D3 (Holtrop et al., 1981; Marie and Travers, 1983) and prostaglandins (VanderWiel, 1979).

At the EM level more changes in morphology can be distinguished, but it is also more difficult to quantify changes. Quantitation is an absolute necessity. Since so little area of the cell is perceived in sections of cells, one cell profile is not representative of the whole cell. One therefore has to work with averages of a great number of cell profiles, a task that the human eye and mind cannot accomplish without the help of random sampling, counting or measuring, and statistics (Holtrop, 1977). A good example of misinterpretation of information can be found in an early descriptive EM study of the effects of parathyroid hormone on osteoclasts *in vivo*, in which no difference was seen in the extent and appearance of ruffled borders in treated osteoclasts compared to controls (Lucht and Maunsbach, 1973). In contrast, later EM studies in rats using either counting methods (% cell profiles with ruffled borders) (Holtrop *et al.*, 1974; Miller, 1978) or a method of random sampling and measuring ruffled border areas and clear zone areas in cell profiles and the entire cell profile, showed unequivocally that osteoclast ruffled borders as well as clear zones, and subsequently the cell, increase dramatically when osteoclasts are exposed to parathyroid hormone and bone resorption is increased, either in tissue culture (King *et al.*, 1978; Holtrop and Raisz, 1979) or *in vivo* (Holtrop *et al.*, 1979). Changes in cell morphology *in vivo* preceded changes in serum calcium and were statistically significant as early as thirty minutes after injection of the hormone (Fig. 15) (Holtrop *et al.*, 1979). This rapid response to parathyroid hormone was also demonstrated in avian osteoclasts (Japanese quail) (Miller *et al.*, 1984). Such activated osteoclasts can also be rapidly deactivated. In tissue culture, after administration of calcitonin, the ruffled border membrane loses its cytoplasmic coating (Kallio *et al.*, 1972), and ruffled borders flatten out or disappear completely (Kallio *et al.*, 1972; Holtrop *et al.*, 1974).

A significant increase in ruffled borders and clear zones was also seen after injection of $1,25(OH)_2D_3$ into rats (Holtrop *et al.*, 1981) and after exposure of rat bones in culture to PGE_2 and OAF (Holtrop and Raisz, 1979). These findings demonstrate clearly the morphological responsiveness of the osteoclast to specific environmental influences.

Osteoclastic and Other Cells

Until fairly recently the osteoclast was considered the only cell capable of bone resorption. Other multinucleated giant cells were recognized, but these showed subtle cytoplasmic differences and, more importantly, they showed no

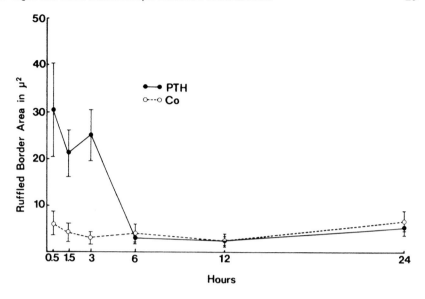

15

Fig. 15 Changes in the average size of ruffled border area as a function of time in bones from thyroparathyroidectomized rats after injection with parathyroid hormone (PTH) or buffer (Co). Each point represents the mean area of ruffled borders in 23-26 cell profiles pooled from 3 rats/group. The vertical bars represent SEM. (Holtrop *et al.*, 1979)

ruffled borders or clear zones. These cells were considered incapable of resorbing bone.

In an effort to find a model of resorption that would generate a large number of osteoclasts in a small delineated area of mineralized tissue in order to study differentiation and function of these cells, several investigators turned to implants of devitalized bone matrix (Glowacki *et al.*, 1981; Krukowski and Kahn, 1982). Small bone fragments prepared from the long bones of adult rats implanted into cranial defects elicited a great number of multinucleated giant cells and resorption of the bone (Glowacki *et al.*, 1981), and the cells that resembled osteoclasts in LM caused fraying of the particle surface as viewed by EM. However, no ruffled borders were present (Fig. 16) (Holtrop *et al.*, 1982; Walters and Schneider, 1985; Popoff and Marks, 1986). This finding revealed that multinucleated cells other than classical osteoclasts have the potential to resorb bone. It is conceivable that cells without ruffled

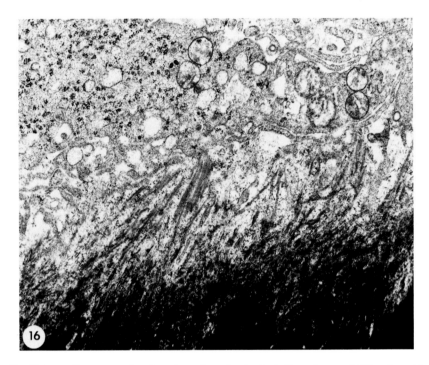

Fig. 16 Area of bone resorption along the surface of an implanted bone fragment. Mineral crystals and collagen fibers can be recognized. The cell opposing the resorption area does not have a ruffled border. (Holtrop *et al.*, 1982) × 19,400

borders resorbing normal live bone have escaped attention in the EM, and have been mistaken for osteoclasts whose ruffled border is just outside the plane of section. However, subsequent work by Glowacki, using the same model but somewhat different circumstances, revealed that the multinucleated giant cells could develop ruffled borders and clear zones and showed other characteristics of osteoclasts, such as the presence of tartrate-resistant acid phosphatase (Glowacki and Cox, 1986), receptors for calcitonin (Goldring *et al.*, 1988) and presence of an antibody against rat bone purple acid phosphatase (Glowacki *et al.*, 1988). These cells were therefore named osteoclastic cells (Glowacki and Cox, 1986). Subsequently, it became clear from studies of different types of mineralized implants on the chorioallantoic membranes of chicken eggs (Krukowski and Kahn, 1982), and subcutaneous implants of particulate bone, polyethylene or polymethylmethacrylate (Glowacki *et al.*,

1986) or particulate hydroxyapatite (Glowacki *et al.*, 1989), that the elicited multinucleated cells only develop ruffled borders and clear zones when in contact with mineralized bone. Other multinucleated cells developed, at best, only clear zones. The development of ruffled borders was even impaired in osteoclasts on particles of defective (osteocalcin-deficient) bone matrix (Lian *et al.*, 1984; Glowacki and Lian, 1987). This is interesting in view of the lack of resorption and the presence of abnormal osteoclasts in some mutant rats and mice (see Chapter 8). It had never been realized that such abnormal osteoclasts might be capable of resorbing bone, to some extent.

These studies show that the structure of the classical osteoclast is specific for normal mineralized bone, but that other multinucleated cells are also capable of the degradation of bone matrix, in all likelihood at a much slower rate. The question remains whether such cells function in normal bone metabolism or are found only under pathological conditions.

There are other cells that may participate in bone resorption: mononuclear phagocytes (blood monocytes and macrophages). In cultures of nonvital bone, monocytes are capable of matrix resorption (Kahn *et al.*, 1978; McArthur *et al.*, 1980; Teitelbaum *et al.*, 1979). By EM, macrophages in such cultures have been seen with contact areas resembling clear zones (Rifkin *et al.*, 1979) and mononuclear cells have been seen with ingested collagen fibrils and clumps of mineral crystals (Rifkin *et al.*, 1980). In resorption of devitalized implants *in vivo*, mononuclear cells with ingested bone matrix were identified as macrophages (Holtrop *et al.*, 1982). In experimental periodontitis the acute inflammatory response led to vigorous osteoclastic resorption of the alveolar bone and a close association of mononuclear cells with osteoclasts, some containing intracellular collagen fibrils (Rifkin and Heijl, 1979). Three functions have been suggested for mononuclear cells in bone resorption: (1) participation in the resorption of bone by ingestion of partially degraded collagen fibrils (Heersche, 1978); (2) participation by local release of factors that activate osteoclasts (Yoneda and Mundy, 1979; Rutherford and Trummel, 1983); (3) participation as a precursor for osteoclasts (see Chapter 2).

In this chapter on the structure of osteoclasts it suffices to say that osteoclasts are the primary bone resorbing cells, but that they are not alone.

References

Addison, W. C. (1980) The effect of parathyroid hormone on the numbers of nuclei in feline osteoclasts *in vivo. J. Anat.* **130**: 479-486.

Anderson C. E., and Parker, J. (1966) Invasion and resorption in enchondral ossification. *J. Bone Joint Surg.* **48**: 899-914.

Bingham, J., Brazell I. A., and Owen M. (1969) The effect of parathyroid extract on cellular activity and plasma calcium levels *in vivo*. *J. Endocr.* **45**: 387-400.

Cameron, D. A. (1968) The Golgi apparatus in bone and cartilage cells. *Clin. Orthop.* **58**: 191-211.

Cooper, R. R., Milgram, J. W., and Robinson R. A. (1966) Morphology of the osteon. An electron microscopic study. *J. Bone Joint Surg.* **48**: 1239-1271.

Cox, K. A., Wilson, S., Dethlefsen, S. and Glowacki J. (1988) Detailed transmission electron-microscopy and immunohistological characteristics of vessels of rat, mouse and human growth plates. *J. Bone and Mineral Res.* **3**: S183.

Daems, W., Wisse, E., and Brederoo, P. (1969) Electron microscopy of the vacuolar apparatus. In: *Lysosomes in Biology and Pathology 1.* (Dingle and Fell, Eds.) : Amsterdam-London. North Holland Publishing Co., pp. 64-112.

Doty, S. B., and Schofield, B. H. (1972) Electron microscopic localization of hydrolytic enzymes in osteoclasts. *Histochem. J.* **4**: 245-258.

Elias, H. (1971) Three-dimensional structure identified from single sections - Misinterpretation of flat images can lead to perpetuated errors. *Science* **174**: 993-1000.

Fetter, A. W. and Capen, C. C. (1971) The fine structure of bone in the nasal turbinates of young pigs. *Anat. Rec.* **171**: 329-346.

Freilich, L. S. (1971) Ultrastructure and acid phosphatase cytochemistry of odontoclasts: Effects of parathyroid extract. *J. Dent. Res.* **50**: 1047-1055.

Gaillard, P. J. (1961) Parathyroid and bone in tissue culture. In: *The Parathyroids.* (Greep and Talmage, Eds.) : Springfield, Charles C Thomas, p. 20-48.

Glowacki, J., Altobelli, D., and Mulliken, J. B. (1981) Fate of mineralized and demineralized osseous implants in cranial defects. *Calcif. Tissue Int.* **33**: 71-76.

Glowacki, J., Cox, K. A. (1986) Osteoclastic features of cells that resorb bone implants in rats. *Calcif. Tissue Int.* **39**: 97-103.

Glowacki, J., Jasty, M. and Goldring S. (1986) Comparison of multinucleated cells elicited in rats by particulate bone, polyethylene, or polymethyl-methacrylate. *J. Bone Min. Res.* **1**: 327-331.

Glowacki, J. and Lian, J. B. (1987) Impaired recruitment and differentiation of osteoclast progenitors by osteocalcin-deplete bone implants. *Cell Diff.* **21**: 247-254.

Glowacki, J., Wilcon, S., Clark, S., Anderson, T., and Toverud, S. (1988) Discrimination between induced osteoclasts and giant cells with an antibody against rat bone purple acid phosphatase. *J. Bone Mineral Res.* **3**: S98.

Glowacki, J., Rey, C., Cox, K. and Lian, J. (1989) Effects of bone matrix components on osteoclast differentiation. In: *Third Symposium on Chemistry and Biology of Mineralized Tissues.* (M. J. Glimcher Ed.). *Connective Tissue Research* **20**: 121-129.

Goldhaber, P. (1961) Oxygen-dependent bone resorption in tissue culture. In: *The Parathyroids.* (Greep and Talmage, Eds.) : Springfield, Charles C Thomas, p. 243-255.

Goldring, S. R., Roelke, M. and Glowacki, J. (1988) Multinucleated cells elicited in response to implants of devitalized bone particles possess receptors for calcitonin. *J. Bone Mineral Res.* **3**: 117-120.

Gonzales, F. and Karnovsky, M. J. (1961) Electron microscopy of osteoclasts in healing fractures of rat bone. *J. Biophys. Biochem. Cytol.* **9**: 299-316.

Gothlin, G. and Ericsson, J. L. (1972) Observations on the mode of uptake of thorium dioxide particles by osteoclasts in fracture callus. *Calc. Tissue Res.* **10**: 216-222.

Hancox, N. M. and Boothroyd, B. (1961) Motion picture and electron microscope studies on the embryonic avian osteoclast. *J. Biophys. Biochem. Cytol.* **11**: 651-661.

Heersche, J. N. M. (1978) Mechanism of osteoclastic bone resorption: a new hypothesis. *Calcif. Tissue Res.* **26**: 81-84.

Holtrop, M. E. (1977) Quantitation of the ultrastructure of the osteoclast for the evaluation of cell function. In: *Bone Histomorphometry, Second Int. Workshop, Lyon, France.* (P. J. Meunier, Ed.), Societe de la Nouvelle Imprimerie Fournie, pp 133-145.

Holtrop, M. E., Cox, K. A., Clark, M. B., Holick, M. F., and Anast, C. S. (1981) 1,25 Dihydroxycholecalciferol stimulates osteoclasts in rat bones in the absence of parathyroid hormone. *Endocrinology* **108**: 2293-2301.

Holtrop, M. E., Cox, K. A. and Glowacki, J. (1982) Cells of the mononuclear phagocytic system resorb implanted bone matrix: a histologic and ultrastructural study. *Calcif. Tissue Int.* **34**: 488-494.

Holtrop, M. E. and King, G. J. (1977) The ultrastructure of the osteoclast and its functional implications. *Clin. Orthop.* **123**: 177-196.

Holtrop, M. E., King, G. J., Cox, K. A. and Reit, B. (1979) Time related changes in the ultrastructure of osteoclasts after injection of parathyroid hormone in young rats. *Calcif. Tissue Int.* **27**: 129-135.

Holtrop, M. E. and Raisz, L. G. (1979) Comparison of the effects of 1,25 dihydroxy-cholecalciferol, prostaglandin E₂, and osteoclast-activating factor with parathyroid hormone on the ultrastructure of osteoclasts in cultured long bones of fetal rats. *Calcif. Tissue Int.* **29**: 201-205.

Holtrop, M. E., Raisz, L. G. and Simmons, H. A. (1974) The effects of parathyroid hormone, colchicine, and calcitonin on the ultrastructure and the activity of osteoclasts in organ culture. *J. Cell Biol.* **60**: 346-355.

Jones, S. J. and Boyd A. (1977) Some morphological observations on osteoclasts. *Cell Tissue Res* **185**: 387-397.

Kahn, A. J., Stewart, C. and Teitelbaum, S. L. (1978) Contact-mediated bone resorption by human monocytes *in vitro*. *Science* **199**: 988-990.

Kallio, D. M., Garant, P. R. and Minkin, C. (1971) Evidence of coated membranes in the ruffled border of osteoclasts. *J. Ultrastr. Res.* **37: 169-177.**

Kallio, D. M., Garant, P. R. and Minkin, C. (1972) Ultrastructural effects of calcitonin on osteoclasts in tissue culture. *J. Ultrastr. Res.* **39**: 205-216.

Kanehisa, J. and Heersche, J. N. (1988) Osteoclastic bone resorption: *in vitro* analysis of the rate of resorption and migration of individual osteoclasts. *Bone* **9**: 73-79.

King, G. J. and Holtrop, M. E. (1975) Actin-like filaments in bone cells of cultured mouse calvaria as demonstrated by binding to heavy meromyosin. *J. Cell Biol.* **66**: 445-451.

King, G. J., Holtrop, M. E. and Raisz, L. G. (1978) The relation of ultrastructural changes in osteoclasts to resorption in bone cultures stimulated with parathyroid hormone. *Metab. Bone Dis. Rel. Res.* **1**: 67-74.

Krukowski, M. and Kahn, A. J. (1982) Inductive specificity of mineralized bone matrix in ectopic osteoclast differentiation. *Calcif. Tissue Int.* **34**: 474-479.

Kolliker, A. *Die normale resorption des knochengewebes in ihre bedeutung fur die entstehung der typischen knochenformen.* Leipzig, F. C. W. Vogel, 1873; p. 86.

Landis, W. J., Paine, M. C. and Glimcher, M. J. (1977) Electron microscopic observations of bone tissue prepared anhydrously in organic solvents. *J. Ultrastr. Res.* **59**: 1-30.

Lehninger, A. L. (1970) Mitochondria and calcium ion transport. *Biochem J.* **119**: 129-138.

Lian, J. B., Tassinari, M. and Glowacki J. (1984) Resorption of implanted bone prepared from normal and warfarin-treated rats. *J. Clin. Invest.* **73**: 1223-1226.

Lucht U. (1972a) Osteoclasts and their relationship to bone as studied by electron microscopy. *Z. Zellforsch. Mikrosk. Anat.* **135**: 211-228.

Lucht, U. (1972b) Cytoplasmic vacuoles and bodies of the osteoclast. *Z. Zellforsch. Mikrosk. Anat.* **135: 229-244.**

Lucht, U. (1972c) Absorption of peroxidase by osteoclasts as studied by electron microscope histochemistry. *Histochemie* **29**: 274-286.

Lucht, U. (1973) Electron microscope observations of centrioles in osteoclasts. *Z. Anat. Entwicklungs Gesch.* **140**: 143-152.

Lucht, U. and Maunsbach, A. B. (1973) Effects of parathyroid hormone on osteoclasts *in vivo*. An ultrastructural and histochemical study. *Z. Zellforsch.* **141**: 529-544.

MacArthur, W., Yaari, A. M. and Shapiro, I. M. (1980) Bone solubilization by mononuclear cells. *Lab. Invest.* **42**: 450-456.

Malkani, K., Luxembourger, M. M. and Rebel, A. (1973) Cytoplasmic modifications at the contact zone of osteoclasts and calcified tissue in the diaphyseal growing plate of fetal guinea pig tibia. *Calc. Tissue Res.* **11**: 258-164.

Marchisio, P. C., Cirillo, D., Naldini, L., Primavera, M. V. Teti, A. and Zambonin-Zallone, A. (1984) Cell-substratum interaction of cultured avian osteoclasts is mediated by specific adhesion structures. *J. Cell Biol.* **99**: 1696-1705.

Marie, P. J. and Travers, R. (1983) Continuous infusion of 1,25 dihydroxyvitamin D$_3$ stimulates bone turnover in the normal young mouse. *Calcif. Tissue Int.* **35**: 418-425.

Matthews, J. L., Martin, J. H. and Race, G. J. (1967) Giant-cell centrioles. *Science* **155**: 1423-1424.

Miller, S. C. (1977) Osteoclast cell-surface changes during the egg-laying cycle in Japanese quail. *J. Cell Biol.* **75**: 104-118.

Miller, S. C. (1978) Rapid activation of the medullary bone osteoclast cell surface by parathyroid hormone. *J. Cell Biol.* **6**: 615-618.

Miller, S. C., Bowman, B. M. and Myers, R. L. (1984) Morphological and ultrastructural aspects of the activation of avian medullary bone osteoclasts by parathyroid hormone. *Anat. Rec.* **208**: 223-231.

Mundy, G. R., Altman, A. J., Gondok, M. D. and Bandelin, J. G. (1977) Direct bone resorption by human monocytes. *Science* **196**: 1109-1111.

Pierce, A. and Lindskog, S. (1988) Coated pits and vesicles in the osteoclast. *J. Submicrosc. Cytol. Pathol.* **20**: 161-167.

Popoff, S. N. and Marks, S. C., Jr. (1986) Ultrastructure of the giant cell infiltrates of subcutaneously implanted bone particles in rats and mice. *Am. J. Anat.* **177**: 491-503.

Rifkin, B. R. and Heijl, L. (1979) The occurrence of mononuclear cells at sites of osteoclastic bone resorption in experimental periodontitis. *J. Periodont.* **50**: 638-640.

Rifkin, B. R., Baker, R. L., Somerman, M. J., Pointon, S. E., Coleman, S. J. and Au, W. Y. W. (1980) Osteoid resorption by mononuclear cells *in vitro*. *Cell Tissue Res.* **210**: 493-500.

Rowe, D. J. and Hausmann, E. (1977) Quantitative analyses of osteoclast changes in resorbing bone organ cultures. *Calcif. Tissue Res.* **23**: 283-289.

Rutherford, B. and Trummel, C. L. (1983) Monocyte mediated bone resorption involves release of nondialyzable substances in addition to prostaglandin. *J. Reticuloendothelial Soc.* **33**: 175-184.

Ryder, M. I., Jenkins, S. D. and Horton, J. E. (1981) The adherence to bone by cytoplasmic elements of osteoclasts. *J. Dent. Res.* **60**: 1349-1355.

Sapp, J. P. (1976) An ultrastructural study of nuclear and centriolar configurations in multinucleated giant cells. *Lab. Invest.* **34**: 109-114.

Schenk, R., Spiro, D. and Weiner, J. (1967) Cartilage resorption in tibial epiphyseal plate of growing rats. *J. Cell Biol.* **34**: 275-291.

Scott, B. L. and Pease, D. C. (1956) Electron microscopy of the epiphyseal apparatus. *Anat. Rec.* **126**: 465-495.

Scott, B. L. (1967) The occurrence of specific cytoplasmic granules in the osteoclast. *J. Ultrastr. Res.* **19**: 417-431.

Singer, F. R., Melvin, K. W. and Mills, B. G. (1976) Acute effects of calcitonin on osteoclasts in man. *Clin. Endocrinology* **5 Suppl**: 335-340S.

Soskolne, W. A. (1978) Phagocytosis of osteocytes by osteoclasts in femora of two-week old rabbits. *Cell Tissue Res.* **195**: 557-564.

Soskolne, W. A. (1979) The osteoclast-endothelium interface during bone resorption in the femurs of young rabbits. *Cell Tissue Res.* **203**: 487-492.

Tatevossian, A. (1973) Effect of parathyroid extract on blood calcium and osteoclast count in mice. *Calcif. Tissue Res.* **11**: 251-257.

Teitelbaum, S. L., Stewart, C. C. and Kahn, A. J. (1979) Rodent peritoneal macrophages as bone resorbing cells. *Calcif. Tissue Int.* **27**: 255-261.

Teitelbaum, S. L. and Kahn, A. J. (1980) Mononuclear phagocytes, osteoclasts, and bone resorption. *Mineral Electrol. Met.* **3**: 2-9.

Thompson, E. R., Baylink, D. J. and Wergedal, J. E. (1975) Increases in number and size of osteoclasts in response to calcium and phosphorus deficiency in the rat. *Endocrinology* **97**: 283-289.

Thyberg, J. (1975) Electron microscopic studies on the uptake of exogenous marker particles by different cell types in guinea pig metaphysis. *Cell Tissue Res.* **156**: 301-315.

Thyberg, J., Nilsson, S. and Friberg, U. (1975) Electron microscopic and enzyme cyto-chemical studies on the guinea pig metaphysis with special reference to the lysosomal system of different cell types. *Cell Tissue Res.* **156**: 273-299.

TranVan, P., Vignery, A. and Baron, R. (1982) An electron-microscopic study of the bone-remodeling sequence in the rat. *Cell Tissue Res.* **225**: 283-292.

VanderWiel, C.J. and Talmage, R. V. (1979) Comparison of the effects of prostaglandin E_2 and parathyroid hormone on plasma calcium concentration and osteoclast function. *Endocrinology* **105**: 588-594.

Vignery, A. and Baron, R. (1978) Effects of parathyroid hormone on the osteoclastic pool, bone resorption and formation in rat alveolar bone. *Calcif. Tissue Res.* **26**: 23-28.

Walters, L. M. and Schneider, G. B. (1985) A functional and morphological study of cells adjacent to ectopic bone implants in rats. *Am. J. Anat.* **173**: 287-297.

Wezeman, F. H., Kuettner, K. E. and Horton, J. E. (1979) Morphology of osteoclasts in resorbing fetal rat bone explants: effects of PTH and AIF *in vitro*. *Anat. Rec.* **194**: 311-323.

Yaeger, J. A. and Kraucunas, E. (1969) Fine structure of the resorptive cells in the teeth of frogs. *Anat. Rec.* **164**: 1-13.

Yoneda, T. and Mundy, G. R. (1979) Monocytes regulate osteoclast-activating factor production by releasing prostaglandins. *J. Exp. Med.* **150**: 338-350.

Zambonin-Zallone, A., Teti, A., Primavera, M. V., Naldini, L. and Marchisio, P. C. (1983) Osteoclasts and monocytes have similar cytoskeletal structures and adhesion property *in vitro*. *J. Anat.* **137**: 57-70.

Zambonin-Zallone, A., Teti, A., Carano, A. and Marchisio, P. C. (1988) The distribution of podosomes in osteoclasts cultured on bone laminae: effect of retinol. *J. Bone Min. Res.* **3**: 517-523.

Zurier, R. B., Hoffstein, S. and Weissman, G. (1973) Mechanisms of lysosomal enzyme release from human leukocytes. I. Effect of cyclic nucleotides and colchicine. *J. Cell Biol.* **58**: 27-41.

2

Cellular Origin and Theories of Osteoclast Differentiation

E. H. BURGER
Department of Oral Cell Biology
Academic Center of Dentistry, ACTA
De Boelelaan 1115
NL 1081 HV Amsterdam
The Netherlands

AND

P. J. NIJWEIDE
Laboratory for Cell Biology and Histology
University of Leiden
Rijnsburgerweg 10
NL 2333 AA Leiden
The Netherlands

List of Abbreviations

BME   bone microenvironment
CAM   chorioallantoic membrane
CFU   colony forming unit
CSF   colony stimulating factor
CT   calcitonin
G-CFC   granulocyte-colony forming cell
GM-CFC   granulocyte-macrophage-colony forming cell
(r)IL-3   (recombinant) interleukin-3
M-CFC   macrophage-colony forming cell
M-CSA   macrophage-colony forming activity
MNC   multinucleated cell
OC   osteoclast
OCP   osteoclast precursor/progenitor
PTH   parathyroid hormone
TRAP   tartrate-resistant acid phosphatase

Introduction

The cellular origin of the osteoclast, the multinucleated cell responsible for the physiological removal of calcified matrix in the skeleton and dentition, has intrigued researchers ever since its discovery, more than 100 years ago, by Kölliker (1873). A number of excellent reviews on this subject have appeared over the last decade which summarize the published evidence and discuss possible interpretations (Loutit and Nisbet, 1982; Marks, 1983; 1984; Chambers, 1985; Nijweide et al., 1986; Mundy and Roodman, 1987; Vaes, 1988, Marks and Popoff, 1988). Here we will try not to repeat an old discussion, but instead to incorporate recent evidence into the still incomplete picture of the osteoclast lineage. Before we do so, however, we should briefly discuss the specific difficulties which are encountered when studying osteoclast formation and origin and which continue to frustrate students of this devious cell. The most important one is probably that an osteoclast is not a cell of fixed morphology and location in the tissue, but instead may be described as a temporary state of fusion of a number of (mononuclear) precursors (see Chapter 1, this volume). Fusion occurs in correlation with resorbing activity (Makris and Saffar 1982) and the number of osteoclast (OC) nuclei may vary from 1 to more than 20. In addition, osteoclasts actively move over mineralized surfaces and through the connective tissue surrounding hard matrix. As a result, histological sections offer very diverse pictures of osteoclasts and no conclusions whatever can be drawn from such observations as to the size and location of the cell a few days or even hours earlier. To make it worse, the mononuclear precursors which fuse to form OC show a lamentable lack of easily detected specific features, and also seem to have no fixed location in skeletal tissues. Compared with, for instance, the chondrocytes of the growth plate, where each stage of development is precisely located in a certain zone of the epiphyseal plate, it is clear that unequivocal data on the identity of the cells which unite to form osteoclasts is very hard to obtain.

As a consequence of these difficulties, only experiments which interfere with the normal biological process of OC formation may offer clues to the origin of OC. However, by their very nature such experiments may be questioned as to the extent to which they represent the physiological situation. To give an example: parabiosis studies of inbred rats have shown without doubt that OC precursors can be transported *via* the blood circulation. However, to what extent circulation of OC precursors occurs under physiological conditions cannot be answered by these studies.

Rather, the available evidence suggests that in the absence of specific demands the percentage of OC precursors among circulating leukocytes is very low (Tinkler *et al.*, 1981, Stanka and Bargsten, 1983).

Notwithstanding these difficulties, data on the subject of osteoclast origin and the factors which regulate OC (precursor) formation have been and are being obtained, often using sophisticated methods. In the following we will discuss first the experimental systems which have been most rewarding and the data they have provided. Secondly, we will discuss the features of OC precursors which have emerged from these and other studies. Lastly we will focus on the importance of the bone microenvironment and local growth factors for OC and OCP development. From the available data a lineage of development of OC's and their progenitor/precursors emerges.

Experimental Evidence on the Origin of Osteoclasts

Evidence for Circulating OC Precursors

Evidence for the existence of circulating osteoclasts precursors in newts appeared as early as 1962 (Fischman and Hay), but conclusive demonstration of this phenomenon in mammals and birds was published only some 10 years later. Göthlin and Erikson (1973), using parabiosed rats, showed osteoclast formation from circulating cells in fracture callus. Walker (1973), using osteopetrotic mice, showed lasting reversal of the disease and sustained

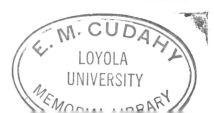

presence of normal osteoclasts by temporary parabiotic union with normal siblings. These parabiosis studies were followed by transplantation of bone marrow or spleen cells to show that the circulating OC precursors were derived from haematopoietic tissue (Walker, 1975; Loutit and Sansom, 1976).

In birds, the existence of circulating OC precursors was demonstrated in quail-chick chimaera consisting of embryonic bone rudiments grafted onto the chorioallantoic membrane (CAM), using the specific quail nuclear morphology as marker to distinguish host- and graft-derived cells (Kahn and Simmons, 1975, Jotereau and LeDouarin, 1978, Simmons and Kahn, 1979). In such grafts, OC developed readily from host-derived cells, without specific measures to induce OC formation. In contrast, grafts of embryonic mouse bone on the quail CAM induced host-derived OC formation only after removal of the local mesenchyme surrounding the bone rudiments (Thesingh and Burger, 1983). This latter study provided evidence for early homing of OC progenitors in the long bone mesenchyme followed by local expansion of the OC precursor pool prior to OC formation. A similar conclusion for quail mesenchyme may be drawn from a study by Yabe and Hanaoka (1985), who demonstrated the formation of donor-derived OC from embryonic limbs transplanted in diffusion chambers.

Evidence for the Haematopoietic Origin of OC Precursors

Evidence for the relationship of OC precursors with the haemopoietic cell family has accumulated in two experimental systems: the *in vivo* system which uses cure of osteopetrosis, usually in mice, to monitor OC formation from transplanted cell suspensions (Walker, 1975; Loutit and Sansom, 1976) and *in vitro* systems which use invasion and resorption of osteoclast-free bone rudiments of fetal mice and rats to monitor OC formation from cocultured cell suspensions (Ko and Bernard, 1981, Burger *et al.*, 1982, Schneider and Relfson, 1988). To obtain OC-free desmal bone, the embryonic anlage of mouse calvaria has been precultured, resulting in osteoblast but not OC development, followed by coculture with non-adherent bone marrow cells to allow OC formation (Ko and Bernard, 1981). The periost-free long bone rudiment system makes use of the two days time lag between onset of mineralisation in the cartilaginous metatarsal bone and its subsequent invasion by OC's and OC precursors. Removal of the periosteum-perichondrium before invasion prevents the formation of OC during organ culture, while coculture of such stripped bones with OC precursors induces formation of OC which excavate the primitive marrow cavity (Burger *et al.*,

1982, 1984; Löwik et al, 1988). A criticism of this technique may be that chondroclasts rather than osteoclasts are formed, as mineralized cartilage matrix rather than bone is resorbed. However neither ultrastructural nor enzyme-histochemical differences have been detected between OC resorbing bone or cartilage (Bromley and Woolley, 1984) while in the long bone metaphysis one and the same clast may be seen resorbing both cartilage and bone. Thus the term "osteoclast" seems justified for all multinuclear cells engaged in the physiological resorption of both cartilage and bone.

The two systems, cure of osteopetrosis *in vivo* and osteoclastic invasion of bone organ cultures *in vitro*, have provided evidence on the origin of OC which agree to a remarkable extent. In 1975, Walker provided roentgenographic and histologic evidence that cell infusions prepared from normal bone marrow or spleen cure osteopetrosis in mutant mice after total body irradiation, while osteopetrotic transplants induce the disease in ir-radiated normal recipients. Similar observations were made by Loutit and coworkers (Barnes *et al.*, 1975; Loutit and Samsom, 1976) who subsequently used nuclear (Nisbet *et al.*, 1979) and cytoplasmic (Ash *et al.*, 1980) markers to demonstrate without doubt that the effective OC indeed developed from the transplanted cells and not as the result of some short-range influence of normal marrow cells on the defective host OC. A similar conclusion was drawn from human osteopetrotic patients treated with marrow transplant, using sex chromatin as the marker to distinguish male donor cells from treated females (Coccia *et al.*, 1980; Sorell *et al.*, 1981). This data indicated that OC are part of the large and diverse haemopoietic cell family. Most authors also agreed that the cell line likely to be closely related to OC is the monocyte/macrophage line. However, evidence against this concept was also published. Marshall *et al.* (1982) by comparing normal bone marrow with defective marrow from mice mutant at the W locus obtained evidence against CFU, (Colony Forming Units in the mouse spleen assay) as giving rise to OC. In 1983 Schneider and Byrnes showed that cellular suspensions of newborn rat liver, juvenile spleen and adult bone marrow are effective in curing osteopetrosis in i.a. rats while suspensions from lymph node, thymus and blood as well as adherent peritoneal and spleen cells were not. This same group subsequently showed that isolated pluripotent haemopoietic stem cells cure osteopetrosis (Schneider, 1985), that bone marrow fractions enriched for M-CFC are ineffective, while fractions enriched for G-CFC or GM-CFC were effective (Schneider and Relfson, 1988a). As their cell fractions were by no means pure, the exact cellular source of the OC remains uncertain, but the data argues against M-CFC, the committed progenitor of the macrophage lineage, as the stem cell for OC.

The *in vitro* approach developed somewhat later, starting with the observation of Ko and Bernard (1981) that non-adherent cells of 7 day mouse bone marrow cultures caused OC formation in precultured embryonic calvarial anlagen. In 1982 Burger *et al.* introduced the stripped metatarsal long bone system and showed OC formation in cocultures with fetal mouse liver as well as non-adherent radiosensitive cells from bone marrow which had been precultured in the presence of M-CSA (Van der Meer *et al.*, 1980). Blood leukocytes or peritoneal cells did not form OC after 7 days coculture (Burger *et al.*, 1982) but the inflammatory peritoneal exudate did, be it only after 11 days and to a lesser extent than bone marrow cells (Burger *et al.*, 1984). The origin of the OC from cocultured, not endogenous bone cells was verified using ^{3}H thymidine labeling (Burger *et al.*, 1984) and by Löwik *et al.* (1988) using filters of varying pore size placed between the OC source and the bone explant. By means of this coculture technique Thesingh (1983) demonstrated that OC could be obtained from the early mouse yolk sac. She showed that OC progenitors were distributed from there to embryonic tissues through the vascular circulation, coincident with the beginning of the haemopoietic capacity of the liver bud. OC formation from human fetal bone marrow in the stripped mouse rudiments has also been described, while human blood leukocytes were ineffective (Helfrich *et al.* 1987). Also, rat bone marrow fractions enriched for G-CFC or GM-CFC but not M-CFC did form OC in coculture with stripped bone rudiments from fetal rats (Schneider and Relfson, 1988b). Lastly, the direct descendance of OC from pluripotent hemopoietic stem cells (PHSC) has recently been demonstrated using the stripped long bone coculture assay. Scheven *et al.* (1986) showed that OC derived from a mouse bone marrow fraction highly enriched in hemopoietic stem cells, while Schneider and Relfson (1989) obtained OC from rat bone marrow PHSC separated according to high Thy 1.1 antigen expression. Lastly, Hagenaars *et al.* (1989) demonstrated the actual generation of OC from the progeny of single cloned PHSC which also gave rise to granulocytes, monocytes and erythrocytes.

Thus, both the *in vivo* approach using osteopetrotic mutants and the *in vitro* approach using osteoclast-free bone explants reach similar conclusions. OC are derived from the haematopoietic stem cell but not from populations of mature macrophages. Both models further provide evidence that OC are formed from populations also containing actively growing mononuclear phagocytes but that M-CFC themselves do not form OC. In line with these observations, pretreatment of bone marrow with M-CSF did not stimulate but rather inhibited OC formation in stripped bones, suggesting that differentiation along the mononuclear phagocyte pathway reduces the capacity of cells to form OC (Van de Wijngaert et al. 1987a). It seems then that OC and monocyte/macrophages do share a common progenitor, but that this progenitor is an early derivative of the pluripotent haemopoietic stem cell, not (yet) committed to the monocyte/macrophage line.

Blood Monocytes as Putative OC Precursors

After it became apparent that OC precursors may circulate in the bloodstream, at least under experimental conditions, several authors have tried to demonstrate OC formation from circulating monocytes, using a variety of techniques. Tinkler et al. (1981) studied OC nuclear labeling after injecting ^{3}H thymidine-labeled leukocytes into recipient syngeneic mice also receiving 1-αhydroxycholecalciferol to stimulate OC formation. Although they did obtain OC with labeled nuclei, the evidence that monocytes were the precursors is not convincing in the light of the very low percentage labeling (18 out of 10,000 OC counted) and the huge doses of labeled monocytes administered (4 × the buffy coat of 3 labeled mice into 1 recipient mouse). In a follow up study (Tinkler et al., 1983) no correlation was found between the time course of monocyte and OC labeling after a single injection of ^{3}H thymidine, again indicating that blood monocytes are not immediate OC precursors. Stanka and Bargsten (1983) found enhanced presence of Barr bodies in OC nuclei after repeated transfusions of female leukocytes in syngeneic male rats, but again the cell type which fused with recipient OC was not identified.

On the other hand, as already discussed above, experiments on osteopetrotic mice and rats as well as coculture studies have failed to demonstrate that blood monocytes and tissue macrophages form OC (Schneider and Byrnes, 1983; Burger et al., 1982). In addition multinuclear giant cells (MNC) formed by fusion of blood monocytes (Sutton and Weiss, 1966) are different from OC in ultrastructural complexity (Osdoby et al., 1982) enzyme pattern (Sundquist et al., 1987; Hermans, 1987), surface antigens (Horton et al., 1986) and location in the tissue (Van de Wijngaert et al., 1988). In a recent study, Helfrich et al. (in press) have demonstrated the formation of OC from mouse blood leukocytes after prolonged coculture with periost-free bone rudiments. However as OC also formed from leucocyte fractions which had been depleted of adherent cells, monocytes do not seem to be the source of OC in their study, in line with earlier work (Burger *et al.* 1982, 1984). This same group had shown earlier (Helfrich *et al.* 1987) that human blood monocytes failed to form OC in cocultures with fetal mouse rudiments while fetal human bone marrow cells did form OC. Lastly, the group of Zambonin-Zallone (Zambonin-Zallone and Teti, 1985; Teti *et al.*, 1988; and Chapter 4, this volume) studied fusion of blood cells with OC in birds. To cultures of OC, isolated from medullary bone of egg-laying chicks maintained on a low calcium diet, they added precultured adherent blood leukocytes from similar animals. Some 8% of the blood cells fused with OC, a phenomenon not modulated by parathyroid hormone or vitamin D3. Thus, in egg-laying hens a subset of peripheral leukocytes with characteristics of monocytes behaves as OC precursors.

In conclusion, the bulk of experimental evidence indicates that in most conditions the circulating OC precursor is a rare cell among the blood leukocytes, in contrast to the abundance of monocytes. It seems however quite conceivable that the level of circulating OC precursors is increased in certain physiological and pathological situations. The egg laying chick may be an example, especially when kept on a low calcium diet. Egg laying hens secrete 1 g calcium per egg shell, of which the skeleton contributes more than half (Mueller *et al.*, 1974). The extremely high medullary bone turnover which is involved may also lead to abnormal high OC turnover and increased OC precursor levels in the circulation.

In this respect it is of interest to consider the blood circulation in the skeleton, and the anatomic relation of haemopoietic marrow and surrounding bone. In cancellous bone the close spatial relationship between haemopoietic marrow and endost is quite obvious. In addition, microangiographic studies on the blood supply of diaphyseal compact bone (Brookes 1971, Rhinelander 1972) have shown that the flow of blood through the diaphyseal cortex is almost entirely centrifugal, *i.e.* flowing from medullar cavity to periosteum. Marrow derived sinusoids and capillaries traverse the diaphyseal compacta *via* vascular channels and empty in capillaries and venules of the periosteum (Brookes, 1971). This applies to the normal situation as well as to the later repair and remodeling phases of diaphyseal fracture repair (Rhinelander 1972). Thus, even in compact bone the endosteal surface is functionally situated next to the bone marrow. Although the precise route whereby OC precursors reach a given bone surface is as yet unknown it is conceivable that cells which are born in the bone marrow may be carried *via* marrow sinusoids and intracortical vascular channels directly to the cutting cones of Haversian systems. As a result, even in compact bone, most OC precursors may already have left the circulation before the blood stream leaves the bone, leading to low levels of circulating OC precursors. In addition, as OC are cells of low frequency, high numbers of circulating precursors are not to be expected in adult animals, unless in specific situations of abnormal high demand for mineral mobilizing cells. It should be noted that the *in vivo* evidence for a circulating OC precursor (see above) was indeed obtained under pathological conditions (fracture repair, osteopetrosis) or in prenatal animals (embryonic birds).

Characteristics of Osteoclast Precursors

Although the precise identity of the proliferating stages of the osteoclast lineage remains in many ways unclear, immature preosteoclast have been described in several morphological studies, mostly of rat tissue. The classical paper by Scott (1967) revealed the existence of two morphologically distinct proliferating cell populations in fetal rat spongiosa. One of them was recognized as representing precursor stages of OC, containing many mitochondria and extensive Golgi apparatus but no accumulation of glycogen or RER. The latter two were considered characteristics of osteoblast precursors.

Similar OC precursor cells were identified by Luk (1974) in rabbit endosteum and by Rifkin *et al.* (1980) in fetal rat calvaria. Ejiri (1983) reported that these cells are negative for peroxidase in contrast to monocytes. A similar observation in alveolar bone of newborn rats was made by Tanaka and Tanaka (1988) who also reported that the preosteoclasts do not exhibit phagocytic function, again unlike mononuclear phagocytes. Cells with preosteclastic phenotype (mononuclear but with similar cytoplasmic features as OC) have been chiefly observed in the inner, osteogenic layer of the periosteum among osteoblasts and close to the bone mineral surface, while mononuclear phagocytes were found in the outer, non-osteognic layer of the periosteum (Ejiri 1983; Van de Wijngaert *et al.*, 1986). This means that the final differentiation of the osteoclastic phenotype occurs in the same cell layer which maintains osteoblastic differentiation. The implications of this observation will be discussed later in this chapter (bone microenvironment).

Tartrate-resistant Acid Phosphatase (TRAP) as Marker of (pre-)osteoclasts

In histological sections of normal bone, acid phosphatase activity which is resistant to 20-50 mM tartrate is a convenient marker for OC which stain very strongly for this enzyme (Minkin, 1982; Chappard *et al.*, 1983; Bianco *et al.*, 1987; Cole and Walters, 1987). Scheven *et al.* (1986b) and Van de Wijngaert *et al.* (1986, 1989) have used this marker to show that mononuclear cells positive for TRAP appear in the periosteum-perichondrium of fetal mouse bones prior to the formation of invading multinucleate OC. Baron *et al.* (1986) using tooth extraction in the rat to induce the formation of multinucleated OC at a predictable and reproducible site and time (Tran Van *et al.*, 1982a, b) found a local increase of mononuclear cells positive for nonspecific esterase activity (a marker enzyme of mononuclear phagocytes), some of which also expressed TRAP, prior to the appearance of multinucleated OC. Scheven *et al.* (1985, 1986b) studied the formation kinetics of OC precursors in the fetal mouse periosteum and demonstrated the local proliferation of TRAP negative cells prior to their differentiation as TRAP positive postmitotic mononuclear OC precursors.

These findings suggest that TRAP activity is a late marker of OC differentiation *in vivo* and discriminates between mononuclear phagocytes and OC precursors under normal conditions (Bianco *et al.*, 1987). However, TRAP activity as marker of OC differentiation under experimental conditions must be used with caution. First, TRAP activity is not specific for OC, and is expressed by human bone marrow mononuclear phagocytes under certain pathologic conditions (Bianco *et al.*, 1987). Some punctate cytoplasmic TRAP activity has even been found in rat osteoblasts and osteocytes at sites of intense osteoclastic mineral resorption (Bianco *et al.*, 1988). Second, TRAP activity is induced in human monocytes during culture, although the enzyme is not expressed by freshly isolated monocytes (Razdun *et al.*, 1983; Weinberg *et al.*, 1984; Snipes *et al.*, 1986). Helfrich *et al.* (1987) studied the capacity of human monocytes to form OC as well as express TRAP. Within 3-5 days in culture, isolated monocytes formed multinucleated giant cells, which like the mononuclear cells, expressed TRAP activity. However, isolated monocytes did not form OC in coculture with fetal mouse rudiments, although fetal human bone marrow did. These authors also showed that TRAP activity was lost from cultured monocytes and giant cells after dehydration and embedding in glycolmethacrylate, unlike OC which kept their strong reactivity. The same group (Helfrich *et al.*, in press) also studied the capacity of mouse blood leukocytes to express TRAP activity and form OC. Unlike human monocytes, mouse leukocyte cultures did not form giant cells and did not express TRAP. Still, leukocyte suspensions did form OC in coculture with stripped bone rudiments, be it after prolonged (10-14 day) coculture time. As the OC also formed from the non-adherent leukocyte fraction, blood monocytes did not seem the precursors of the OC.

Seven days-cultured mouse bone marrow mononuclear phagocytes formed no (Van de Wijngaert *et al.*, 1987a) or very few (Takahashi *et al.*, 1988) multinucleated giant cells, unless cultured in the presence of vitamin D or PTH (Takahashi *et al.*, 1988). In both studies a small number of mononuclear, strong TRAP positive cells were present in non-hormone-treated cultures, which differed from the many mononuclear phagocytes by a low expression of macrophage-specific antigens and low phagocytosis activity (Van de Wijngaert *et al.*, 1987b). Löwik *et al.* (1988) in a study of mouse haemopoietic cell migration and differentiation found that loss of the capacity of the cells to form OC coincided with loss of TRAP activity but not tartrate-sensitive AcP or expression of macrophage-specific antigens.

In chicks, Teti *et al.* (1988) reported that low numbers of multinucleate giant cells are formed in 5 day blood monocyte cultures, while about 60% of the monocytes were slightly positive for TRAP.

So, human, mouse and chick monocyte-macrophages differ in the readiness with which they fuse and express TRAP in culture. Only in tissue sections of normal bone and bone marrow does TRAP seem to be a reliable marker of OC and probably also of OC precursors. In cultures of isolated cells however TRAP staining should always be used in combination with other characterizations, preferably resorption of mineralized tissue. In mice TRAP activity seems to be a better indicator of osteoclastic differentiation than in human and chick cells.

Osteoclast-specific Surface Antigens

Over the last few years there has been a growing interest in the antigenic phenotype of the osteoclast, which stemmed largely from the continuing study of OC ontogeny. Macrophage-specific antigens were found absent (Hume *et al.*, 1984; Horton *et al.*, 1984; 1985a, b) and present (Sminia and Dijkstra, 1986; Athanasou *et al.*, 1986) on OC, findings which were interpreted as arguments for a divergence as well as a similarity of the developmental pathways of OC and mononuclear phagocytes. In addition, monoclonal antibodies have been produced by direct immunization of mice with human (Horton *et al.*, 1985c) chick (Oursler *et al.*, 1985) or quail (Nijweide *et al.*, 1985) OC. Some of these antibodies were able to discriminate between OC and other bone marrow cells or osteoblasts.

In principle, OC specific antibodies offer great possibilities for the experimental analysis of the ontogeny of the osteoclast from its earlier precursors, but up to now very few studies have been reported which were based on this approach (Horton *et al.*, 1986; Fuller and Chambers, 1987). Nijweide *et al.* (1985) found a small number of mononuclear cells in isolates of quail medullary bone which showed surface antigens recognized by OC-specific antibodies not cross-reacting with bone marrow macrophages. They speculated that these cells might represent the immediate precursors of the osteoclast, but have not otherwise characterized them.

Receptors for Hormones and Cytokines

The majority of hormones and factors which stimulate bone resorption, such as parathyroid hormone (PTH), 1,25 dihydroxy vitamin D_3 and inter-leukin-1, do not seem to act on osteoclasts directly but rather affect the synthesis (presumably by osteoblasts) of "factors" which in turn stimulate osteoclasts. These osteoblast-derived factors might also interact with osteoclast precursors, but both the factors and their receptors are at present ill-defined and their presence on OC precursors is unknown.

Receptors for calcitonin (CT), which inhibits bone resorption, have been demonstrated in abundance on rat (Warshawsky *et al.*, 1980; Nicholson *et al.*, 1986) but not chicken (Arnett and Dempster 1987; Nicholson *et al.*, 1987) osteoclasts. In a recent study of osteoclast-like multinucleated cell (MNC) formation from mouse bone-marrow, 1-α, 25(OH)$_2$ vit D_3-induced expression of CT receptors by mononuclear cells was linked to induction of TRAP in the same cell (Takahashi *et al.*, 1988b). In addition, receptors for PTH have recently been described on hemopoietic blast cells giving rise to osteoclast-like multinucleated cells, while MNC formation was stimulated by PTH (Hakeda *et al.*, 1989). Interestingly, the MNC themselves did not show specific binding of PTH. These studies suggest that in the course of differentiation from multipotential cells to specific OC precursors, PTH receptors are lost while CT receptors are induced, together with TRAP expression.

Although reactivity to CT is a strong argument in favour of cells in culture being of the osteoclastic lineage, other haemopoietic cells also respond to CT. In rat thymocytes (Macmanus and Whitfield, 1970) and in haemopoietic stem cells (Gallien-Lartigue and Carrez, 1974) CT inhibited the mitogenic action of PTH. Whether CT and PTH act similarly on OC progenitors is still uncertain, although there is some evidence to support this (Krieger *et al.*, 1982).

Osteoclast Differentiation in Bone Marrow Cultures, Effects of Colony-stimulating Factors (CSF)

Based on the accumulating evidence that the osteoclast is of haemopoietic origin, several groups have tried to obtain osteoclast formation in cell cultures of isolated whole bone marrow or bone marrow fractions. Such an approach offers great advantages for the study of OC formation and its regulation by hormones, CSF etc. The key problem with this technique has been and still is to provide convincing proof that the cells detected as OC or OC precursors are indeed of osteoclast lineage, and to distinguish them from mononuclear phagocytes and foreign body giant cells.

The first studies claiming OC generation in bone marrow cultures were those by the group of Testa and Allen (Testa *et al.*, 1981; Allen *et al.*, 1981; Suda *et al.*, 1983) using cat bone marrow. The multinucleated cells which formed in monolayer liquid cultures were identified as OC based on their ultrastructural morphology and high acid phosphate activity (Testa *et al.*, 1981; Allen *et al.*, 1981) but tartrate inhibition was not studied. However, the cells did not resorb calcified matrix when seeded on thin slices of dentin but avidly phagocytosed particles of bone matrix as well as latex spheres. The latter is a property of foreign body giant cells rather than OC. These studies were elaborated by other groups, all using cat marrow. Ibbotson *et al.* (1984) reported that PTH stimulated the formation of multinucleated cells (MNC) as well as the TRAP activity per cell and that CT inhibited both effects of PTH. Prostaglandin E2 and 1,25 (OH)2 vitamin D3 (Pharoah and Heersche, 1985) also stimulated MNC formation. Pharoah and Heersche (1986) showed that CT induced these cells to contract, a phenomenon which had been described by Chambers and Magnus (1982) to be OC specific. Still the authors remained cautious, stating that the evidence obtained was insufficient to distinguish OC from inflammatory giant cells.

Apart from cat bone marrow, baboon (Roodman *et al.*, 1985), human (MacDonald *et al.*, 1987; Takahashi *et al.*, 1986a, b), rabbit (Horton *et al.*, 1986; Fuller and Chambers, 1987) and mouse (Van de Wijngaert *et al.*, 1987a, b; Takahashi *et al.*, 1988) bone marrow have been used to generate mono- and multinucleated osteoclast-like cells in culture. In the studies on baboon and human marrow, the osteoclastic nature of the relevant cells was deduced from

their multinuclearity, sensitivity for osteotropic hormones (especially calcitonin) and TRAP activity. Also, their formation was increased in response
to bone resorption stimulatory agents such as PTH, interleukin 1, and Transforming Growth Factor α in combination with 1,25(OH)2 vit. D3 (Takahashi
et al., 1989). About 50% of the MNC formed in long-term (3 weeks) marrow
cultures contracted in response to calcitonium while 1-10% of the MNC
formed resorption lacunae on dentine slices (Takahashi *et al.*, 1989). Interestingly, cultured peripheral blood cells also formed MNC in response to
1,25(OH)2 vit D3, but these cells did not show similar responses to the
osteotropic factors as MNC from bone marrow. Staining with a panel of
monoclonal antibodies revealed no clear cut separation between MNC's from
peripheral blood and bone marrow as to expression of OC - or macrophage -
specific antigens. Still, expression of OC-specific antigens was higher in
MNC from bone marrow than from blood, while the expression of a monocyte
related antigen, absent from authentic OC, was high in blood derived MNC
but low in bone marrow derived MNC (Kukita *et al.* 1989). Some of the
anti-human OC specific antibodies cross react with rabbit OC and have been
used to characterize MNC in rabbit marrow cultures, (Horton *et al.*, 1986;
Fuller and Chambers, 1987). In the absence but not in the presence of horse
serum, 1,25 (OH)2 vitamin D3 strongly stimulated the formation of TRAP
positive MNC in such cultures, as it does in human bone marrow cultures (*e.g.*
MacDonald *et al.*, 1987). However, application of osteoclast-specific
monoclonal antibodies stained only a minority of the multinucleated cells,
specifically those with a small number of nuclei and not the giant cells
(Horton *et al.*, 1986; Fuller and Chambers, 1987). This suggests that the giant
MNC were foreign body giant cells rather than OC. In addition cultures
devoid of antibody-staining cells but containing MNC were unable to form
pits in slices of bone mineralized matrix.

Studies using mouse bone marrow have the advantage that contrary to
avian, rabbit and human monocytes, mouse leukocytes do not express TRAP
in culture (see above). Mononuclear cells showing strong TRAP were obtained from mouse bone marrow by Van de Wijngaert *et al.* (1987a) which
differed from the far more numerous macrophages in antigen expression and
(low) phagocytosis activity (Van de Wijngaert *et al.*, 1987b). Their presence
in marrow cultures correlated positively with the formation of OC when
marrow cultures were added to stripped bone rudiments, while the presence
of macrophages correlated negatively (Van de Wijngaert *et al.*, 1989). Very
few multinucleated cells were found, in agreement with a study by Takahashi

et al. (1988a) who reported that addition of 1,25 (OH)$_2$ vitamin D$_3$ or PTH is obligatory for the formation of TRAP positive MNC, similar to human bone marrow MNC. Formation of MNC but not mononuclear TRAP cells was sensitive to calcitonin. Although monoclonal antibodies specific for mouse OC are not yet available, and direct testing of the TRAP cells for OC specific antigen expression is not yet possible, they did express CT receptors (Takahashi *et al.*, 1988b).

Thus MNC formed in cultures of haemopoietic tissue from several species show many of the characteristics of OC, but they also show certain differences with authentic OC, formed *in vivo*. This is probably the result of an inadequate tissue culture environment compared with local conditions *in vivo*, and stresses the need for studies of the local regulatory factors in OC development.

As the osteoclast in all probability originates from the haemopoietic stem cell, haemopoietic growth factors which regulate the proliferation and differentiation of blood cell lineages may also be important for OC formation. The effect of haemopoietic growth factors or colony stimulating factors (CSF) may be general or more lineage specific (Metcalf, 1984; Nicola and Vadas, 1984). CSF's such as interleukin 3 stimulate stem cell proliferation and renewal, while factors such as GM-CSF, G-CSF and M-CSF specifically stimulate granulocytes and/or macrophages. Growth and differentiation CSF's which specifically stimulate certain haemopoietic cell lines may positively or negatively influence OC formation by either propagating a cell line which also produces OC or diverting the cell flow to another line which does not spawn OC.

The information on CSF's as modulators of OC formation or the production of CSF by bone tissue is still scanty. Shiina-Ishimi *et al.* (1986) reported the production of CSF-activity by the osteoblastic murine cell line MC 3T3-E1 (Kodama *et al.*, 1981) but the type of CSF was not clarified. Elford *et al.* (1987) showed that MC3T3-E1 and calvarial cells isolated from neonatal mice release M-CSF like activity. Its production could be stimulated by bacterial lipopolysaccharide (LPS) and 1,25 (OH)$_2$ vitamin D$_3$. In a later study the same group (Felix *et al.*, 1988) showed that LPS-treated calvaria released GM-CSF, G-CSF and some IL-3, while isolated calvarial cells produced GM-CSF and some G-CSF. As the calvaria and calvaria-derived cell populations are contaminated with non-osteogenic cells such as macrophages and lymphocytes, the cellular origin of these products is not yet clear, but their production in or by bone tissue seems likely.

As to effects of CSF on OC formation, recombinant human GM-CSF and highly purified M-CSF increased the number of MNC in baboon marrow cultures (MacDonald *et al.*, 1986). However, GM-CSF which acts on a less differentiated myeloid progenitor than M-CSF stimulated MNC formation more consistently than M-CSF. In murine fetal bones in organ culture, interleukin 3 (IL-3) increased the number of OC in young rudiments but decreased it in older bones (Nijweide *et al.*, 1987) while IL-3 and GM-CSF decreased the percentage of recently replicated OC nuclei in rudiments treated with PTH (Lorenzo *et al.*, 1987). In mouse bone marrow cultures M-CSF decreased the number of TRAP positive cells and reduced the capacity of the bone marrow culture to generate OC in stripped bone (Van de Wijngaert *et al.*, 1987a). These studies suggest that M-CSF is an inhibitor rather than a stimulator of OC formation. The same group (Van de Wijngaert *et al.*, 1989) also showed that conditioned media of periost free long bone rudiments stimulated the formation of TRAP-positive cells in mouse bone marrow cultures, but did not stimulate macrophage growth. Kurihara *et al.* (1989) recently described a culture system of spleen cells enriched for primitive hemopoietic progenitors by treatment of mouse donors with a high dose of 5-fluorouracil. The hemopoietic blast cells which developed *in vitro* could be induced to form TRAP positive bone-resorbing MNC's, by treatment with $1,25(OH)_2$ vit D_3 and rIL-3 or GM-CSF. Mature macrophages did not form MNC. Interestingly, rG-CSF or rM-CSF had much less OC-inducing capacity than rGM-CSF.

So, the subject of local regulation of (pre-)OC differentiation by growth factors and cytokines is still only in its infancy, but holds great promises for the future. Bone marrow cultures have in principle great advantages for the study of OC formation from primitive progenitors, but the identification of OC in such cultures and, more important, of their mononuclear progenitor/precursors, is not always certain. The same holds for the influence of haemopoietic growth factors in OC formation. All available evidence however suggests that M-CSF is not a stimulator of OC formation. This observation alone has already important implications for the (dis-)similarity of the OC and macrophage differentiation process, and thus for the interrelationship of these two cell types.

The Bone Microenvironment (BME) and Osteoclast Differentiation

More than 20 years ago, Young (1962) in a study of cell kinetics in the metaphysis of growing long bones observed that incorporation of recently divided nuclei in OC occurred mainly in a zone close to the junction of growth cartilage and metaphysis. This same zone also contained the highest concentration of proliferating osteoblast precursors. This observation was confirmed by a more recent study of Kimmel and Jee (1980). After flash labeling of growing rats with ^{3}H-thymidine, appearance of labeled nuclei in OC occurred in the same zone which contained the highest concentration of newly formed osteoblasts, although the cell kinetics of osteoblasts and osteoclast nuclei were quite different.

The implication of these observations for the existence of a local microenvironment at specific sites in a bone organ which permits osteoblast and OC formation was not elaborated by the authors although the data is suggestive. Over the last few years, a growing body of experimental evidence has been published which supports the concept that local interaction between OC progenitors/precursors and the stromal compartment of skeletal tissue, including osteoblasts/osteocytes, growth plate chondrocytes and their matrices, is of crucial importance for OC differentiation.

Ejiri (1983) studied OC development in fetal rat calvaria *in vivo* and *in vitro*, and found preosteoclasts (identified by the criteria of Scott, 1967) located in the inner endocranial periosteum, in contact with osteoblasts and/or osteoblast-like cells. He concluded that osteoblasts might either serve as inducers of OC formation or even as constituents of the forming OC, and that direct contact of OC precursors with mineralized bone matrix might induce their final cytodifferentiation into OC. The importance of matrix factors is also stressed by a study of Krukowski and Kahn (1982) who showed that cells with OC-like characteristics developed in response to implants of intact bone matrix onto the chorioallantoic membrane of chick embryo's but not to implants of other mineralized materials. Glowacki and co-workers (1986) implanted particles of various materials into subcutaneous pockets in rats and found that only cells adjacent to bone particles stained positive for TRAP while multinucleate cells adjacent to other materials were TRAP negative. Löwik *et al.* (1988) showed that mouse haemopoietic cells cocultured with periost-free bone rudiments expressed TRAP only after direct contact with the bone explant. Addition of bisphosphonate (dimethyl-APD) prevented TRAP expression and OC formation, which was interpreted by the authors as interference of the bisphosphonate with a matrix factor required for attachment and maturation of OC precursors. Lastly, Fuller and Chambers (1989) found that culture of rabbit bone marrow mononuclear cells on bone slices instead of plastic stimulated the differentiation of mono- and multinucleated cells expressing OC-specific antigens.

While these studies stipulate the importance of (mineralized) matrix in OC development, other studies suggest a regulating role of bone stromal cells in OC differentiation. Burger *et al.* (1984) reported that live but not devitalized long bone rudiments stripped of periosteum-perichondrium induced the formation of OC from bone marrow cultures. This observation was confirmed by Boonekamp *et al.* (1986) who used fetal liver instead of bone marrow as source of OC. Employing ^{3}H-thymidine prelabeling to demonstrate the bone marrow origin of OC formed in cocultures, Burger *et al.* (1984) found the labeling index of the OC nuclei to exceed that of the mononuclear phagocytes which were also present in the cocultures, but outside the bone rudiment. This might either reflect a selective origin of OC from proliferative bone marrow cells, or alternatively a selective expansion of the OC precursor pool during coculture with bone rudiments. The authors suggested that viable cells of the bone rudiment might act as regulators of OC generation, similar to their role as regulators of OC function (Rodan and Martin, 1981). The latter hypothesis has now been convincingly demonstrated in a number of studies (McSheehy *et al.*, 1986; Braidman *et al.*, 1986; Thomson *et al.*, 1986) but the role of bone stromal cells in OC generation from primitive progenitors has not yet received much attention. This may be partly due to the difficulties encountered when unequivocally demonstrating OC generation *in vitro* (see above).

The importance of the bone anlage in inducing OC differentiation during ontogeny has been demonstrated by Thesingh (1986). In cocultures of stripped bone rudiments and various fetal or postnatal tissues, she obtained OC formation from all fetal tissues tested, including heart, kidney and brain. In the adult mouse, OC progenitor/precursors were confined to haematopoietic tissues. Apparently, cells capable of OC formation are widely distributed throughout the fetal mouse body, and confrontation with the developing bone rudiment induced their differentiation as OC. An earlier study (Thesingh and Burger, 1983) had shown that during embryonic ontogeny primitive proliferative OC progenitors home in the mesenchyme of the mouse limb bud long before OC formation is due. Scheven *et al.* (1985, 1986b) demonstrated that in the course of development of a long bone rudiment the population of OC progenitors in the perichondrium-periosteum shifts from mainly proliferating cells to mainly postmitotic precursors before expression of TRAP and cell fusion occur.

Further experimental support for the importance of stromal bone cells in regulating OC formation derives from the following studies. Marshall *et al.* (1986) grew cells from neonatal rat long bones and bone marrow, and observed that confluent primary cultures of osteoblast-like cells permitted the formation of multinucleate osteoclast-like cells from a second addition of bone- or marrow cells seeded on top of the confluent layer. Confluent layers of skin fibroblasts were ineffective in inducing OC formation. Jilka (1986) grew cells from neonatal mouse calvaria released by sequential digestion. In monolayers derived from the inner periosteum, cells responsive to PTH by strongly increased resorptive activity were only maintained if the cells were initially seeded at confluent density. If seeded at normal, 10x lower density the response to PTH and PTH-stimulated development of TRAP-positive cells was lost within 5 days. Others (Burger *et al.*, 1986) showed that these low density-seeded monolayers still formed OC as well as many osteoblasts in co-culture with stripped rudiments, while monolayer cells from the outer periosteum formed neither OC nor osteoblasts. These studies suggest that the OC phenotype present in bone cell populations is only expressed in an environment also containing a high concentration of osteoblasts or, in the coculture assay, calcifying growth plate cartilage.

Lastly, radiation injury resulting from irradiating stripped bone rudiments reduced their capacity to induce OC formation from (non-irradiated) haemopoietic cells (Scheven *et al.* 1987). The authors compared this phenomenon with the well known disturbances of blood cell generation resulting from radiation damage of the stromal haemopoietic microenvironment. Van de Wijngaert *et al.* (1988) showed that live bone rudiments had a much stronger capacity for OC recruitment than dead bones, when transplanted in syngeneic hosts. Recently this group showed (Van de Wijngaert *et al.*, 1989) that conditioned media of live but not dead bone rudiments increased the number of TRAP positive cells in mouse bone marrow cultures but had no effect on the growth of mononuclear phagocytes.

In conclusion, several recent studies, using *in vitro* as well as *in vivo* methods, provide evidence for a crucial role of signals elaborated by skeletal stroma (cells and matrix) during growth and differentiation of OC and OC precursors. The identification of these factors and clarification of their precise role during OC ontogeny is an obvious challenge for future research.

Conclusion

Although many details of the osteoclast lineage are still unclear, present published data limits the possible lines of osteoclast development to a restricted number of options which we have tried to summarize in Fig. 1.

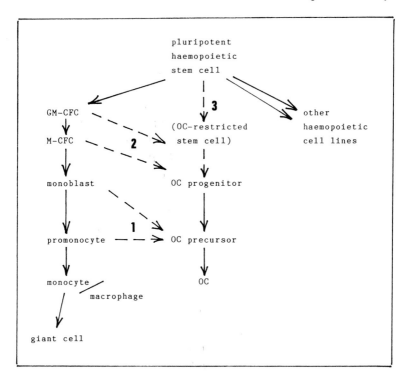

Fig. 1 Schematic representation of possible routes of osteoclast differentiation which are compatible with present knowledge. In route 1, OC precursors develop from early cells of the mononuclear phagocyte lineage. In route 2 the ties between osteoclasts and macrophages lie at the level of committed stem cells. In route 3, the osteoclast lineage is a separate derivative of the pluripotent haemopoietic stem cell, unrelated to mononuclear phagocytes. This latter hypothesis requires, in analogy with other myeloid lineages, a stem cell restricted to osteoclasts, but to date there is no experimental support for such a cell.

There is general agreement that OC are derived from the haemopoietic stem cell and should be included in the haemopoietic cell family. The ties of the OC lineage with the mononuclear phagocyte pathway are however still unclear. Recent data favour the concept that these ties only relate to (very) early stages of cellular differentiation, and not to the mature end cells. At one end of the spectrum, OC are considered full blown members of the mononuclear phagocyte system and to develop from immature monoblasts or promonocytes. At the other end, OC are not even related to committed monocyte/granulocyte stem cells but derive from a cell, as yet hypothetical, which develops directly from the pluripotent stem cell and which is restricted

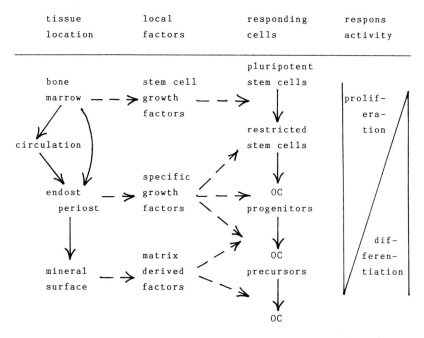

Fig. 2 Cells and factors involved in osteoclast generation, and their possible location in bone.

to OC development. In between these extreme views, OC share a committed stem cell with granulocytes and/or macrophages.

For further study on the lineage of the osteoclast, work on the (un)responsiveness of OC development to lineage-specific growth factors seems particularly fruitful, as this approach may provide evidence on the (dis)similarity of OC and macrophage development even if the cells in question cannot yet be identified with certainty. Granulocyte and macrophage growth factors are of particular importance, as well as other, recently identified factors with differentiative capacity (Abe *et al.*, 1986). In addition, the fact that osteoclasts are tissue-specific cells, unlike macrophages, deserves closer attention. Multinucleated osteoclasts are only found in mineralized tissues. A growing body of evidence supports the important role of skeletal stroma in directly or indirectly regulating the physiological resorption of mineralized matrices. Indeed, the influence of stromal cells and calcified matrix on osteoclasts seems so important that in a sense OC could be regarded as hired hands, recruited at a certain location and time to fulfill local and temporary needs of mineral removal. In this concept local factors are crucial in determining OC activity and probably OC generation.

As a framework of thought we have listed in Fig. 2 the hypothetical factors and cells which may be involved in OC formation. In particular we have tried to connect the separate steps of OC development with factors regulating these processes, as well as their likely place of action in bone organs. Although largely speculative, it may help in defining unknown areas and generating new questions about the OC lineage.

In this concept, osteoclasts derive from cells born in the bone marrow. Their further differentiation occurs in spatial and chemical relation to mineralized tissue surfaces. The more mature the developmental step, the closer its relation to the mineralized matrix surface. Osteoclast growth factors may either be secreted directly from stromal cells of the endost/periost/perichondrium or they may be set free from the matrix after having been deposited there at an earlier time. In this view, the question of osteoclast and macrophage relationship is reduced to the question of overlap in growth requirements of their respective progenitor/precursors.

References

Abe, E.,Tanaka, H., Ishimi, Y., Miyaura, C., Hagashi, T., Hagasawa, T., Tomida, W., Yamaguchi, Y., Hozumi M. and Suda, T. (1986) Differentiation inducing factor purified from conditioned medium of mitogen-treated spleen cell cultures stimulates bone resorption. *Proc. Natl. Acad. Sci. USA* **83**: 5958-62

Allen, T. D., Testa, N. G., Suda, T., Schor, S. L., Onions, D., Jarret O. and Boyde A. (1981) The production of putative osteoclasts in tissue culture: ultrastructure, formation and behavior. *Scanning Electron Microsc.* **3**: 347-354

Arnett T. R. and Dempster, D. W. (1987) A comparative study of disaggregated chick and rat osteoclasts *in vitro*, effects of calcitonin and prostaglandins. *Endocrinology* **120**: 602-608

Ash, P., Loutit J. F. and Townsend, K. M. S. (1980) Osteoclasts derived from haematopoietic stem cells. *Nature Lond.* **283**: 669-670

Athanasou, N. A., Heryet, A., Quinn, J., Gatter, K. C., Mason D. Y. and McGee J. O'D (1986) Osteoclasts contain macrophage and megakaryocyte antigens. *J. Pathol.* **150**: 239-246

Barnes, D. W. H., Loutit J. F. and Samson, J. W. (1975) Histocompatible cells for the resolution of osteopetrosis in microphthalmic mice. *Proc. Roy. Soc. Ser. B* **188**: 501-505

Baron, R., Neff, L., Tran Van, P., Nefussi J. R. and Vignery, A. (1986)Kinetic and cytochemical identification of osteoclast precursors and their differentiation into multinucleated osteoclast. *Am. J. Pathol.* **122**: 363-78

Bianco, P., Costantini, M., Dearden L. C. and Bonucci, E. (1987) Expression of tartrate-resistant acid phosphatase in bone marrow macrophages. *Basic Appl. Histochem.* **31**: 433-40

Bianco, P., Ballant P. and Bonucci, E., (1988) Tartrate-resistant acid phosphatase activity in rat osteoblasts and osteocytes. *Calcif. Tissue Int.* **43**: 167-171

Boonekamp, P. M., van der Wee-Pals, L. J. A., van Wijk-van Lennep, M. M. L., Thesingh C. W. and Bijvoet, O. L. M. (1986) Two modes of action of bisphosphonates on osteoclastic resorption of mineralized matrix. *Bone Mineral* 1: 27-39

Braidman, I. P., St. John, J. G., Anderson D. C. and Robertson, W. R. (1986) Effect of physiological concentrations of parathyroid hormone on acid phosphatase activity in cultured rat bone cells. *J. Endocrinol.* 111: 17-26

Brookes, M. (1971) *The blood supply of bone.* Butterworths, London (1971).

Bromley, M. and Woolley, D. E. (1974) Chondroclast and osteoclasts at subchondral sites of erosion in the rheumatoid joint. *Arthritis Rheum.* 27: 968-75

Burger, E. H., van der Meer, J. W. M., van de Gevel, J. S., Gribnau, J. C., Thesingh C. W. and van Furth, R. (1982) *in vitro* formation of osteoclasts from longterm culture of bone marrow mononuclear phagocytes. *J. Exp. Med.* 156: 1604-1614

Burger, E. H., van der Meer J. W. M and Nijweide, P. J. (1984) Osteoclast formation from mononuclear phagocytes, role of bone-forming cells. *J. Cell Biol.* 99: 1901-1906

Burger, E. H., Bonekamp P. M. and Nijweide, P. J. (1986) Osteoblast and osteoclast precursors in primary cultures of calvarial bone cells. *Anat. Rec.* 214: 32-40

Chambers, T. J. and Magnus, C. I. (1982) Calcitonin alters behaviour of isolated osteoclasts. *J. Pathol.* 136: 27-39

Chambers, T. J. (1985) The pathobiology of the osteoclast. *J. Clin. Pathol.* 38: 241-252

Chappard, D., Alexandre C. and Riffat, G. (1983) Histochemical identification of osteoclasts. Review of current methods and reappraisal of a simple procedure for routine dianosis on undecalcified human iliac bone biopsies. *Basic Appl. Histochem.* 27: 75-85

Coccia, P. F., Krivit, W., Cervenka, J., Clawson, C., Kersey, J. H., Kim, T. H., Nesbit, M. E., Ramsay, N. K. C., Warkentin, P. I., Teitelbaum, S. L., Kahn A. J. and Brown, D. M. (1980) Successful bone-marrow transplantation for infantile malignant osteopetrosis. *N. Engl. J. Med.* 302: 701-708

Cole, A. A. and Walters, L. M. (1987) Tartrate-resistant acid phosphatase in bone and cartilage following decalcification and cold-embedding in plastic. *J. Histochem. Cytochem.* 35: 203-206

Ejiri, S. (1983) The preosteoclast and its cytodifferentiation into the osteoclast, ultrastructural and histochemical studies of rat fetal parietal bone. *Arch. Histol. Jpn.* 46: 533-557

Elford, P. R., Felix, R., Cecchini, M., Trechsel U. and Fleisch, H. (1987) Murine osteoblast-like cells and the osteogenic cell MC 3T3-Ei release a macrophage colony-stimulating activity in culture. *Calcif. Tissue Int.* 41: 151-156

Felix, R., Elford, P. R., Stoerckle, C., Cecchini, M., Wetterwald, A., Trechsel, U., Fleisch H. and Stadler, B. M (1988) Production of hemopoietic growth factors by bone tissue and bone cells in culture. *J. Bone Min. Res.* 3: 27-36

Fischman D. A. and Hay,, E. D. (1962) Origin of osteoclasts from mononuclear leukocytes in regenerating newt limbs. *Anat. Rec.* 143: 329-337

Fuller K. and Chambers, T. J. (1987) Generation of osteoclasts in cultures of rabbit bone marrow and spleen cells. *J. Cell Phys.* 132: 441-452

Fuller K. and Chambers, T. J. (1989) Bone matrix stimulates osteoclastic differentiation in cultures of rabbit bone marrow cells. *J. Bone Min. Res.* 4: 179-183

Gallien-Lartique O. and Carrez, D. (1974) Induction *in vitro* de la phase S dans les cellules souches multipotentes de la moelle osseuse par l'hormone parathyro dienne. *C.R. Seances Acad. Sci. Ser. III Sci. Vie* 278: 1765-68

Glowacki, J., Jasty M., and Goldring, S. (1986) Comparison of multinucleated cells elicited in rats by particulate bone, polyethylene, or polymethyl-methacrylate. *J. Bone Min. Res.* 1: 327-331

Göthling G. and Ericsson, J. L. E. (1973) On the histogenesis of the cells in fracture callus. *Virchows Arch. Abt. B Zellpathol.* **12**: 318-329

Hagenaars, C. E., van der Kraan, A. A. M., Kawilarang-de Haas, E. W. M., Visser J. W. M. and Nijweide, P. J. (1989) Osteoclast formation from cloned pluripotent hemopoietic stem cells. *Bone Mineral* **6**: 179-189

Hakeda, Y., Hiura, K., Sato, T., Okazaki, R., Matsumoto, T., Ogata, E., Ishitani R. and Kumegawa, M. (1989) Existence of parathyroid hormone binding sites on murine hemopoietic blast cells. *Biochem. Biophys. Res. Com.* **163**: 1484-1486

Helfrich, M. H., Thesingh, C. W., Mieremet R. H. P. and van Iperen-van Gent, A. S. (1987) Osteoclast generation from human fetal bone marrow in coculture with murine fetal long bones. A model for *in vitro* study of human osteoclast formation and function. *Cell Tissue Res.* **249**: 125-136

Helfrich, M. H., Mieremet R. H. P. and Thesingh, C. W. (1990) Osteoclast formation *in vitro* from progenitor cells present in the adult mouse circulation. *J. Bone Min. Res.* in press.

Hermans, W. (1987) Identification of osteoclasts and their differentiation from mononuclear phagocytes by enzyme histochemistry. *Histo Chemistry* **86**: 225-7

Horton, M. A., Rimmer, E. F., Lewis, D., Pringle, J. A. S., Fuller K. and Chambers, T. J. (1984) Cell surface characterisation of the human osteoclast, phenotypic relationship to other bone marrow cell types. *J. Pathol.* **144**: 281-294

Horton, M. A., Lewis, D., McNulty, K., Pringle J. A. S. and Chambers, T. J. (1985a) Human fetal osteoclasts fail to express macrophage antigens. *Br. J. Exp. Pathol.* **66**: 103-108

Horton, M. A., Rimmer, E. F., Moore A. and Chambers, T. J. (1985b) On the origin of the osteoclast: the cell surface phenotype of rodent osteoclasts. *Calcif. Tissue Int.* **37**: 46-50

Horton, M. A., Lewis, D., McNulty, K., Pringle J. A. S. and Chambers, T. J. (1985c) Monoclonal antibodies to osteoclastomas (giant cell bone tumors): definition of osteoclast-specific antigens. *Cancer Res.* **45**: 5663-5669

Horton, M. A. and Chambers, T. J. (1986) Human osteoclast-specific antigens are expressed by osteoclasts in a wide range of non-human species. *Br. J. Exp. Path.* **67**: 95-104

Horton, M. A., Rimmer E. F. and Chambers, T. J. (1986) Giant cell formation in rabbit long-term bone marrow cultures: immunological and functional studies. *J. Bone Min. Res.* **1**: 5-14

Hume, D. A., Loutit J. F. and Gordon, S. (1984) The mononuclear phagocyte system of the mouse defined by immunohistochemical localization of antigen F4/80: macrophages of bone and associated connective tissue. *J. Cell Sci.* **66**: 189-194

Ibbotson, K. J., Roodman, G. D., McManus L. M. and Mundy, G. R. (1984) Identification and characterization of osteoclast-like cells and their progenitors in cultures of feline marrow mononuclear cells. *J. Cell Biol.* **99**: 417-480

Jilka, R. L. (1986) Parathyroid hormone-stimulated development of osteoclasts in cultures of cells from neonatal murine calvaria. *Bone* **7**: 29-40

Joterau F. V. and Le Douarin, N. M. (1978) The developmental relationship between osteocytes and osteoclasts: a study using the quail-chick nuclear marker in endochondral ossification. *Dev. Biol.* **63**: 253-265

Kahn A. J. and Simmons, D. J. (1975) Investigation of cell lineage in bone using a chimaera of chick and quail embryonic tissue. *Nature Lond.* **258**: 325-327

Kimmel D. B. and Jee, W. S. S. (1980) Bone cell kinetics during longitudinal bone growth in the rat. *Calcif. Tissue Int.* **32**: 123-133

Ko J. S. and Bernard, G. W. (1981) Osteoclast formation *in vitro* from bone marrow mononuclear cells in osteoclast free bone. *Am. J. Anat.* **161** 415-425

Kodama, H., Amagai, Y., Sudo, H., Kasai S. and Yamamoto, S. (1981) Establishment of a clonal osteogenic cell line from new born mouse calvaria. *Jap. J. Oral Biol.* **23**: 899-901

Kölliker, A. (1873) *Die normale Resorption der Knochengewebes und ihre Bedeutung für die Entstehung der typischen Knochenformen*. Leipzig, GDR, Vogel (1873).

Krieger, N. S., Feldman R. S. and Tashjian, A. H. (1982) Parathyroid hormone and calcitonin interactions in bone: irradiation-induced inhibition of escape *in vitro*. *Calcif. Tissue Int.* 34: 197-203

Krukowski M. and Kahn, A. J. (1982) Inductive specificity of mineralized bone matrix in ectopic osteoclast differentiation. *Calcif. Tissue Int.* 34: 474-479

Kukita, T., McManus, L. M., Miller, M., Civin C. and Roodman, G. D. (1989) Osteoclast-like cells formed in long-term human bone marrow cultures express a similar surface phenotype as authentic osteoclasts. *Lab. Invest.* 60: 532-538

Kurihara, N., Suda, T., Miura, Y., Nakauchi, H., Kodama, H., Hiura, K., Hakeda Y. and Kumegawa, M. (1989) Generation of osteoclasts from isolated hematopoietic progenitor cells. *Blood* 74: 1295-1302

Lorenzo, J. A., Sousa, S. L., Fonseca, J. M., Hock, J. M. and Medlock, E. S. (1987) Colony stimulating factor regulate the development of multinucleated osteoclasts from recently replicated cells *in vitro*. *J. Clin. Invest.* 80: 160-164

Loutit J. F. and Nisbet, N. W. (1982) The origin of osteoclasts. *Immunobiology* 161: 193-203

Loutit J. F. and Sansom, J. S. (1976) Osteopetrosis of microphthalmic mice - a defect of the hematopoietic stem cell. *Calcif. Tissue Res.* 20: 251-259

Löwik, C. W. G. M., van der Pluijm, G., van der Wee-Pals, L. J. A., Bloys van Treslong-de Groot H. and Bijvoet, O. L. M. (1988) Migration and phenotypic transformation of osteoclast precursors into mature osteoclasts: the effect of a bisphosphonate. *J. Bone and Min. Res.* 3: 185-192

Luk, S. C., Nopajaroonsri C. and Simon, G. T. (1974) The ultrastructure of endosteum: a topographic study in young adult rabbits. *J. Ultrastruct. Res.* 46: 165-183

MacDonald, B. R., Mundy, G. R., Clark, S., Wang, E. A., Kuehl, T. J., Stanley E. R. and Roodman, G. D. (1986) Effects of human recombinant GSF-GM and highly purified CSF-1 on the formation of multinucleated cells with osteoclast characteristics in long-term bone marrow cultures. *J. Bone Min Res.* 1: 227-233

MacDonald, B. R., Takahashi, N., McManus, L. M., Holahan, J., Mundy, G. R. and Roodman, G. D. (1987) Formation of multinucleated cells which respond to osteotropic hormones in long-term human bone marrow cultures. *Endocrin.* 120: 2326-2333

MacManus, J. P. and Whitfield, J. W. (1970) The inhibition by thyrocalcitonin of the mitogenic actions of parathyroid hormone and cyclic adenosine 3151-monophosphate on the rat thymocytes. *Endocrinology* 86: 934-939

Makris, G. P. and Saffar, J. L. (1982) Quantitative relationship between osteoclasts, osteoclast nuclei and the extent of the resorbing surface in hamster periodontal disease. *Archs. Oral Biol.* 27: 965-69

Marks, S. C. (1983) The origin of osteoclast: evidence, clinical implications and investigative challenges of an extra-skeletal source. *J. Oral Pathol.* 12: 226-256

Marks, S. C. (1984) Congenital osteopetrotic mutations as probes of the origin, structure, and function of osteoclasts. *Clin. Orthop.* 189: 239-263

Marks, S. C. and Popoff, S. N. (1988) Bone cell biology: The regulation of development structure and function in the skeleton. *Am. J. Anat.* 183: 1-44

Marshall, M. J., Nisbet, N. W., Menage J. and Loutit, J. F. (1982) Tissue repopulation during cure of osteopetrotic (mi/mi) mice using normal and defective (We/Wv) bone marrow. *Exp. Haematol.* 10: 600-608

Marshall, M. J., Nisbet, N. W., Green, P. M. (1986) Evidence for osteoclast production in mixed bone cell culture. *Calcif. Tissue Int.* 38: 268-274

McSheehy, P. M. J. and Chambers, T. J. (1986) Osteoblastic cells mediate osteoclastic responsiveness to parathyroid hormone. *Endocrinology* **118**: 824-828

Metcalf, D. (1984) *The hemopoietic colony-stimulating factors.* Elsevier, Amsterdam, pp. 277-307 (1984).

Minkin, C. (1982) Bone acid phosphatase: tartrate-resistant acid phosphatase as a marker of osteoclast function. *Calcif. Tissue Int.* **34**: 285-290

Mueller, W. J., Schraer, H. and Schraer, R. (1974) Calcium metabolism and skeletal dynamics of laying pullets. *J. Nutr.* **84**: 20-26

Mundy, G. R. and Roodman, G. D. (1987) Osteoclast ontogeny and function. In: *Bone and Mineral Research 5*, W. A. Peck, editor. Elsevier Science Publ. 209-279 (1987).

Nicola, N. A. and Vadas, M. (1984) Hemopoietic colony-stimulating factors. *Immunology Today* **5**: 76-80

Nicholson, G. C., Moseley, J. M., Sexton, P. M., Mendelson, F. A. O. and Martin, T. J. (1986) Abundant calcitonin receptors in isolated rat osteoclasts: Biochemical and autoradiographic characterisation. *J. Clin. Invest.* **78**: 355-360

Nicholson, G. C., Moseley, J. M., Sexton, P. M. and Martin, T. J (1987) Chick osteoclasts do not express calcitonin receptors. *J. Bone Min. Res.* **2**: 53-59

Nijweide, P. J., Vrijheid-Lammers, T., Mulder, R. J. P. and Blok, J. (1985) Cell surface antigens on osteoclasts and related cells in the quail studied with monoclonal antibodies. *Histochemistry* **83**: 315-324

Nijweide, P. J., Burger, E. H. and Feyen, J. H. (1986) Cells of bone: proliferation, differentiation, and hormonal regulation. *Physiol. Rev.* **66**: 855-886

Nijweide, P. J., Scheven, B. A. A. and Visser, J. W. M. (1987) Proliferation and differentiation of osteoclast progenitor and precursor cells. In: *Calcium regulation and bone metabolism: bone and clinical aspects.* (D. V. Cohn, T.J. Martin and P.J. Meunier, Eds.) Exerpta Medica, Amsterdam, 9, 301-307 (1987).

Nisbet, N. W., Menage, J. and Loutit, J. F. (1979) Resolution and relapse of osteopetrosis in mice transplanted with myeloid tissue of variable histocompatibility. *Transplantation* **28**: 285-290

Osdoby, P., Martini, M. C. and Caplan, A. I. (1982) Isolated osteoclasts and their presumed progenitor cells, the monocyte in culture. *J. Exp. Zool.* **224**: 331-344

Oursler, M. J., Bell, L. V., Clevinger, B. and Osdoby, P. (1985) Identification of osteoclast-specific monoclonal antibodies. *J. Cell Biol.* **100**: 1592-1600

Pharoah, M. J. and Heersche, J. N. M. (1985) 1,25-Di-hydroxy vitamin D_3 causes an increase in the number of osteoclast-like cells in cat bone marrow cultures. *Calcif. Tissue Int.* **37**: 276-281

Pharoah, M. J. and Heersche, J. N. M. (1986) Dexamethasone inhibits formation of osteoclast-like cells in bone marrow cultures. *J. Dent. Res.* **65**: 1006-1009

Razdun, H. J., Kreipe, H. and Parwaresch, M. R. (1983) Tartrate-resistant acid phosphatase as a differentiation marker for the human mononuclear phagocyte system. *Hematol. Oncol.* **1**: 321-327

Rhinelander, F. W. (1972) Circulation in bone. In: *The biochemistry and physiology of bone.* (G. H. Bourne Ed.) Sec. ed., Vol. II, p.2-77, Academic Press, N.Y.

Rifkin, B. R., Brand, J. S., Cushing, J. E., Coleman, S. J. and Sanavi, F. (1980) Fine structure of fetal rat calvarium: provisional identification of preosteoclasts. *Calcif. Tissue Int.* **31**: 21-28

Rodan, G. A. and Martin, T. J. (1981) Role of osteoclasts in hormonal control of bone resorption - a hypothesis. *Calcif. Tissue Int.* **33**: 349-351

Roodman, G. D., Ibbotson, K. J., MacDonald, B. R., Kuehl, T. J. and Mundy, G. R. (1985) 1,25-Dihydroxyvitamin D_3 causes formation of multinucleated cells with several osteoclast characteristics in cultures of primate marrow. *Proc. Natl. Acad. Sci. USA* **82**: 8213-8217

Scheven, B. A. A., Burger, E. H., Kawilarang-de Haas, E. W. M., Wassenaar, A. M. and Nijweide, P. J. (1985) Effects of ionizing irradiation on formation and resorbing activity of osteoclasts *in vitro*. *Lab. Invest.* **53**: 72-79

Scheven, B. A. A., Visser, J. W. M. and Nijweide, P. J. (1986a) *in vitro* generation from different bone marrow fractions including a highly enriched hematopoietic stem cell population. *Nature (London)* **321**: 79-81

Scheven, B. A. A., Kawilarang-de Haas, E. W. M., Wassenaar, A. W. and Nijweide, P. J. (1986b) Differentiation kinetics of osteoclasts in the periosteum of embryonic bones *in vivo* and *in vitro*. *Anat. Rec.* **214**: 418-423

Scheven, B. A. A., Wassenaar, A. M., Kawilarang-de Haas, E. W. M. and Nijweide, P. J. (1987) Comparison of direct and indirect radiation effects on osteoclast formation from progenitor cells derived from different hemopoietic sources. *Radiat. Res.* **111**: 107-118

Schneider, G. B. and Byrnes, J. E. (1983) Cellular specificity of the cure for neonatal osteoporosis in the ia rat. *Exp. Cell Biol.* **51**: 44-50

Schneider, G. B. (1985) Cellular specificity of the cure for osteopetrosis: Isolation of and treatment with pluripotent hemopoietic stem cells. *Bone* **6**: 241-247

Schneider, G. B. and Relfson, M. (1988a) The effects of transplantation of granulocyte-macrophage progenitors on bone resorption in osteopetrotic rats. *J. Bone Min. Res.* **3**: 225-232

Schneider, G. B. and Relfson, M. (1988b) A bone marrow fraction enriched for granulocyte-macrophage progenitors gives rise to osteoclasts *in vitro*. *Bone* **9**: 303-308

Schneider, G. B. and Relfson, M. (1989) Pluripotent hemopoietic stem cells give rise to osteoclasts *in vitro*: effects of rGM-CSF. *Bone Mineral* **5**: 129-138

Scott, B. L. (1967) Thymidine-^{3}H electron microscope radioautography of osteogenic cells in the fetal rat. *J. Cell Biol.* **35**: 115-126

Shiina-Ishimi, Y., Abe, E., Tanaka, H. and Suda, T. (1986) Synthesis of colony-stimulating factor (CSF) and differentiation-inducing factor (D-factor) by osteoblastic cells, clone MC 3T3-E1. *Biochem. Biophys. Res. Commun.* **134**: 400-406

Simmons, D. J. and Kahn, A. J. (1979) Cell lineage in fracture healing in dimeric bone grafts. *Calcif. Tissue Int.* **27**: 247-253

Sminia, T. and Dijkstra, C. D. (1986) The origin of osteoclasts: an immunohistochemical study on macrophages and osteoclasts in embryonic rat bone. *Calcif. Tissue Int.* **39**: 263-266

Snipes, R. G., Lam, K. W., Dodd, R. C., Gray, T. K. and Cohen, M. S. (1986) Acid phosphatase activity in mononuclear phagocytes and the U937 cell line: monocyte-derived macrophages express tartrate-resistant acid phosphatase. *Blood* **67**: 729-34

Sorell, M., Kapoor, N., Kirkpatrick, D., Rosen, J. F., Chaganti, R., Lopez, C., Dupont, B. O., Pollack, M. S., Terrin, N., Harris, M. B., Vine, D., Rose, J. S., Goossen, C., Lane, J., Good, R. A. and O'Reilly, R. J. (1981) Marrow transplantation for juvenile osteopetrosis. *Amer. J. Med.* **70**: 1280-1287

Stanka, P. and Bargsten, G. (1983) Experimental study on the haematogenous origin of multinucleated osteoclasts in the rat. *Cell Tissue Res.* **233**: 125-132

Suda, T., Testa, N. G., Allen, T. D., Onions, D. and Jarret, O. (1983) Effect of hydrocortisone on osteoclasts-generated in cat bone marrow cultures. *Calcif. Tissue Int.* **35**: 82-86

Sundquist, K. I., Leppilampi, M., Järvelin, K., Kumpulainen, T. and Vaananen, H. K. (1987) Carbonic anhydrase isoenzymes in isolated rat peripheral monocytes, tissue macrophages and osteoclasts. *Bone* **8**: 33-38

Sutton, J. S. and Weiss, L. (1966) Transformation of monocytes in tissue culture into macrophages, epithelioid cell, and multinucleated giant cells. *J. Cell Biol.* **28**: 303-332

Takahashi, N., MacDonald, B. R., Hon, J., Winkler, M. E., Derynck, R., Mundy, G. A and Roodman, G. D. (1986) Recombinant human transforming growth factor alpha stimulates the formation of osteoclast-like cells in long term human marrow cultures. *J. Clin. Invest.* **78**: 894-898

Takahashi, N., Mundy, G. R. and Roodman, G. D. (1986) Recombinant human gamma-interferon inhibits information of human osteoclast-like cells by inhibiting the fusion of their precursors. *J. Immunol.* **137**: 3544-3550

Takahashi, N., Yamana, H., Yoshiki, S., Roodman, G.D., Mundy, G. R., Jones, S. J., Boyde, A. and Suda, T. (1988) Osteoclast-like cell formation and its regulation by osteotropic hormones in mouse bone marrow cultures. *Endocrinology* **122**: 1373-1382

Takahashi, N., Akatzu, T., Sasahi, T., Nicholson, G. C., Moseley, J. M., Martin, J. T. and Suda, T. (1988b) Induction of calcitonin receptors by 1α,25-dihydroxy vitamin D_3 in osteoclast-like multinucleated cells formed from mouse bone marrow cells. *Endocrinology* **123**: 1504-1510

Takahashi, N., Kukita, T., MacDonald, B. R., Bird, A., Mundy, G. R., McManus, L. M., Miller, M., Boyde, A., Jones, S. J. and Roodman, G. D. (1989) Osteoclast-like cells form in long-term human bone marrow but not in peripheral blood cultures. *J. Clin. Invest.* **83**: 543-550

Tanaka, T. and Tanaka, M. (1988) Cytological and functional studies of preosteoclasts and osteoclasts in the alveolar bone from neonatal rats using microperoxidase as a tracer. *Calcif. Tissue Int.* **42**: 267-72

Testa, N. G., Allen, T. D., Lajtha, L. G., Onions, D. and Jarret, O. (1981) Generation of osteoclasts *in vitro*. *J. Cell Sci.* **47**: 127-137

Teti, A., Volleth, G., Carano, A. and Zambonin Zallone, A. (1988) The effects of parathyroid hormone and 1,25 dihydroxyvitamin D_3 on monocyte-osteoclast fusion. *Calcif. Tissue Int.* **42**: 302-308

Thesingh, C. W. and Burger, E. H. (1983) The role of mesenchyme in embryonic long bones as early deposition site for osteoclast progenitor cells. *Dev. Biol.* **95**: 429-438

Thesingh, C. W. (1986) Formation sites and distribution of osteoclast progenitor cells during the ontogeny of the mouse. *Dev. Biol.* **117**: 127-134

Tinkler, S. M. B., Linder, J. E., Williams, D. M. and Johnson, N. W. (1981) Formation of osteoclasts from blood monocytes during 1α-OH vit D stimulated bone resorption in mice. *J. Anat.* **133**: 389-396

Tinkler, S. M. B., Williams, D. M., Linder, J. E. and Johnson, N. W. (1983) Kinetics of osteoclast formation: the significance of blood monocytes as osteoclast precursors during 1α-hydroxycholecalciferol-stimulated bone resorption in the mouse. *J. Anat.* **137**: 335-340

Thomson, B. M., Saklatvala, J. and Chambers, T. J. (1986) Osteoblasts mediate interleukin 1 stimulation of bone resorption by rat osteoclasts. *J. Exp. Med.* **164**: 104-112

Tran Van, P., Vignery, A. and Baron, R. (1982a) An electron microscopic study of the bone remodeling sequence in the rat. *Cell Tissue Res.* **225**: 283-292

Tran Van, P., Vignery, A. and Baron, R. (1982b) Cellular kinetics of the bone remodeling sequence in the rat. *Anat. Rec.* **202**: 445-51

Vaes, G. (1988) Cellular biology and biochemical mechanism of bone resorption. *Clin. Orthop. Rel. Res.* **231**: 239-271

Van der Meer, J. W. M., van de Gevel, J. S., Diesselhoff-den Dulk, M. M. C., Beelen, R. H. L. and van Furth, R. (1980) Long-term culture of murine bone marrow mononuclear phagocytes. In: *Mononuclear Phagocytes: Functional Aspects*. (R. van Furth, Ed) The Hague: Nijhoff, 343-356 (1980).

Van de Wijngaert, F. P. and Burger, E. H. (1986) Demonstration of tartrate-resistant acid phosphatase in un-decalcified, glycolmethacrylate-embedded mouse bone: a possible marker for (pre)osteoclast identification. *J. Histochem. Cytochem.* **34**: 1317-1323

Van de Wijngaert, F. P., Tas, M. C., van de Meer, J. W. M. and Burger, E. H. (1987a) Growth of osteoclast precursor like cell from whole mouse bone marrow: inhibitory effect of CSF-1. *Bone and Mineral* **3**: 97-110

Van de Wijngaert, F. P., Tas, M. C. and Burger, E. H. (1987b) Characteristics of osteoclast precursor-like cells grown from mouse bone marrow. *Bone Mineral* **3**: 111-123

Van de Wijngaert, F. P., Schipper, C. A., Tas, M. C. and Burger, E. H. (1988) Role of mineralizing cartilage in osteoclast and osteoblast recruitment. *Bone* **9**: 81-88

Van de Wijngaert, F. P., Tas, M. C. and Burger, E. H. (1989) Conditioned medium of fetal mouse long bone rudiments stimulated the formation of osteoclast precursor like cells from mouse bone marrow. *Bone* **10**: 61-68

Walker, D. G. (1973) Osteopetrosis cured by temporary parabiosis. *Science* **180**: 875-881

Walker, D. G. (1975) Control of bone resorption by hematopoietic tissue. *J. Exp. Med.* **142**: 651-663

Warshawsky, H., Goltzman, D., Rouleau, M. F. and Bergeron, J. J. M. (1980) Direct *in vivo* demonstration by autoradiography of specific binding sites for calcitonin in skeletal and renal tissues of the rat. *J. Cell Biol.* **85**: 682-694

Weinberg, J. B., Hobbs, M. M. and Misukonis, M. A. (1984) Recombinant human gamma-interferon induces human monocyte polykaryon formation. *Proc. Natl. Acad. Sci. USA* **81**: 4554-57

Yabe, H. and Hanaoka, H. (1985) Investigation of the origin of the osteoclast by use of transplantation on chick chorioallantoic membrane. *Clin. Orthop. Rel. Res.* **187**: 255-265

Young, R. W. (1962) Cell proliferation and specialization during endochondral osteogenesis in young rats. *J. Cell Biol.* **14**: 357-370

Zambonin Zallone, A. and Teti, A. (1985) Autoradiographic demonstration of *in vitro* fusion of blood monocytes with osteoclasts. *Basic Appl. Histochem.* **29**: 45-48

3

Histochemistry and Enzymology of Osteoclasts

STEPHEN B. DOTY
Research Building
Hospital for Special Surgery
New York, New York

Introduction
Sugars, carbohydrates and osteoclasts
The histochemical distribution of acid glycerophosphatase activity in the
   osteoclast
The distribution of other histochemical activities in the osteoclast
   The golgi complex
   The lysosome
   The mitochondria
   The ruffled border
Secretion of acid phosphatase activity by the osteoclast
Summary
References

Introduction

The mechanisms involved in bone resorption by the osteoclast have, until recently, been studied by techniques which were applied only to *in vivo* experiments. Cytochemical techniques and electron microscopic histochemistry provided most of the information regarding osteoclastic functions. Today, with the ability to isolate osteoclasts and to carry out *in vitro* experiments, the function of these cells is becoming better understood. In this chapter the descriptions of enzymatic activities found in osteoclasts will be derived from numerous sources including my own histochemical studies.

There is a tremendous amount of published literature on bone resorption and the biochemical events involved (see the excellent review by Vaes, 1988). The intent of this chapter is to restrict discussion to histochemical or cytochemical findings which can then be related to organelles or structures

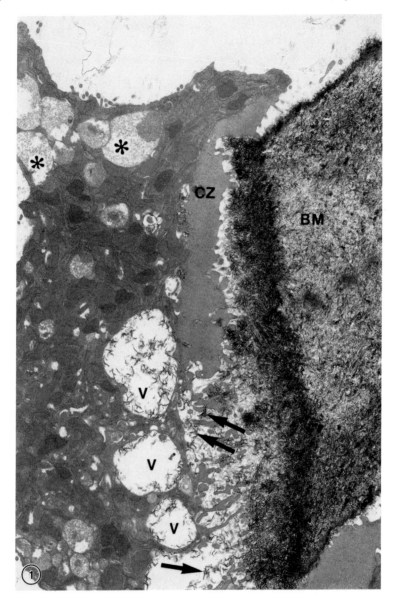

Fig. 1 An electron micrograph of an osteoclast resorbing mineralized bone matrix (BM). The infoldings of the ruffled border contain crystals of bone mineral (arrows) which are also seen loose in the underlying matrix and within large vacuoles (V) associated with the ruffled border. The clear zone (CZ) next to the ruffled border shows no infoldings. Large cytoplasmic vacuoles (*) opposite the bone surface being resorbed do not contain crystals of mineral. Mag: 11,500 ×

within the osteoclast. The morphological characteristics of the osteoclast have already been discussed (see Chapter 1, this volume) however several concepts of osteoclastic activity should be remembered. In Fig. 1 it can be seen that bone derived crystallites have accumulated within the cytoplasmic infoldings of the ruffled border. The presence of these large crystals is probably artefactually created during tissue fixation. The bone mineral is likely to be dissolved by the acidic environment associated with the ruffled border (more on this later). Therefore, when samples of bone are exposed to large volumes of neutral buffer during the fixation process, the crystals may re-precipitate to produce the results seen in Fig. 1. This photograph then suggests that there is no evidence for phagocytosis of bone crystals into the osteoclast's cytoplasm. However, the presence of phagocytic vacuoles at some distance from the ruffled border suggests that the osteoclast breaks down some intracellular material. We will add to this story in the following sections.

Sugars, Carbohydrates and Osteoclasts

It was observed in 1954 (Kroon, 1954) that bone resorbing osteoclasts contained periodic-acid Schiff stainable granules in their cytoplasm but no such granules in the ruffled border. There followed for several years an ongoing argument as to whether the collagen in bone was resorbed extracellularly or intracellularly (for example, see Bonucci, 1974). Even though electron microscopy showed disruption of the collagen under the osteoclast, the inability to find a collagenase associated with bone resorption led to much speculation about the degradative process (Vaes, 1988). In 1972, (Lucht, 1972) the uptake of intravenous injected horseradish peroxidase was studied in osteoclasts. Lucht concluded that since this tracer was taken up so quickly into the ruffled border and cytoplasmic vacuoles, the bone organic material was certain to follow the same pathway during the resorption process. A later study (Takagi et al., 1982) in which complex carbohydrates in bone were stained for electron microscopy, seems to have clarified some of these questions. By using a differential staining method for sulfated vs. vicinal glycol containing glycoconjugates, it was shown that sulfated extracellular material was phagocytized by the osteoclast and degraded intracellularly. Further, it appeared that collagen degradation was confined to the extracellular compartment beneath the osteoclast.

An additional source of information concerning carbohydrate chemistry in the osteoclast comes from studies of the gastric mucosa. The gastric parietal cell, which secrets hydrochloric acid, was shown to bind to peanut lectin (Sato

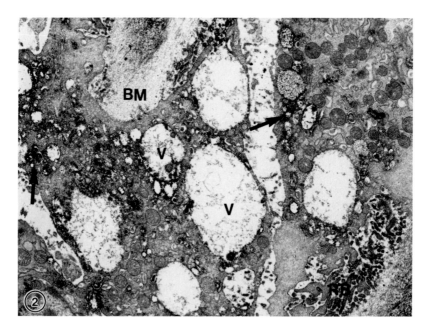

Fig. 2 These osteoclasts have been reacted with peanut lectin which was conjugated to horse-radish peroxidase. A dense black organic deposit is produced by a peroxidase-diaminobenzidine reaction. This reaction product is found in the ruffled border (RB), the underlying bone matrix (BM) and the cytoplasmic vacuoles (V), or areas adjacent (arrows) to these vacuoles. Mag: 7,500 ×

and Spicer, 1982),a lectin which complexes with galactosyl/galactosamine groups on carbohydrates (Kessiman *et al.*, 1986). When we apply peanut lectin (*Arachis hypogaea*) conjugated with horseradish peroxidase to os-teoclasts, lectin binding occurs along the infoldings of the ruffled border and within the large and small cytoplasmic vacuoles (Fig. 2). This lectin binding ability has been used to identify osteoclasts for light and electron microscopy (Vaananen *et al.*, 1986; Takagi *et al.*, 1988). It is interesting that the bone surface undergoing resorption shows a strong binding affinity for this lectin, suggesting that the osteoclast secrets a carbohydrate with a high concentration of galactosyl/galactosamine groups.

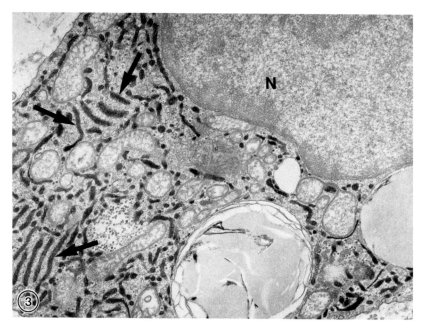

Fig. 3 Small osteoclasts on the bone surface may contain significant enzyme activity in the endoplasmic reticulum (arrows). This particular example shows the distribution of aryl sulfatase in the cytoplasmic but not in the nuclear (N) endoplasmic reticulum. Mag: 25,000 ×

The Histochemical Distribution of Acid Glycerophosphatase Activity in the Osteoclast

Acid phosphatase was localized to osteoclasts in the light microscope in 1960 (Burstone, 1960a) and by electron microscopy in 1967 (Doty et al., 1967). Although the function of acid phosphatase in this cell is unknown it has been a useful marker for osteoclasts for many years. In fact it has recently been shown that if osteoclastic acid phosphatase activity is inhibited with molybdate or neutralized with a specific antibody, there is a significant reduction in bone resorption (Zaidi et al., 1989). We showed in our early studies (Doty et al., 1967; also see Figs 12A & 12B) that this enzyme activity was also found attached to the bone matrix being resorbed beneath the ruffled border. This was confirmed by Lucht (1971); later, using H^3-leucine, he showed that this label passed through the osteoclast and was secreted onto the resorbed bone surface (Lucht and Norgaard, 1976). Secretion of acid phosphatase from the osteoclast is under some control by calcitonin but appeared

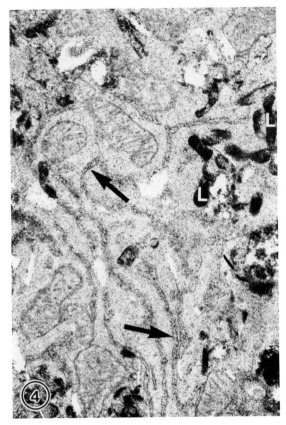

Fig. 4 In the fully differentiated osteoclast, the lysosomes (L) are always reactive for acid glycerophosphatase activity but a low level of activity can also be seen in the endoplasmic reticulum (arrows). Mag: 27,000 ×

to be unresponsive to parathyroid hormone or 1,25(OH) vitamin D3 (Chambers *et al.*, 1987).

The fine structural location of acid glycerophosphatase provides some interesting insights into the biology of the osteoclast. When the osteoclast is small in size with only a few nuclei present, the endoplasmic reticulum often shows enzyme activity for acid glycerophosphatase (Fig. 3), aryl sulfatase (Doty and Schofield, 1972; Baron *et al.*, 1988), beta glucuronidase (Baron *et al.*, 1988) and para-nitrophenyl phosphatase (Akisaka *et al.*, 1989). As the cell matures and becomes more fully differentiated the acid glycerophosphatase activity is difficult to find in the cytoplasmic ER (Fig. 4) even though the

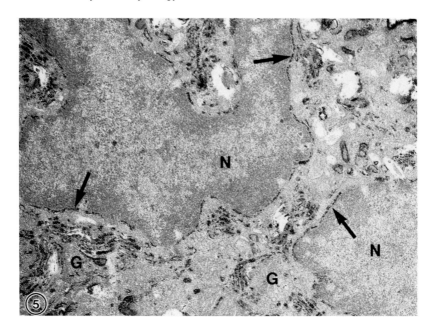

Fig. 5 In this osteoclast, acid glycerophosphatase activity can be found in the endoplasmic reticulum (arrows) associated with the nuclei (N). Much of the cytoplasmic activity seen in this photograph appears associated with the Golgi complex (G) adjacent to the nuclei. It cannot be determined whether there are any elements of the endoplasmic reticulum associated with these Golgi membranes . Mag: 32,000 ×

nuclear envelope may continue to show histochemical reactivity (Fig. 5). Such variations in acid phosphatase activity in the Golgi or lysosomes are not so evident, if in fact they occur. The Golgi saccules usually contain a strong acid phosphatase reaction in all saccules from the cis to trans face (Fig. 6). In the Golgi area there are numerous small vesicles, 60-80 nm in diameter, which contain reaction product. Some vesicles appeared to be coated (Doty and Schofield, 1972) whereas many others are not (Figs 7 and 16). So the vesicles could be used to shuttle products between Golgi saccules or to carry acid glycerophosphatase activity to the lysosomes or the ruffled border. The mature lysosome in the osteoclast consists of a round or a rod-shaped membrane bound body (Figs 8-10). We previously referred to the rod shaped lysosome as "serpentine" because it could be found as an elongated structure which had an appearance similar to agranular endoplasmic reticulum. The two lysosomal types contain high concentrations of acid glycerophosphatase activity. Al-

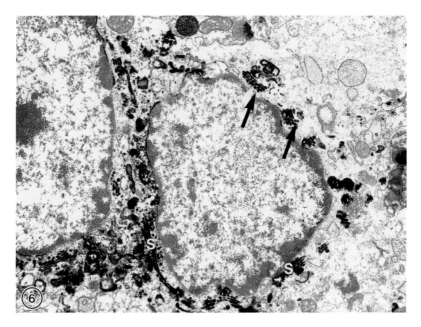

Fig. 6 The Golgi complex extends around the circumference of each nucleus in an osteoclast. Acid glycerophosphatase activity can usually be found in all the saccules (S) and within many of the small vesicles (arrows) associated with the saccules of the Golgi complex. Mag: 18,500 ×

though we have not found any histochemical differences between these two types of lysosomes, Touw *et al.* (1980) found that the rod shaped structures stained for lactate dehydrogenase activity. Both types of lysosomes contain tartrate resistant acid phosphatase activity. These lysosomes persist as the osteoclast ages (Fig. 11) and may be used to degrade intra-cellular organelles (Figs 17 A and B). In the actively resorbing osteoclast the large vacuoles adjacent to the ruffled border as well as those near the free surface of the osteoclast should be considered as phagolysosomes or at least as secondary lysosomes (Figs 12, 13, 15). The lysosomal bodies accumulate around these vacuoles and release their hydrolytic enzymes into these structures. The large vacuoles may or may not contain acid glycerophosphatase activity at any particular moment (Figs 12 and 13). Those vacuoles which are connected with the infoldings of the ruffled border are part of the extracellular space and will contain phosphatase activity only if the enzyme has been released into that space. The suggestion by Baron *et al.* (1985) that the bone resorbing ruffled border region should be considered as a secondary lysosome may not be

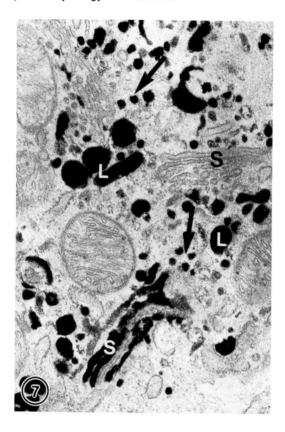

Fig. 7 Acid glycerophosphatase and aryl sulfatase activity are similarly localized within the Golgi complex. Some saccules (S), lysosomes (L), and 60-80 nm vesicles (arrows) are strongly reactive for these enzyme activities. Mag: 30,000 ×

totally accurate since some phagocytosis also occurs in this region (Lucht, 1972; Takagi *et al.*, 1988). Some of the large vacuoles in the cell opposite the ruffled border, and apparently not connected to the ruffled border may be true phagolysosomes where degradation of extra-cellular matrix material can occur. Fig. 15 shows that these large vacuoles which contain cellular and non-cellular debris are surrounded by numerous acid phosphatase containing lysosomes. The final structure where we localize acid glycerophosphatase is in the ruffled border and the underlying matrix which is being resorbed (Figs 12A and B). It appears that lysosomal bodies which contain phosphatase activity fuse with the infolded membranes of the ruffled border and release the

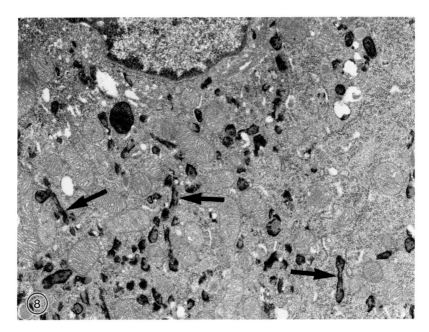

Fig. 8 A relatively brief incubation for acid glycerophosphatase activity can be used to stain the mature lysosomal population without producing reaction in the Golgi complex. The mature lysosomes, distributed between numerous mitochondria, are rounded or rod-shaped (arrows) membrane bound bodies. Mag: 20,000 ×

enzyme to the extracellular space (Figs 12 and 14). It is apparent that if there are no well defined channels in the ruffled border, then no extra-cellular release of enzyme activity can be found (Fig. 13). It is interesting that the rod-shaped lysosomes are always found in abundance at the cytoplasmic/ruffled border interface (Fig. 14).

The Distribution of Other Histochemical Activities in the Osteoclast

The Golgi Complex

Thiamine pyrophosphatase activity in most cells is confined to the "trans" saccules of the Golgi apparatus (Rambourg *et al.*, 1987). In the osteoclast (Fig. 16) there is histochemical reactivity showing this pyrophosphatase distribution in the saccules on the "trans" face of the Golgi as well as in small vesicles in the cytoplasm or budding off terminal ends of saccules. We showed

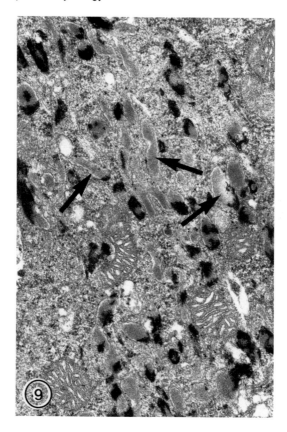

Fig. 9 Brief incubation times results in incomplete reaction product forming within the lysosomal bodies. The morphology of the rod-shaped lysosomes (arrows) can be appreciated in this photograph. Mag: 30,000 ×

with the acid glycerophosphatase reaction that all saccules of the Golgi contained reaction as well as the small vesicle population. The Golgi also reacts with cytidine monophosphate, trimetaphosphate, aryl sulfatase, and many other substrates with activity optima near pH 5.0. It is interesting that nicotinamide adenine dinucleotide phosphatase which is strongly reactive in the medial saccules of Golgi in osteoblasts (refer to the chapter in Volume 1 of this series by Doty and Schofield) is not reactive in the Golgi of the osteoclast.

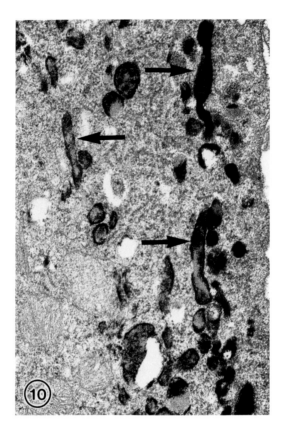

Fig. 10 The rod-shaped lysosomes (arrows) in the osteoclast stain for aryl sulfatase and many of the same enzymes found in the typical round shaped lysosome. Mag: 32,000 ×

The Lysosomes

One of the earliest histochemical studies of the osteoclast (Warner, 1964) showed that there were numerous granules in the cytoplasm which stained for leucine aminopeptidase, beta- glucuronidase and acid phosphatase activities. Warner concluded that all three enzymes were in the same granule and that these granules were lysosomes. The histochemical studies using electron microscopy would come to a similar conclusion; that is, that each lysosomal granule probably contains more than one enzyme activity. Lysosomal bodies in osteoclasts are strongly reactive for aryl sulfatase, beta-glucuronidase, glycerophosphatase, tri-metaphosphatase, thiamine pyrophosphatase, and p-

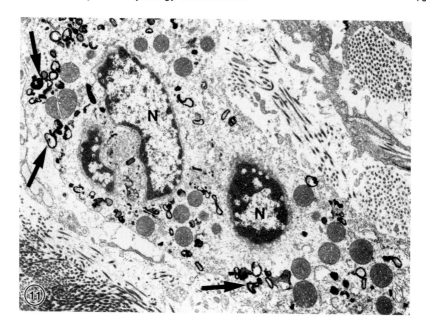

Fig. 11 Osteoclasts appear to undergo an aging process; the nuclei become pyknotic or densely heterochromatic, and the cytoplasmic organelles are not as numerous as more active osteoclasts. These cells will continue to demonstrate a strongly reactive lysosomal population (arrows). Mag: 13,000 ×

nitrophenylphosphatase at pH optima of 5.0. The lysosomal histochemistry at neutral pH produces strong lysosomal staining but the enzymes involved are difficult to characterize. In 1967 (Doty *et al.*) we demonstrated that the osteoclast's lysosomes and ruffled border contained the ability to hydrolyze adenosine triphosphate following a fixation regime which destroyed the mitochondrial and transport ATPase activities. We subsequently showed that phosphoprotein phosphatase activity at neutral pH could explain these ATPase results (Doty and Schofield, 1972). Lysosomal activity with either one of these substrates is stimulated by 4mM cysteine and inhibited by 3 mM zinc. When the thiamine pyrophosphatase activity is determined in osteoclasts at neutral pH, the reactivity of the lysosomes is also inhibited in the presence of zinc. This result and recent studies by Goshi *et al.* (1980) would suggest that this particular ATPase reaction (which still occurs after mitochondrial and transport ATPase have been destroyed by chemical fixation) is probably due to a pyrophosphatase. The important point to be made however is that

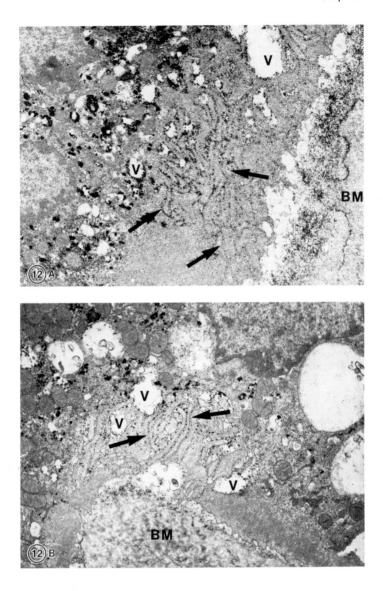

Fig. 12 The ruffled border, during active bone resorption, consists of numerous narrow infoldings of the cell membrane which penetrate into the organelle-rich region of the cytoplasm. In 12A, acid glycerophosphatase activity is found along the infoldings (arrows), within some of the vacuoles (V) which are connected to the infoldings, and deposited along the bone surface being resorbed (BM). In 12B, an ATPase reaction at pH 7.0 shows the same histochemical result as the acid glycerophosphatase reaction at pH 5.0. Mag: (12A) 13,000 ×   (12B) 13,000 ×

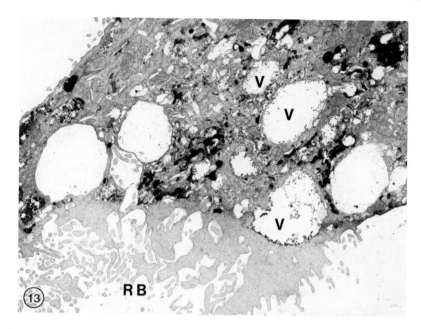

Fig. 13 The aryl sulfatase and p-nitrophenyl phosphatase reactions are seldom found in the ruffled border or on the bone surface being resorbed. This aryl sulfatase reaction is present in lysosomes and some of the cytoplasmic vacuoles (V) but is not seen in the ruffled border. Mag: 10,000 ×

osteoclasts contain lysosomes, vacuoles and a ruffled border which show extremely strong staining for some hydrolytic enzymes at neutral pH. Both the rod shaped and round membrane bound lysosomes show the same histochemical staining characteristics.

Lysosomes in connective tissue cells have been shown biochemically to contain cathepsins which could degrade collagen (Wang, 1982; Burleigh *et al.*, 1974). Attempts to histochemically localize cathepsin B, dipeptidyl peptidase I, and dipeptidyl peptidase II in bone have shown very little reactivity in osteoclasts (Sannes *et al.*, 1986). However, samples of frozen bone which were not chemically fixed, showed cathepsin B activity in osteoclasts (Van Noorden *et al.*, 1989). Unfortunately, this technique does not provide enough resolution to determine which structures contain the enzyme activity.

Non-specific esterase activity has been difficult to localize in osteoclasts. Baron *et al.* (1986) showed a diminution in esterase activity as the osteoclast precursor differentiated into a well recognized multinucleated cell on the surface of bone. Doty and Schofield (1972) could not find a nonspecific

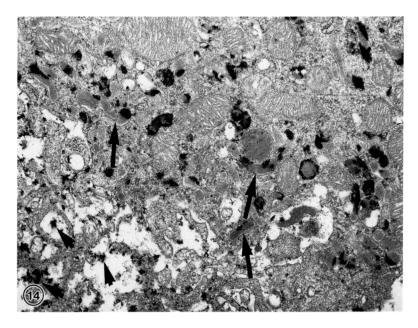

Fig. 14 This region demonstrates a area of infoldings of ruffled border which have been cut in cross section. Reaction to acid glycerophosphatase is seen between the infoldings (arrowheads) and in the lysosomes. Note the presence of numerous rod shaped lysosomes (arrows) in the area where the infoldings intersect with the osteoclast's cytoplasm. Mag: 27,800 ×

esterase in osteoclasts by electron microscopy. This was confirmed by Hermanns (1987) by light microscopy even though he showed strong esterase activity in macrophages. Ries (1984) has obtained an esterase reaction in osteoclasts which were freshly isolated from bone. The reasons for these variable results in bone by different investigators is unclear, although all investigators obtain a nonspecific esterase in macrophages.

It was mentioned earlier that lactate dehydrogenase activity has been localized to the rod shaped lysosomes in osteoclasts (Touw, *et al.*, 1980) as well as to the cytoplasmic vacuoles (Coleman *et al.*, 1976). This enzyme is sensitive to fixation and apparently diffuses during fixation, so its exact location may have to await improvements in technique.

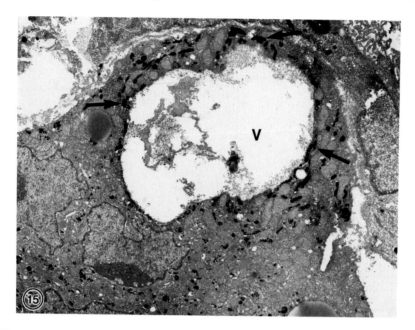

Fig. 15 Frequently there are large cytoplasmic vacuoles at the osteoclast's surface opposite the bone matrix. These vacuoles (V) usually contain some debris and are surrounded by lysosomes (arrows). These vacuoles would appear to have a function in the phagocytic and degradative activity of the osteoclast. Mag: 6,000 ×

The Mitochondria

Light microscopy has shown the presence of succinic dehydrogenase and cytochrome oxidase in high concentrations in osteoclasts (Burstone, 1960b, 1960c). Recently the cytochrome oxidase within mitochondrial cristae was shown to be altered following calcitonin treatment of osteoclasts (Noda, 1988). When tissues are fixed by perfusion the cytochrome oxidase is localized to the cristae of the mitochondria, but with *en bloc* fixation there is some diffusion of the enzyme into the intercristae spaces (Fig. 18). Nevertheless this enzyme provides a useful histochemical marker of cellular energy levels.

The Ruffled Border

Many of the lysosomal enzymes found by histochemical methods in the osteoclast can also be found in the ruffled border and on the bone matrix beneath the infoldings of the ruffled border. Acid glycerophosphatase (Fig.

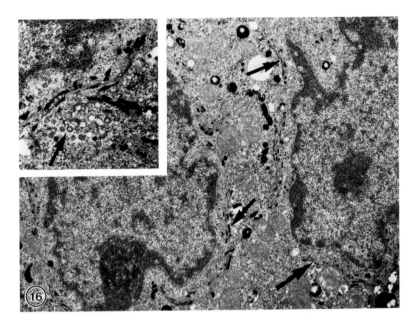

Fig. 16 Thiamine pyrophosphatase is a useful marker for the saccules on the "trans" face of the Golgi. In this osteoclast the enzyme activity is found in these saccules (arrows) and in lysosomes. Insert: There are coated and uncoated vesicles in the Golgi region which may or may not contain lysosomal enzyme activity. For example, the uncoated vesicles in Fig. 7 contained reaction product, whereas the uncoated vesicle in this photograph (arrows) does not show lysosomal enzyme activity. Mag: 17,500 × (Insert) 40,000 ×

12A), trimetaphosphatase (Doty and Schofield, 1984), and the hydrolysis of ATP at pH 7.0 (Fig. 12B) are examples of enzyme activities found in the ruffled border and underlying bone matrix. Akisaka et al. (1989) found that p-nitrophenyl phosphatase activity was also found in these same locations but was similar to aryl sulfatase in showing a strong reaction in the endoplasmic reticulum of the osteoclast. However, aryl sulfatase seems to be different than these other lysosomal enzymes in that our studies and those of Baron et al. (1985) have not shown aryl sulfatase activity in the underlying matrix or within the ruffled border. There seem to be two morphological requirements which are necessary if the ruffled border is going to demonstrate any enzyme activity: (1) The infoldings of the border must be numerous and must invaginate into the cytoplasmic region containing the lysosomal population (Figs 12A and 12B). (2) There will be large numbers of rod shaped lysosomes

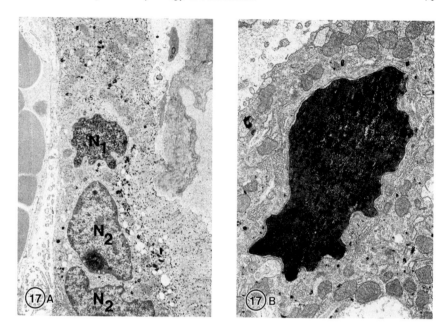

Fig. 17 Some lysosomal activity in the osteoclast is used for its own maintenance. In 17A a nucleus (N-1) contains acid glycerophosphatase activity in one pyknotic nucleus whereas adjacent normal nuclei(N-2) appear without reaction product. In 17B, a nucleus within an osteoclast contains acid glycerophosphatase activity suggesting the eventual degradation of this structure. Mag: 17A, 5,000 × 17B, 11,000 ×

at the zone where the infoldings intersect with the cytoplasmic compartment of the osteoclast (Fig. 14).

The significance of the lectin binding at the ruffled border and along the bone surface being resorbed is unknown. If the analogy between osteoclasts and gastric parietal cells is valid, then these lectin binding sugars may have something to do with acid secretion by the osteoclast. The presence of an acidic compartment beneath the ruffled border has been established by the use of pH markers (Cretin, 1951; Neuman et al., 1960; Baron et al., 1985) and by microelectrode measurements (Silver et al., 1988).

Our previous discussion of ATP hydrolysis by the osteoclast suggested that lysosomal ATPase activity remained following routine fixation regimens which would normally inactivate mitochondrial or ion transport ATPases. Using a mild fixation technique an ATPase and a ouabain sensitive p-nitrophenyl phosphatase activity were localized to the ruffled border region

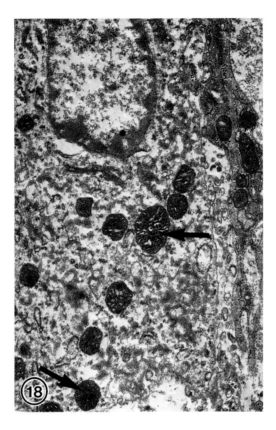

Fig. 18 Cytochrome oxidase activity appears as dark spots (arrows) within the mitochondria of the osteoclast. Because of diffusion of the enzyme during en bloc fixation, the reaction product is not found within the cristae where it is normally located. This reaction is a sensitive indicator of mitochondrial energy levels. Mag: 14,000 ×

and thought to be involved in a proton pump mechanism (Akisaka and Gay, 1986). This study involved the use of lead capturing methods on calcified tissues so the results were not always easily interpreted. However the histochemical activity was magnesium dependent and inhibited by parachloromercuricbenzoic acid, which strongly implicated an ATPase enzyme. Studies by Baron *et al.* (1986) utilized a monoclonal antibody to a (Na-K)ATPase and showed by immunocytochemistry that this ATPase was found in the ruffled border and plasma membrane of the osteoclast. This

ATPase could act as a sodium or calcium exchanger for hydrogen ions and thus regulate the acidity of the ruffled border region.

Carbonic anhydrase is another important enzyme which plays a role in the acidification of the area beneath the ruffled border. This enzyme has been localized within the cytosol of the osteoclast (Anderson *et al.*, 1982) and appears by immunocytochemistry to be the type II isoenzyme (Vaanann, 1984). This enzyme activity can be inhibited by sulfonamides (Gay and Mueller, 1974) and as a result of the inhibition, bone resorption is reduced (Dulce *et al.*, 1960). In addition, it has been shown in other systems that bicarbonate can stimulate ATPase activity (Kinne-Saffron and Kinne,1979; Sener *et al.*, 1979). Thus the production of hydrogen ion and bicarbonate by carbonic anhydrase activity and the transport of hydrogen ions across the membrane by ATPase (which may also be stimulated by presence of bicarbonate ion) would appear to be an efficient mechanism for production of an acidic environment.

Secretion of Acid Phosphatase Activity by the Osteoclast

In 1971 (Hammarstrom *et al.*, 1971) it was histochemically determined that the acid phosphatase activity in osteoclasts was different from other acid phosphatases because it was resistant to inhibition by tartrate. Later it was shown by biochemical separation that two acid phosphatases existed in bone (Anderson and Toverud, 1977) one of which was tartrate sensitive and the other tartrate resistant. At this same time, Schofield *et al.* (1977) demonstrated that acid phosphorylcholine phosphatase activity was a marker for secreted acid phosphatase. This enzyme activity was inhibited by L(+) tartaric acid and was localized to lysosomes in the osteoclast. In 1982 it was suggested that tartrate resistant acid phosphatase (TRAP) could be used as a marker for osteoclasts (Minkin, 1982). More recently however TRAP has been shown to exist in non-bone cells (Efstrakadis and Moss, 1985) and under culture conditions, marrow and peritoneal cells switched from TRAP negative to TRAP positive cells but did not show more osteoclastic activity (Hattersley and Chambers, 1989). Thus the specificity of TRAP has been questioned although among cells on the surface of bone it may still be a useful marker for osteoclasts. It has been suggested that tartrate resistant acid ATPase might be a better marker for osteoclasts (Anderson and Marks, 1989) however this reaction does not stain the resorbing bone surface beneath the osteoclast and may not represent a secreted enzyme activity.

Summary

Studies of histochemical activities of osteoclasts are made difficult by the complex nature of the techniques. Worthwhile histochemical results require that the tissue retain significant enzyme activity and at the same time the morphological results must be of highest quality. These are almost mutually exclusive requirements and lead to many compromises. However the information we have gained from histochemistry provides a good foundation for the coming wave of immunocytochemical studies to be made possible by modern molecular biology. We can then attack such problems as which lysosomes contain specific enzymes or combination of enzymes. Where is the extracellular matrix degraded? What components of the extracellular matrix are actually transported through the osteoclast? Are enzyme activities released through the ruffled border in a specific sequence? Can we follow the life and death of an osteoclast? Can we evaluate the "activity" of an osteoclast relative to other osteoclasts? All these and many more questions will be researched as the histochemical methods of today are replaced by the immunocytochemical methods of tomorrow.

References

Akisaka, T. and Gay, C. V. (1986) Intracytochemical Evidence for a Proton Pump Adenosine Triphosphatase in Chick Osteoclasts. *Cell Tiss. Res.* **245**: 507-512

Akisaka, T., Subita, G. P., Kawaguchi, H., and Shigenaga, Y. (1989) Different Tartrate Sensitivity and pH Optimum for two Isoenzymes of Acid Phosphatase in Osteoclasts. An Electron-microscopic Enzyme-Cytochemical Study. *Cell Tiss. Res.* **255**: 69-76

Anderson, R. E., Schraer, H., and Gay, C. V. (1982) Ultrastructural Immunocytochemical Localization of Carbonic Anhydrase in Normal and Calcitonin-Treated Chick Osteoclasts. *Anat. Rec.* **204**: 9-20

Anderson, T. R.and Toverud, S. U. (1977) Chromatographic Separation of Two Acid Phosphatases from Rat Bone. *Calcif. Tiss. Res.* **24**: 187-190

Andersson, G. N. and Marks, S. C. (1989) Tartrate-resistant Acid ATPase as a Cytochemical Marker for Osteoclasts. *J. Histochem. Cytochem.* **37**: 115-117

Baron, R., Neff, L., Brown, W., Courtoy, P. J., Louvard, D. and Farquhar,M. G. (1988) Polarized Secretion of Lysosomal Enzymes:Co-Distribution of Cation-Independent Mannose-6-Phosphate Receptors and Lysosomal Enzymes along the Osteoclast Exocytic Pathway. *J. Cell Biol.* **106**: 1863-1871

Baron, R., Neff, L, Louvard, D. and Courtoy, P. J. (1985) Cell- mediated Extracellular Acidification and Bone Resorption: Evidence for a Low pH in Resorbing Lacunae and Localization of a 100-kD Lysosomal Membrane Protein at the Osteoclast Ruffled Border. *J. Cell Biol.* **101**: 2210-2222

Baron, R., Neff, L.,Roy, C.,Boisvert, A. and Caplan, M. (1986) Evidence for a High and Specific Concentration of (Na,K)ATPase in the Plasma Membrane of the Osteoclast. *Cell* **46**: 311-320

Baron, R.,Neff, L., Tran Van, P., Nefussi, J-R. and Vignery, A. (1986) Kinetic and Cytochemical Identification of Osteoclast Precursors and Their Differentiation Into Multinucleated Osteoclasts. *Am. J. Pathol.* **122**: 363-378

Bonucci, E. (1974) The Organic-inorganic Relationships in Bone Matrix Undergoing Osteoclastic Resorption. *Calcif. Tiss. Res.* **16**: 13-36

Burleigh, M. C.,Barrett, A. J. and Lazarus, G. S. (1974) Cathepsin B1. A Lysosomal Enzyme That Degrades Native Collagen. *Biochem. J.* **137**: 387-395

Burstone, M. S. (1960a) Histochemical Observations in Enzymatic Processes in Bones and Teeth. *Ann. NY Acad. Sci.* **85**: 431-444

Burstone, M. S. (1960b) Histochemical Demonstration of Succinic Dehydrogenase Activity in Osteoclasts. *Nature* **185**: 866-867

Burstone, M. S. (1960c) Histochemical Demonstration of Cytochrome Oxidase Activity in Osteoclasts. *J. Histochem. Cytochem.* **8**: 225-226.

Chambers, T. J., Fuller, K. and Darby, J. A. (1987) Hormonal Regulation of Acid Phosphatase Release by Osteoclasts Disaggregated From Neonatal Rat Bone. *J. Cell. Physiol.* **132**: 90-96

Coleman, R. A., Ramp, W. K., Toverud, S. U. and Hanker, J. S. (1976) Electron Microscopic Localization of Lactate Dehydrogenase in Osteoclasts of Chick Embryo Tibia. *Histochem. J.* **8**: 543-558.

Cretin, A. (1951) Contribution Histochemique a l'Etude de la Construction et de las Destruction Osseuse. *Presse Med.* **59**: 1240-1251

Doty, S. B. and Schofield, B. H. (1972) Electron Microscopic Localization of Hydrolytic Enzymes in Osteoclasts. *Histochem. J.* **4**: 245-258.

Doty, S. B. and Schofield, B. H. (1984) Ultrahistochemistry of Calcified Tissues. In: *Methods of Calcified Tissue Preparation* (G. R. Dickson, Ed.), Elsevier Science Publisher,pp.149-198.

Doty, S. B., Schofield, B. H. and Robinson, R. A. (1967) The Electron Microscopic Identification of Acid Phosphatase and Adenosinetriphosphatase in Bone Cells Following Parathyroid Extract or Thyrocalcitonin Administration. In: *Parathyroid Hormone and Thyrocalcitonin (Calcitonin). Proceedings of the Third Parathyroid Conference.* (R. V. Talmage, L. F. Belanger and I. Clark, Eds.), Excerpta Medica Foundation, pp.169-181

Dulce, H. J., Siegmund, P., Korber, F. and Schutte, E. (1960) Zur Biochemie der Knochenauflosung II. Uber das Vorkommen Carboahnydratase in Knochen. *Hoppe-Seyler Z. Physio. Chem.* **320**: 163-167

Efstrakadis, T. and Moss, D. W. (1985) Tartrate-resistant Acid Phosphatase of Human Lung: Apparent Identity with Osteoclastic Acid Phosphatase. *Enzyme* **33**: 34-42

Gay, C. V. and Mueller, W. J. (1974) Carbonic Anhydrase and Osteoclasts: Localization by Labeled Inhibitor Autoradiography. *Science* **183**: 432-435

Goshi, N.,Hayakawa, T. and Kosugi, K. (1980) Behavior of ATPase Activity in Rat Osteoclasts Under the Effect of Calcitonin, or Following Pretreatment with $MgCl_2$ or Ouabain. *Acta. Histochem. Cytochem.* **13**: 508-520

Hammarstrom, L. E., Hanker, J. S. and Toverud, S. U. (1971) Cellular Differences in Acid Phosphatase Isoenzymes in Bone and Teeth. *Clin. Orthop. Rel. Res.* **78**: 151-167

Hattersley, G. and Chambers, T. J. (1989) Generation of Osteoclastic Function in Mouse Bone Marrow Cultures: Multinuclearity and Tartrate-resistant Acid Phosphatase are Unreliable Markers for Osteoclastic Differentiation. *Endocrinology* **124**: 1689-1696

Hermanns, W. (1987) Identification of Osteoclasts and Their Differentiation from Mononuclear Phagocytes by Enzyme Histochemistry. *Histochem.* **86**: 225-227

Kessiman, N., Langner, B. J.,McMillan, P. N., and Jauregiri, H. O. (1986) Lectin Binding to Parietal Cells of Human Gastric Mucosa. *J. Histochem. Cytochem.* **34**: 237-245

Kinne-Saffran, E. and Kinne, R. (1979) Further Evidence for the Existence of an Intrinsic Bicarbonate-stimulated Mg-ATPase in Brush Border Membranes Isolated from Rat Kidney Cortex. *J. Membrane Biol.* **49**: 235-244

Kroon, D. B. (1954) The Bone Destroying Function of Osteoclasts. *Acta. Anat.* **21**: 1-11

Lucht, U. (1971) Acid Phosphatase of Osteoclasts Demonstrated by Electron Microscopic Histochemistry. *Histochemie* **28**: 103-117

Lucht, U. (1972) Absorption of Peroxidase by Osteoclasts as Studied by Electron Microscope Histochemistry. *Histochemie* **29**: 274-286

Lucht, U. and Norgaard, J. O. (1976) Export of Protein from the Osteoclast as Studied by Electron Microscopic Autoradiography. *Cell Tiss. Res.* **168**: 89-99

Minkin, C. (1982) Bone Acid Phosphatase: Tartrate-resistant Acid Phosphatase as a Marker of Osteoclast Function. *Calcif. Tiss. Res.* **34**: 285-290

Neuman, W. F., Mulryan, B. J. and Martin, G. R. (1960) Clinical View of Osteoclasis Based on Studies with Yttrium. *Clin. Orthop. Rel. Res.* **17**: 124-134

Noda, K. (1988) Localization of Cytochrome C Oxidase Activity in Osteoclasts Treated with Calcitonin During Experimental Tooth Movement. *Acta. Histochem. Cytochem.* **21**: 301-315

Rambourg, A., Clermont, Y., Hermo, L. and Segretain, D. (1987) Tridimensional Architecture of the Golgi Apparatus and Its Components in Mucous Cells of Brunner's Glands of the Mouse. *Am. J. Anat.* **179**: 95-107

Ries, W. L. (1984) Osteogenic Periosteum Esterase Activity: A Comparative Morphological and Cytochemical Study of Bone Cells *in situ* on Rat Proximal Tibiae and in Smears. *J. Histochem. Cytochem.* **32**: 55-62

Sannes, P. L., Schofield, B. H., and McDonald, D. F. (1986) Histochemical Localization of Cathepsin B,Dipeptidyl Peptidase I and Dipeptidyl Peptidase II in Rat Bone. *J. Histochem. Cytochem.* **34**: 983-988

Sato, A. and Spicer, S. S. (1982) Ultrastructural Visualization of Galactose in Glycoprotein of Gastric Surface Cells with a Peanut Lectin Conjugate. *Histochem. J.* **14**: 125-137

Schofield, B. H., Mulhern, H. L. and McDonald, D. F. (1977) Acid Phosphorylcholine Phosphatase of Sebaceous Glands and Osteoclasts. *J. Histochem. Cytochem.* **25**: 309-310

Sener, A., Valverde, I. and Malaisse, W. J. (1979) Presence of a HCO3-activated ATPase in Pancreatic Islets. *FEBS Lett.* **105**: 40-51

Silver, I. A., Murrills, R. J. and Etherington, D. J. (1988) Microelectrode Studies on the Acid Microenvironment Beneath Adherent Macrophages and Osteoclasts. *Exptl. Cell Res.* **175**: 266-276

Takagi, M., Parmley, R. T., Toda, Y.,and Denys, F. R. (1982) Extracellular and Intracellular Digestion of Complex Carbohydrates by Osteoclasts. *Lab. Invest.* **46**: 288-297

Takagi, M., Yagasaki, H., Baba, T. and Baba, H. (1988) Ultrastructural Visualization of Selective Peanut Agglutinin Binding Sites in Rat Osteoclasts. *J. Histochem. Cytochem.* **36**: 95-107

Touw, J. A., Hemrika-Wagner, A. M.,and Vermeiden, J. P. W. (1980) An Electron Microscopic,Enzyme Cytochemical Study on the Localization of Lactate Dehydrogenase (LDH) in Osteoclasts and Peritoneal Macrophages of the Rat and Its Implication for the Process of Bone Resorption and the Origin of Osteoclasts. *Cell Tiss. Res.* **209**: 111-116

Vaananen, H. K. (1984) Immunohistochemical Localization of Carbonic Anhydrase Isoenzymes I and II in Human Bone, Cartilage and Giant Cell Tumor. *Histochem.* **81**: 485-487

Vaananen, H. K., Malmi, R., Tuukanenk, J., Sundquist, K. and Harkonen, P. (1986) Identification of Osteoclasts by Rhodamine Conjugated Peanut Lectin. *Calcif. Tissue Int.* **39**: 161-170

Vaes, G. (1988) Cellular Biology and Biochemical Mechanism of Bone Resorption. *Clin. Orthop. Rel. Res.* **231**: 239-271

Van Noorden, C. J. F., Vogels, I. M. C. and Smith, R. E. (1989) Localization and Cytophotometric Analysis of Cathepsin B Activity in Unfixed and Undecalcified Cryostat Sections of Whole Rat Knee Joints. *J. Histochem. Cytochem.* **37**: 617-624

Wang, H. M. (1982) Detection of Lysosomal Enzymes Derived from Pig Periodontal Ligament Fibroblasts and their Ability to Digest Collagen Fibrils and Proteoglycan. *Archs. Oral Biol.* **27**: 715-720

Warner, S. P. (1964) Hydrolytic Enzymes in Osteoclasts Cultured *In Vitro. J. Roy. Micros. Soc.* **83**: 397-403

Zaidi, M., Moonga, B., Moss, D. W. and MacIntyre, I. (1989) Inhibition of Osteoclastic Acid Phosphatase Abolishes Bone Resorption. *Biochem. Biophys. Res. Comm.* **159**: 68-71

4

Isolation and Behaviour of Cultured Osteoclasts

ALBERTA ZAMBONIN ZALLONE AND ANNA TETI
Institute of Human Anatomy
University of Bari
Bari, Italy

Introduction

The heterogeneity of cell populations located both within and around bone (periosteum, marrow space, haversian channels, etc.) made it very difficult to establish a distinct role for every cell type involved in bone metabolism. In fact, while the resulting net effect of an applied stimulus was demonstrable, the interrelationships between the different cells leading to the final result were merely hypothesized. For these reasons, attempts to isolate and purify the different cellular bone elements were made. Due to the peculiar organization of this hard tissue, the first successful results concerning viable osteoclastic cell cultures only appeared in the literature in 1982. Previously, research had been performed using cell populations merely related to osteoclasts.

Bone Cells from Calvaria

The first efforts to isolate bone cells resulted in mixtures of cellular types (Peck *et al.*, 1964; Rodan and Rodan, 1974), which could be used only immediately after isolation. Attempts to maintain these cells in culture resulted in rapid overgrowth by fibroblasts (Peck *et al.*, 1964).

In 1974, Wong and Cohn published a method for the isolation of selected populations of bone cells from neonatal mouse calvaria which exhibited, and retained in culture for several days, distinct morphological and biochemical characteristics.

The method was based on sequential enzymatic digestions of freshly excised calvaria with collagenase and trypsin. The cells collected from each digestion were cultured in a monolayer and characterized by several criteria. The populations obtained from the first two enzymatic digestions were characterised as osteoclast-like cells (OC). These populations responded to calcitonin by a significant increase of cAMP and to PTH by increasing both the synthesis of hyaluronate and the activity of acid phosphatase. The action of PTH was blocked by calcitonin (Wong and Cohn, 1974; Luben *et al.*, 1976). When cultured on ^{3}H-proline prelabeled devitalized calvaria, a few multinucleated cells appeared in the culture, and the release of the radioisotope in the medium was enhanced with respect to other calvarium cell populations (termed osteoblast-like cells). The release of ^{3}H-proline and ^{3}H-hydroxyproline was stimulated by PTH and inhibited by calcitonin (Luben *et al.*, 1977).

These cells were mostly mononuclear, and actively proliferated in culture. Their features correspond only partially to osteoclast characteristics and for this reason results obtained on these cell populations should not necessarily be considered indicative of the behaviour of differentiated osteoclasts.

Monocytes and Macrophages as Resorbing Cells

Much evidence indicates that osteoclasts arise from the fusion of hematopoietic precursor cells carried within the blood vascular system or present in the bone marrow (Walker, 1973; 1975; Kahn *et al.*, 1975, Jouterau and Le Douarin, 1978, Loutit and Nisbet, 1981; Marks and Walker, 1981; Baron *et al.*, 1984). Because of the ability of monocytes to fuse and form foreign body giant cells which resemble osteoclasts in morphology and in the number of their nuclei, and because macrophages have been shown to directly remove both mineralized and non mineralized skeletal matrices *in vivo* under certain circumstances, monocytes and macrophages have been used as surrogate osteoclasts in order to study the mechanisms of bone resorption in culture.

Monocytes

In 1977 Mundy *et al.* reported that human blood monocytes, without physical contact with the substrate or notable cellular changes resorbed fetal rat bone in tissue culture. On the other hand, Kahn *et al.*, in 1978, demonstrated that these cells adhered avidly to a calcified tissue substrate and assumed some morphological features of osteoclasts (such as polarization of organelles, strong acid phosphatase staining concentrated in the portion of the cell contacting the matrix surface, formation of extensive clear zone) and resorbed adult human or rat bone matrix *in vitro*. Although the cultured monocytes possessed or acquired in culture the osteoclastic features described above, they did not display well-developed ruffled membranes, which represents the major requisite for identification of differentiated active osteoclasts (Gothlin and Ericsson, 1976; King and Holtrop, 1975; Holtrop and King, 1977). More recently, using scanning electron microscopy, Ali *et al.* (1984b) showed that human blood monocytes cultured onto sperm whale dentine for 20 days failed to produce any morphological sign of resorptive activity. The reasons for these contradictions could be the different substrata used for resorption (25-43 μm bone particles versus a flat calcified surface) as well as the different sources of monocytes.

Macrophages

The initial reports describing macrophages as resorbing cells were published in 1979. Rifkin *et al.* (1979, 1980) showed morphologically that macrophages resorbed devitalized fetal rat long bones, disrupting calcified tissue extracellularly and apparently engulfing large fragments of mineralized matrix. They did not display a ruffled border at the resorptive site while a clear zone was well developed.

Teitelbaum *et al.* (1979) studied bone resorption using mouse peritoneal macrophages which were elicited by injection of thyoglycolate and cultured *in vitro* together with ^{45}Ca- or ^{3}H-proline prelabeled devitalized bone particles. Under these conditions macrophages released both isotopes into the medium, in a time-dependent manner. Resorption started 3 hours after addition of bone particles and was preceded by a phase of adhesion to the substrate. Prohibition of contact between bone matrix and cells, by interposition of a hydrophilic ultrafilter with low, non specific binding properties, resulted in a marked reduction of ^{45}Ca mobilization.

After these first reports, many others were published which clarified the mechanism and regulation of bone degradation by macrophages. This activity was inhibited by calcitonin in the presence of parathyroid hormone, while 25(OH)D3 and 1,25(OH)2D3 seemed to modulate the development of resorptive capability (Kahn et al., 1981a). Macrophage-mediated bone degradation was also inhibited by endotoxins from several species of bacteria, was not affected by PGE1 and PGE2 (Kahn and Teitelbaum, 1981b) and was specifically enhanced by glucocorticoid (Teitelbaum et al., 1981). Multinucleation also enhanced this activity. Macrophage polykarions bound and degraded bone particles more efficiently, suggesting that multinucleation produces qualitative changes in the resorptive capacity of macrophages and probably represent not a coincidental but a causal physiological event important in bone resorption (Fallon et al., 1983).

Differentiated Osteoclasts in Culture

Although the use of osteoclast surrogates for studying bone resorption was an important step in the development the field, their use has been superseded by the possibility of utilizing differentiated osteoclasts obtained from different species.

Bones are complex organs composed of different tissues. The cooperation of several kinds of cell populations, as well as of many known and unknown factors, results in correct bone metabolism. Osteoclasts represent only one cellular component of bone and the use of osteoclast culture systems allows insight into their biology and regulation, and presents the possibility of discriminating between a direct effect on these cells and indirect effects due to the activity of other cell types.

Criteria for Obtaining Differentiated Osteoclasts in Culture

Osteoclasts have several peculiar features that have to be considered as specific markers.

(1) They are multinucleated cells;
(2) they resorb bone, displaying specialized membrane structures: the ruffled border, a complicated array of deep membrane folds, and the clear zone, the seal of the resorbing compartment;

(3) they have high content of tartrate resistant acid phosphatase (TRAP);

(4) they derive from fusion of mononuclear precursors.

Isolation of osteoclasts presents many technical difficulties due to the following:

(1) osteoclasts represent only one of the many cell populations found within the bone and bone marrow compartments;

(2) when they are active they adhere strictly to the bony surface, making their safe mechanical detachment very difficult. Moreover, they are irreversibly damaged by enzymatic treatments;

(3) osteoclasts do not proliferate and have a short life span in culture. For these reasons only primary cultures and short term experiments are possible.

Isolation of Mammalian Osteoclasts

The pioneer paper describing the isolation and culture of differentiated osteoclasts appeared in 1977 (Nelson and Bauer, 1977). This method was not suitable for experimental approaches but stimulated new methodologies in this field. Previously, Mears (1971) and Walker (1972) were able to isolating osteoclasts from mammals, utilizable only for histochemical and short-term electrophysiological studies which did not involve cell culture.

A method for isolating and culturing mammalian osteoclasts was introduced by Chambers and Magnus in 1982. It is based on the removal of osteoclasts from the endosteal side of growing rat or rabbit long bones (femurs and tibias) by curetting the bone surface. Pipetting the released fragments and incubating the cell suspension for 30 minutes at 37°C, a mixed cell culture containing adherent osteoclasts is obtained. Observation showed that after rapid adhesion and spreading osteoclasts develop ruffled membranes and broad-fronted lamellipodia. Continuous retraction and formation of lamellipodia indicated a high motility for cultured osteoclasts. In spite of the rapidity of cell adhesion and spreading, the majority of the osteoclasts do not survive overnight incubation. Death occurs abruptly and it is characterized by retraction of cell processes, stopping of the granule movement and rounding off of the cell ending in cell detachment.

The osteoclastic nature of these cells has been verified by their receptor-mediated (Rao *et al.*, 1983; Nicholson *et al.*, 1986) response to calcitonin (Chambers and Magnus, 1982; 1983). At concentrations above 50 pg/ml salmon calcitonin reversibly inhibits lamellipodia formation and ruffling activity, with subsequent cytoplasmic retraction. The specificity of the salmon calcitonin effect on osteoclasts is demonstrated by the lack of inhibition of cellular movement in peritoneal macrophages and inflammatory giant cells.

Osteoclasts prepared by this method are also capable of resorbing bone (Chambers *et al.*, 1984 a, b; 1985; Boyde *et al.*, 1984). Bone resorption assay has been set up using isolated osteoclasts plated onto bone slices and subsequently observed by scanning electron microscopy. The presence of single or multiple excavations (pits) at the site where osteoclasts were settled is considered evidence for resorption. Treatment with salmon calcitonin inhibits pit formation (Chambers *et al.*, 1985).

Although this method provides a good model for studying mammalian osteoclast activity *in vitro*, it has some disadvantages. The number of cells obtained is low, with consequent relatively reliable statistical evaluations. No purification can be carried out; therefore many marrow cells (such as monocyte-macrophages or stromal cells) contaminate the osteoclast preparation. Consequently, it is impossible to perform any biochemical study or to distinguish between agents directly affecting osteoclast activity and effects mediated by other cell types. Finally, the short life-span in culture does not allow long-term experiments.

Attempts have also been made to induce osteoclast formation *in vitro* from a bone marrow population. In 1981 Testa *et al.* described giant cell formation in cat bone marrow cell cultures after 6 weeks of incubation. Ibbotson *et al.*, (1984), Roodman *et al.*, (1985) and Mc Donald *et al.* (1987), characterized giant cell populations obtained using this method from mammalian long-term bone marrow culture. They found that some of the multinucleated cells that formed in these cultures contained tartrate resistant acid phosphatase whose activity was increased by 1,25-dihydroxyvitamin D_3 and parathyroid hormone and inhibited by calcitonin. Morphologically, they resembled differentiated osteoclasts. More recently (Takahashi *et al.*, 1988) it has been demonstrated that the number of osteoclast-like cells formed is increased by 1,25-dihydroxyvitamin D_3 and that, when the formation of these cells is obtained on sperm whale dentin slices, numerous resorption lacunae are formed. Thus, these cells seem to satisfy most of the criteria that distinguish differentiated osteoclasts. With this method osteoclast-like cells have been obtained also from human normal and Pagetic bone marrows and used to study the effects of a number of factors on osteoclast differentiation (Chenu *et al.*, 1988; Kukita *et al.*, 1989a,b; Pfeilschifter *et al.*, 1989; Takasaki *et al.*, 1989).

Giant cells derived from human osteoclastomas (Horton, 1984) or normal human fetal bones have also been isolated. They have been used, for example, in preparing specific monoclonal antibodies capable of recognizing osteoclasts (Horton *et al.*, 1986).

Isolation of Avian Osteoclasts

Isolation of osteoclasts from birds has been developed in several laboratories at the same time as mammalian osteoclast isolation. Chicks or quails of different ages have been used.

Osdoby *et al.* (1982) isolated osteoclasts from the endosteal surface of day 19 embryonic chick tibias by mild trypsinization. Osteoclast enrichment was achieved by passing cell suspensions through Nitex screens of selective sizes or by fractionation on Percoll gradient. The enrichment procedure produced osteoclast population of 50-70% purity based on morphological criteria. However, the authors did not specify the number of cells obtained. Osteoclasts could be maintained in culture for up to 10 days but they gradually lost osteoclast morphology. Freshly isolated osteoclasts produced cytoplasmic blebs and attached to the dish within 5 hours. After 24, hours osteoclasts became flat with smooth surface. During the course of culture they retained acid phosphatase and butyrate esterase activities. After 6 days in culture these osteoclasts became more elongated and underwent reduction in the number of nuclei.

Late stage embryonic chick long bones provide a convenient source of osteoclasts, but cell viability is reduced by the manipulations performed for their purification on Percoll gradients. Percoll itself often damages osteoclasts probably because, as other cells of the phagocytic family (Wakefield *et al.*, 1982) they phagocytise Percoll particles (unpublished observations).

Another source of avian osteoclasts is represented by long bones from 8 week chicks, a stage characterized by rapid growth of the skeleton (Gay *et al.*, 1983a; 1985; Oursler *et al.*, 1985; Baron *et al.*, 1985; 1986; Vaananen *et al.*, 1986). During this stage the endosteal surfaces of long bones, particularly tibia, are very rich in active osteoclasts. However, most of them are buried in resorption lacunae, making their extraction difficult.

The method that, until now, has provided the largest number of osteoclasts uses as its source the medullary bone of laying hens. Medullary bone is a peculiar tissue, present in the marrow cavity of long bones of female birds during reproduction. It is formed by thin, highly mineralized trabeculae, deposited following stimulation by estrogens and androgens, which provide a calcium deposit utilized for the egg shell formation (Bloom et al., 1941; 1958). Medullary bone is surprisingly rich in bone cells. Both osteoblasts and osteoclasts line the trabeculae and undergo functional modifications according to the egg-laying cycle (Zambonin Zallone and Mueller, 1969; Miller, 1977; de Bernard et al., 1980). Osteoclasts display typical clear zone and ruffled border (active form) during the egg-shell secretion, or retract their membrane in folds facing the vascular side (inactive form) during the following resting phase (Miller, 1977; 1978).

Taking advantage of this features, Nijweide et al. (1985) isolated quail osteoclasts during the resting phase of the cycle, when the cells are do not adhere strictly by the clear zone to the bone surface. Purification was achieved by sequential filtration on nylon meshes and Percoll fractionation which, however, for reasons described earlier, reduced their viability.

In our laboratory osteoclasts are isolated and purified from the medullary bone of laying hens fed with a hypocalcaemic diet (Zambonin Zallone et al., 1982). During a period of calcium depletion the osteoclast population undergoes a series of modifications (Zambonin Zallone and Teti, 1981). During the first 48 hours osteoclasts are very active and strictly attached to the bone surface. After a prolonged diet (7 days) calcified trabeculae of the medullary bone are almost completely removed (in order to provide calcium for egg-shell formation). However, new trabeculae are formed by active osteoblasts which, due to the calcium deficiency, calcify only partially (Zambonin Zallone and Mueller, 1969, de Bernard et al., 1980). In this circumstance most of the osteoclasts, in the absence of a calcified surface, move into the inter-trabecular spaces (Zambonin Zallone and Teti, 1981) forming a motile, non resorbing population whose fate in vivo is still uncertain. Cell degeneration has never been observed, leading to the hypothesis that they are migrating toward the endosteal surfaces where resorption still takes place very actively.

The advantage of using medullary bone at this stage as a source of osteoclasts is the availability of a synchronous, rich osteoclast population which can be extracted without the use of proteolytic enzymes.

The method for purifying this population, first published in 1982 (Zambonin Zallone *et al.*, 1982), has been further improved and now provides 1,000,000 to 10,000,000 osteoclasts per animal (70-90% pure, 50-90% viability).

A cell suspension rich in osteoclasts is obtained mechanically by squeezing the medullary bone from femurs and tibias through a 100 μm diameter nylon net or by gently scraping the bone trabeculae with a sharpened needle. Osteoclast enrichment is achieved by the following steps:

(1) sedimentation (1 to 3 depending on the composition of the initial cell suspension) on 75% fetal calf serum in Ca^{2+}, Mg^{2+}-free phosphate buffer saline or in Joklik-MEM;

(2) sequential filtrations through 100 and 50 μm diameter nylon nets for eliminating fibroblasts, bone marrow cell clusters and bone debris;

(3) culture in a nucleotide free medium in the presence of cytosine-1-β-D-arabinofuranoside, an analogue of cytosine which blocks mitosis of proliferating cells;

(4) washing of cell culture after 24-36 hours to eliminate non-adherent bone marrow cells.

A modification of the method has also been introduced recently (Blair *et al.*, 1986; Teti *et al.*, 1989b). Osteoclast enriched cell suspension, after only one sedimentation on 75% FCS, is plated with devitalized bone fragments, which induce selective adhesion of osteoclasts to mineralized matrix. After 24 hours bone particles (with the attached cells) are removed by gentle pipetting of the medium, further sedimented twice for 20 minutes in phosphate buffer saline, and finally cultured. This last modification can be used when the presence of bone particles does not interfere with the experimental protocol.

The cells obtained by the method described above are multinucleated, retain their shape when freshly isolated, and start to adhere to the substrate after 8 hours. The plasma membrane forms typical blebs and then spreads onto the plastic or glass substratum and the cells become disk-shaped within 48-72 hours. The central area contains the cluster of nuclei, mitochondria, lysosomes and vacuoles, while the peripheral area adheres to the substratum with a clear zone-like area (Figs 1 and 2) (Zambonin Zallone *et al.*, 1982; Marchisio *et al.*, 1984).

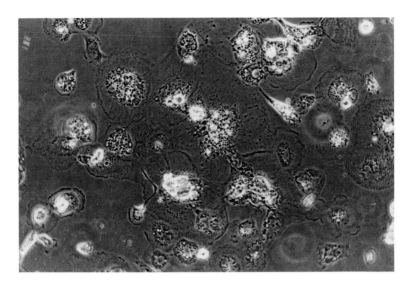

Fig. 1 Phase contrast micrograph of isolated avian osteoclasts from medullary bone after 5 days of culture. The osteoclasts are spread onto the plastic dish. 320×

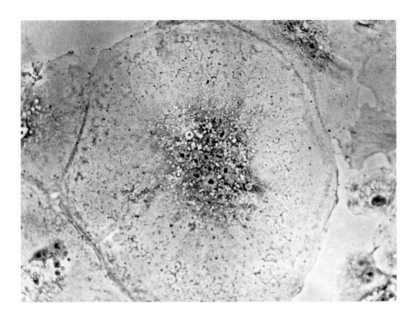

Fig. 2 Phase contrast micrograph of a completely spread avian osteoclast after 4 days in culture. The nuclear cluster and the outer zone apparently devoid of organelles are well evident.900×

A bone resorption assay, performed utilizing ^{3}H-proline or ^{45}Ca prelabeled devitalized bone fragments, shows that they are capable of resorbing bone over a period of 6 days at a rate much higher than those for peritoneal macrophages, skin fibroblasts (Blair *et al.* 1986) and long term cultured bone marrow macrophages (Teti *et al.*, 1988). Morphologically, bone resorption *in vitro* occurs with a modality similar to bone resorption *in vivo*. Osteoclasts are strongly attracted by bone fragments, adhere to the bony surface, and develop a clear zone and ruffled border. After a few hours calcified fragments are found in osteoclast vacuoles or between folds of the ruffled border (Zambonin Zallone *et al.*, 1984).

The osteoclastic nature of these cells has been further confirmed by morphological features, tartrate resistant acid phosphatase positivity, and reaction with a specific monoclonal osteoclast antibody prepared by Oursler *et al.* (1985).

Avian *Versus* Mammalian Osteoclasts

The isolation procedure performed from calcium deficient medullary bone has the advantage of providing a large number of highly purified osteoclasts suitable for both morphological and biochemical studies. However, these osteoclasts derive from a species not related to mammals, from a peculiar bone tissue and after a hypocalcaemic diet that could induce modifications in the cell populations. The concern of some authors is based on the finding that chick osteoclasts lack calcitonin receptors (Nicholson *et al.*, 1986) and, consequently, are not inactivated by the hormone (Dempster *et al.* 1987). However, controversy still exists concerning this problem. De Vernejoul *et al.* (1988) found an inhibitory effect of salmon calcitonin on bone resorption by isolated chick osteoclasts, while Ali *et al.*, (1984a), using rabbit osteoclasts on sperm whale dentin, found that resorption lacunae occurring in the salmon calcitonin-treated cultures were not significantly different in size from those of controls. These last authors however admitted that the number of resorption lacunae could be lower in rat osteoclast cultures treated with calcitonin. The meaning of these data and their importance in the comparison between mammalian and avian osteoclasts need to be discussed. There is now a renewed interest of many laboratories in this problem. Calcitonin has been detected in embryonic chick plasma on day 16 of embryogenesis (1 ng/ml), the level rises until pipping occurs just before hatching (3 ng/ml), then drastically drops (Braimbridge and Taylor, 1980; Abbas *et al.*, 1985). Calcitonin is synthesized by the ultimobranchial body, present also in mature animals. Plasma levels of calcitonin in domestic fowl are high during the inactive phase of egg shell formation, and lower during the active phase (Dacke *et al.*, 1972). Gay (1988) suggests that the lack of calcitonin receptors in chick embryos detected by Nicholson *et al.*, (1986) could be due either to the fact that they have not yet been expressed, since plasma levels of calcitonin are extremely low before hatching, or to the possibility that these cells are chondroclasts rather than osteoclasts. She also suggests that the assessment of cAMP increase in osteoclasts to study their response to calcitonin may be not ideal (Yamamoto and Gay, 1986). However, the possibility that mammalian and avian osteoclasts are regulated differently cannot be excluded. We did not find any modification of intracellular calcium level following calcitonin administration in chicken osteoclasts, while in rat osteoclasts an increase in intracellular calcium was detected (Malgaroli *et al.*, 1989). Other interesting comparative studies on osteoclasts from avian or mammalian sources have been performed. Jones *et al.* (1984) demonstrated that Howship lacunae were formed by both mammalian and avian osteoclasts onto either untreated, unmineralized, anorganic or surface-demineralized mammalian dental tissues. There was no species or substrate specificity. In addition, osteoclasts resorbed avian egg shell and mollusc shell containing calcite and aragonite. The same authors (Jones *et al.*, 1986) showed that the highest resorbing efficiency is displayed by chick osteoclasts, followed by rabbit and rat.

Behaviour of Osteoclasts In Culture

Bone Resorption

Since methods for isolating osteoclasts were established much work has appeared, detailing their features and behaviour in culture. First, studies were designed to establish the mechanism of bone resorption *in vitro*. A morphological evaluation of bone resorption was performed in our laboratory (Zambonin Zallone *et al.*, 1984) using either vital or devitalized bone. Devitalized bone particles were prepared as described by Teitelbaum *et al.* (1979). Alternatively, whole diaphysis of long bones were devitalized by freezing and thawing. Vital bone was obtained from diaphyses of long bones, cleaned of soft tissues (including periosteum and endosteum) in sterile conditions, and cultured for different lengths of time before adding osteoclasts. Quail bone was used in order to distinguish, on the basis of their nucleolar pattern (Kahn and Simmons, 1975; Jouterau and Le Douarin 1978), chicken osteoclasts, added to the culture, from resident quail osteoclasts. In these experiments we established that bone resorption by cultured avian osteoclasts occurred with

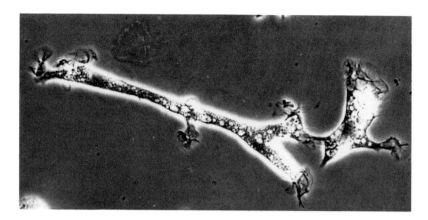

Fig. 3 Motile osteoclasts can be found at any culture time. 900×

morphological features comparable to bone resorption *in vivo*. Clear zone and ruffled border formed at the site of bone-cell attachment, and bone matrix fragments were seen in vacuoles and/or in folds of the ruffled border membrane. When bone particles were added to the osteoclast culture, cells, initially disk-shaped, became polymorphic, migrated toward the bone particles adhering to them and starting to resorb bone within 1 hour (Fig. 5). Ruffled border and clear zone were observable only when bone particles were of sufficiently large size. Small bone fragments did not induce ruffled border organization but were resorbed in deep folds of the osteoclast membrane. If osteoclasts were plated on periosteum-endosteum free freshly prepared vital bone, they also adhered and started resorption. However, if the vital bone was precultured for 24 hours before plating osteoclasts, a newly formed multiple layer of lining cells completely enveloped the bone surfaces, preventing contact of the osteoclasts with the substrate.

A morphological assay for quantitating bone resorption at SEM, by counting the number and measuring the depth of pits excavated by osteoclasts plated on bone slices, has been developed by Chambers *et al.*, (1984 a,b; 1985). The same method has been adopted by Jones *et al.*, (1984), using dentine as substratum. Dempster *et al.* (1987) modified this method, counting the number of toluidine blue-stained pits in the light microscope. An increased number of pits, and enlargement of their size, are considered indicators of stimulated bone resorption. However, this technique has the disadvantage of being time consuming and, due to the low number of osteoclasts utilized, can

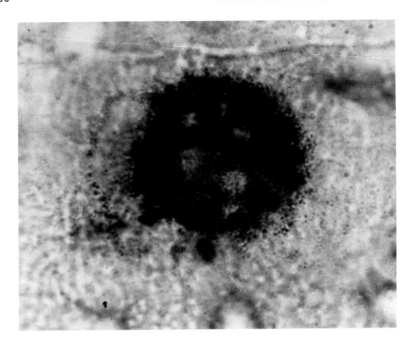

Fig. 4 Intense staining reaction for tartrate resistant acid phosphatase is shown by isolated avian osteoclasts plated on bone slices. 500×

be statistically inaccurate. Statistical variability is further worsened, in our experience, by the high variability in osteoclast size, which in turn, is reflected in differences in pit size.

A biochemical assay for *in vitro* bone resorption has been developed by Blair *et al.*, (1986) using medullary bone osteoclasts. The method, first used for studying macrophage-mediated bone resorption (Teitelbaum *et al.*, 1979), is based on the ability of osteoclasts to remove bone matrix and secrete its digested products into the culture medium. ^{45}Ca or ^{3}H-proline-prelabeled bone fragments are incubated together with cultured osteoclasts and the radioactivity released in the media is measured. With this method Blair *et al.*, demonstrated that ^{45}Ca release precedes that of ^{3}H-proline and ^{3}H-hydroxyproline, indicating that demineralization occurs before degradation of organic matrix. This method provides a good tool for quantitizing bone resorption. ^{45}Ca release results are less indicative than ^{3}H release because a flux of calcium ions continuously occurs between the calcified matrix and the

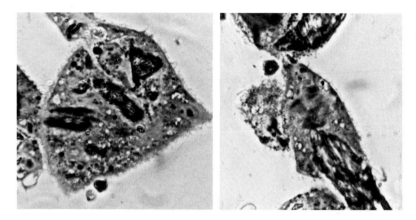

Fig. 5 Micrograph of embedded and sectioned osteoclasts cultured with bone particles. The cells surround the bone. 500×

medium in both directions. The use of ^{3}H-proline prelabeled bone particles is more reliable, with very little variability.

Osteoclast Enzymes in Culture

Some enzymes have been identified in osteoclasts in culture. Acid phosphatase is one of the most representative enzymes in these cells, and its presence has been confirmed also in cultured osteoclasts. Particular attention had been given to tartrate resistant acid phosphatase (TRAP) (Fig. 4). For a long time TRAP has been considered a specific marker for osteoclasts but it has recently been found (Teti *et al.*, 1988) that other cells of the monocyte-macrophage lineage in culture can display the enzyme. Thus, TRAP is not as specific for osteoclasts as previously suggested. The role of acid phosphatase in bone resorption is uncertain. However, it increases in cultured avian osteoclasts following treatment with retinol or retinoic acid, which directly stimulate osteoclast bone resorption (Oreffo *et al.*, 1988).

Carbonic anhydrase is present in osteoclasts in association with the ruffled border, in some vesicles, and also throughout the cytoplasm of chick (Gay and Mueller, 1974; Gay *et al.*, 1974; 1983 a;b Anderson *et al.*, 1982), rat (Vaananen, and Parvinen, 1983; Marie and Hott, 1987; Sundquist *et al.*, 1987), mouse (Jilka *et al.*, 1985) and human (Vaananen, 1984) osteoclasts. Its activity is quite high, similar to that found in kidney tubular cells and pancreatic cells, suggesting a major role in osteoclast function. Type II isoenzyme is particularly abundant in both mammalian and avian osteoclasts.

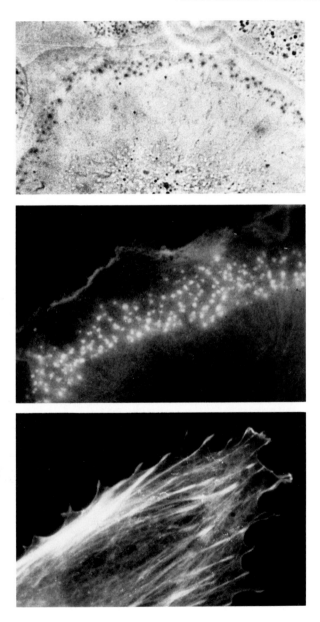

Fig. 6 Phase contrast and fluorescence microscopy pictures of cultured avian osteoclasts. (A) A row of dark spots corresponding to the podosomes are distributed in the paramarginal cytoplasm. 600×. (B) R-PHD staining for F-actin. Fluorescent dots are seen in the same localization. 800×.

It catalyzes the hydration of CO_2 to H_2CO_3, which could represent the source of H^+ for the proton pump responsible for the acidification of the resorbing compartment (see below).

At one time, on the basis of observations by Sakamoto and Sakamoto (1982), the presence of collagenolytic enzymes in osteoclasts was excluded. The lack of neutral collagenase and of convincing morphological evidence of collagen degradation, led to the hypothesis that osteoclasts were unable to resorb the organic matrix of bone and that other cell types, belonging to the phagocytic family, removed demineralized bone components (Heersche, 1978; Rifkin et al., 1979; 1980). Using osteoclasts isolated from the medullary bone of laying hens, Blair et al. (1986) established that, although osteoclasts do not have a neutral collagenase, they are capable of removing both inorganic and organic components of bone matrix. The enzyme responsible for collagen digestion is an acid collagenolytic enzyme (pH optimum, 4.0) which breaks down collagen into fragments of low molecular weight (below 10,000 daltons). The characterization of the enzyme is still under investigation. Delaisse' et al. (1987) demonstrated that inhibitors of cysteine proteinases reduced bone resorption about 75% by isolated osteoclasts in vitro, suggesting a role for these enzymes in bone degradation.

Osteoclast Specializations

Osteoclast plasma membrane is highly complex and is directly involved in bone resorption. Utilizing isolated and purified osteoclasts some of its molecular components and ion transport systems were identified.

The clear zone is present in osteoclasts but it does not represent a specific osteoclast marker. Macrophages and inflammatory giant cells are also capable of organizing a typical clear zone. In osteoclasts this structure appears during bone resorption and provides a strong seal that allows the cell to attach to the bony surface. Studies in vivo (King and Holtrop, 1975; Holtrop and King, 1977) established that the clear zone, devoid of organelles except some ribosomes, presents a filamentous material characterized as actin microfilaments by decoration with heavy meromyosin. The characteristics of the clear zone have been further studied in avian osteoclasts in vitro by immunofluorescence, interference reflection microscopy and electron microscopy (Marchisio et al., 1984; 1987; Zambonin Zallone et al., 1983; 1988; 1989). Osteoclasts cultured onto a glass substratum display a well organized clear zone from the second-third day of culture. It appears as an organelle-free peripherical area which allows osteoclast adhesion to the substrate. Under phase contrast dark spots are visible within this area. They correspond to focal microvillous-like adhesion areas, named podosomes, presenting a core of actin microfilaments colocalized with proteins controlling the polymerized-actin status (fimbrin, alpha-actinin and gelsolin). Vinculin and talin, proteins that in other adhesion structures colocalize with actin, mediating microfilament linkage to the plasma membrane, are found surrounding the actin core in osteoclasts. Podosome formation is not only observed on glass substrate, but also in osteoclasts cultured on bone slices and in the clear zone of osteoclasts *in vivo* (Zambonin Zallone *et al.*, 1988). Their importance as adhesive structures is demonstrated by the fact that their formation is modulated by a number of factors (see below).

The ruffled border represents a complex membrane specialization organized in the sites of active bone resorption. Through the plasma membrane of this area lysosomal enzymes are secreted into the resorbing compartment (Vaes, 1969, Doty *et al.*, 1972; Gothlin and Ericsson, 1971, Lucht, 1971; Baron, 1985) where they digest bone matrix components. Ruffled border membrane plays an important role in driving lysosomal enzyme secretion. Mannose-6-phosphate receptors have been immunolocalized in the osteoclast ruffled border, as well as in the secretory pathway membranes, by Baron *et al.* (1988). Blair *et al.*, (1988), further demonstrated the role played by ruffled border mannose-6-phosphate receptors in the uptake of lysosomal enzymes from the extracellular space.

Bone resorption takes place extracellularly in an acid environment. The acid pH of this compartment has been evaluated using many different probes (Cretin 1951; Fallon, 1984; Baron 1985; Silver *et al.*, 1988). Solubilization of hydroxyapatite requires a substantial proton flux, approximately 6 moles per mole of hydroxyapatite at pH 5 (Fallon *et al.*, 1984). Using osteoclasts from newly hatched chicks both *in vivo* and *in vitro*, Baron *et al.*, (1985) demonstrated, by immunohistochemistry, that the ruffled border membrane contains a 100-kDa integral membrane protein also present in limiting membranes of lysosomes and other related organelles. This 100-kDa protein cross-reacts with antibodies against the K^+-H^+ATPase of pig gastric mucosa.

On the other hand, Blair *et al.* (1989) have recently shown that chicken medullary bone osteoclasts react *in vivo* with polyclonal antibodies raised against the bovine F0F1-like renal tubule proton pump and the reaction is mainly localized at the bone attachment site. Using isolated osteoclasts they confirmed, by western blot, the presence of the 31, 56 and 71 kDa subunits of the F0F1-like proton pump. Incubating acidifying vesicles produced by fractionation of osteoclasts they showed that the vesicles accumulated protons by an ATP-dependent transport that is not inhibited by vanadate. These data, although controversial concerning the exact nature of the H+ pumping system, indicate that an ATP-dependent proton transport mechanism is actively involved in the acidification of the resorbing compartment.

Recently, other mechanisms of ion transport have been identified in osteoclasts. Baron *et al.* (1986), found that the osteoclast plasma membrane is highly enriched in (Na^+, K^+)ATPase compared with other bone cells, monocytes, macrophages, and other blood and bone marrow cells. Using monoclonal antibodies they found that both α and β subunits of the permease are present. The number of binding sites per cell was estimated at 5,070 per osteoclast against about 1,500 in other cell types. The pump is inhibited by ouabain, and its α subunit is identical to that of the (Na^+, K^+)ATPase present in kidney cells (Baron *et al.*, 1988).

H^+ secretion into the resorbing compartment at the rate necessary to maintain the required acidity would cause an equal alkaline load in the cytoplasm of the osteoclast. Measuring the intracellular pH of isolated medullary bone osteoclasts during active bone resorption, we recently demonstrated that osteoclasts have a high capacity for HCO_3^- efflux. This transport is Na and energy independent, but it is sensitive to extracellular Cl and is inhibited by anion exchange inhibitors.

Finally, a Na/H antiport (Teti *et al.*, 1989b) and a Ca^{2+}ATPase (Akisaka *et al.*, 1988) have also been demonstrated in avian osteoclasts.

Cytoskeletal Structures of Isolated Osteoclasts

The cytoskeleton of isolated osteoclasts has been studied in both birds and mammals.

By immunofluorescence techniques the major cytoskeletal components have been studied in chicken osteoclasts (Zambonin Zallone *et al.*, 1983; Marchisio *et al.*, 1984). When fully spread, osteoclasts demonstrated a well developed array of microtubules, radiating from single or multiple microtubule organizing centers toward the cell's outer edge where they end abruptly or turn back toward the cell center. Microtubule organization is affected by treatment with retinol. They are completely depolymerized in 6 hours by 10^{-6} M retinol, with a visible effect already detectable after 2 hours of treatment. The phenomenon is reversible; removal of retinol from the medium allows complete microtubule reorganization within 16 hours. The meaning of these modifications is not completely understood. Certainly they are not due to toxic effect because retinol, at the same dose, increases bone resorption in isolated osteoclasts (Oreffo *et al.*, 1988)

Vimentin intermediate filaments are distributed in a regular array and are particularly abundant in the paramarginal ring (Zambonin Zallone *et al.*, 1983; Marchisio *et al.*, 1984).

The distribution of F-actin has also been investigated with fluorescent phalloidin. Typically, avian osteoclasts do not display stress fibers; instead short bundles of microfilaments are located in the core of podosomes present in the clear zone. Microfilament bundles are also seen intertwining single podosomes (Marchisio *et al.*, 1984). This organization is typical of fully spread osteoclasts and has also been found when these cells are plated on bone slices (Zambonin Zallone *et al.*, 1988). Motile osteoclasts, more numerous in the first hours after plating but always present over the entire culture period, present F-actin organized in a fine network at the level of ruffling membranes.

The cytoskeleton of mammalian osteoclasts has also been studied (Warshafsky *et al.*, 1985) and a similar distribution of microtubules was found. F-actin appeared to be localized mainly in ruffles, while myosin showed a patchy distribution. Both myosin and actin organization changed in cells treated with calcitonin, with the actin distributed in retraction fibers and the myosin in a ring at the cell periphery, demonstrating the active participation of these cytoskeletal proteins to the calcitonin-induced cell retraction.

Cell Substratum Interactions

One of the most fascinating aspects of osteoclast biology is its specific recognition of the bone substratum which, in turn, switches on bone resorption.

Studies performed in our laboratory (Zambonin Zallone *et al.*, 1989) and by Davies *et al.*, (1989), both carried out on osteoclastoma giant cells, revealed peculiar characteristics of osteoclast-substratum interactions.

Osteoclastoma giant cells display several osteoclast features (multinuclearity, TRAP positivity, bone resorption, response to calcitonin) and have successfully been used in these studies. Osteoclastoma cell plasma membrane reacts with specific antibodies directed against membrane proteins belonging to the superfamily of integrins. These are $\alpha\beta$ transmembrane heterodimers capable of linking cytoskeletal structures by their cytoplasmic short tail, and Arg-Gly-Asp (RGD)-containing extracellular matrix proteins by their extracellular domain. Thus, they participate in the recognition of the cell specific substratum. Osteoclastoma giant cells present at least two different integrins whose β-chains are respectively β1 and β3. β1-chain is diffusely organized in the plasma membrane, while β3-chain is specifically localized in the clear zone, at the level of podosomes, as are vinculin and talin (Zambonin Zallone *et al.*, 1989). The features of α-chains linked to the β1 and β3 subunits are still under investigation as well as the RGD-containing bone protein recognized by osteoclast integrins. However, specific data indicating the presence of an α chain belonging to the vitronectin receptor, have recently been published by Davies *et al.* (1989).

Regulation of Isolated Osteoclasts *In Vitro*

The role of calciotropic hormones in the regulation of osteoclast activity has been studied utilizing isolated cells. Despite the clear *in vivo* effect on bone resorption, for many of them no direct effect has been found *in vitro*. The lack of PTH receptors on chicken osteoclasts found by Silve *et al.* (1982), and by Pliam *et al.* (1982) *in vivo*, although not yet directly studied *in vitro*, has been indirectly confirmed by the lack of effect of this hormone on bone resorption by isolated osteoclasts (Chambers and Dunn 1982a; 1984a, 1985, De Vernejoul *et al.*, 1988).

Merke *et al.* (1986) demonstrated that isolated chicken osteoclasts do not display 1,25-dihydroxyvitamin D_3 receptors, but that monocytes isolated from the same animal source do. It has also been found that osteoclasts are not the target cells for cytokines active in bone resorption, such as interleukin 1, transforming growth factor, tumor necrosis factor and prostaglandin E_2 (Martin *et al.*, 1987; Martin and Mundy, 1987). To explain why these factors are only indirectly active in bone resorption, a possible intermediary role played by osteoblasts or by other cells of the immune system has been hypothesized (Rodan and Martin, 1981; Baron *et al.*, 1984; Martin *et al.*, 1987). The only known factors directly affecting isolated osteoclasts are calcitonin, whose action is receptor mediated (Nicholson *et al.*, 1986), and retinoids (Oreffo *et al.*, 1987, 1988).

The effect of calcitonin has been well documented in mammalian osteoclasts that display cell retraction, inhibition of resorbing activity, changes in cytoskeletal pattern and hyperpolarization of membrane potential (Mears, 1971; Chambers and Magnus, 1982; Chambers *et al.*, 1982; 1983 a, b; 1984a; 1985; 1986; Warshafsky *et al.*, 1985; Ferrier *et al.*, 1986; Dempster *et al.*, 1987). Retinol and retinoic acid, active metabolites of vitamin A, play an important role in bone metabolism (Zile *et al.*, 1979), and act directly on both osteoblastic cells (Ng *et al.*, 1985; Oreffo *et al.*, 1985; 1987) and differentiated avian osteoclasts *in vitro* (Oreffo *et al.*, 1987; 1988). A cytosolic retinol binding protein has however been found only in osteoclasts (Oreffo *et al.*, 1987). Isolated avian osteoclasts show reversible depolymerization of microtubules in response to retinoid treatment and a dose-dependent increase of podosome-mediated adhesion, acid phosphatase activity and bone resorption rate as revealed by release of ^{3}H-labeled products of bone collagen degradation.

Bone resorption is initiated only at certain sites and not at others, implying that local factors could also be involved, at least partially, in the regulation of osteoclast activity. Prostaglandin E_2, a potent stimulator of bone resorption in organ culture (Klein and Raisz, 1970) is, because of its lability in the circulation, likely involved as local regulator of bone resorption. *In vitro* it has been shown to act directly on isolated osteoclasts, causing retraction of cytoplasm (Chambers *et al.*, 1985; Arnett and Dempster, 1987), and inhibition of bone resorption (Chambers *et al.*, 1989). The reason why prostaglandin effect leads to two opposite results in organ culture and in isolated osteoclast culture is still unknown. Recently, a biphasic effect characterized by an early inhibition followed by stimulation of bone resorption has been described in prostaglandin E_2-treated rabbit osteoclasts *in vitro* (Okuda *et al.*, 1989).

The microenvironmental ion composition around bone cells could also change. Osteoclasts are exposed to high local levels of calcium ions (Silver *et al.*, 1988). It is not yet clear if, after hydroxyapatite dissolution, calcium ions reach the vascular stream by active transport through the osteoclast cytoplasm, or if they diffuse through the space between bone surface and osteoclast membrane. We do not know if the clear zone is a real sealing structure or if the diffusion into the outer fluid of small molecules or ions is possible independent of cellular transport. An intermittent activity of resorbing osteoclasts might also be possible. After loading of the resorbing compartment with calcium ions deriving from the dissolution of hydroxyapatite (Silver *et al.*, 1988), the cell could change its relationship with the substrate, allowing calcium diffusion into the extracellular fluid. Removal of such a high local concentration of calcium ions, could, in turn, allow the osteoclast to start a new resorption phase.

We extensively studied the presence and characteristics of calcium channels in isolated avian and mammalian osteoclasts and their role in cell regulation. We found that osteoclasts present two different calcium channels, a calcium-operated calcium channel (CaOCC) (Malgaroli *et al.*, 1989), and a voltage operated calcium channel (VOCC) (Miyauchi *et al.*, in press).

CaOCCs are gated by increased concentrations of extracellular calcium, as well as by the presence of other divalent cations (barium and cadmium, but not magnesium or lantanum). The increase in extracellular calcium, together with the opening of the CaOCCs, also stimulates release of calcium from intracellular stores, leading to a transient spike of cytosolic calcium followed by a sustained phase higher than the basal level. CaOCCs are inhibited by lantanum and insensitive to extracellular sodium and to VOCC inhibitors (Miyauchi *et al.*, in press).

VOCCs, gated by K-induced membrane depolarization, have also been found in chicken osteoclasts. They are specifically inhibited by dihydropiridine derivatives, and by phenylalkylamines and benzodiazepines. While CaOCCs still operate during bone resorption, VOCCs are down regulated when the cells are incubated in the presence of bone fragments. The role of the two types of calcium channels have been studied and are discussed below.

Metabolic acidosis has been reported to increase bone resorption *in vivo* (Chan *et al.*, 1985; Kraut *et al.*, 1986), in organ culture (Bushinsky *et al.*, 1985; Goldhaber *et al.*, 1987) and by disaggregated rat osteoclasts (Anderson *et al.*, 1986; Arnett and Dempster, 1986).

Adding permeant weak acid to incubation media and measuring, by fluorescent traces in single cells, intracellular pH and intracellular calcium concentration ($[Ca2^+]_i$), we found that changes in $[Ca2^+]_i$ are coupled to changes in pH_i (Teti *et al.*, 1989a).

In particular, cell acidification leads to reduction in $[Ca^{2+}]_i$ probably by activation of cyanide and vanadate sensitive, ATP-dependent, outward calcium transport. Conversely, cell alkalinization induces $[Ca^{2+}]_i$ increase. Both conditions lead to modifications of osteoclast activity. Thus, a decrease in cell pH and $[Ca^{2+}]_i$ results in an increase in podosome-mediated cell-substratum attachment (Teti *et al.*, 1989a) and in bone resorbing activity (Arnett and Dempster, 1986, Carano *et al.*, 1989).

Other recent data obtained in our laboratory confirm that cytosolic calcium plays a role in controlling osteoclast function. Calcitonin-treated rat osteoclasts show a small cAMP-dependent increase in cytosolic calcium. However, calcitonin treatment synergistically potentiates several fold the cytosolic calcium increase registered when extracellular calcium is augmented (Malgaroli *et al.*, 1989). Calcitonin being an inhibiting hormone, this result suggests that an increase in $[Ca^{2+}]_i$ also plays an inhibiting role in cell function. This has recently been confirmed (Miyauchi *et al.*, in press), in studying the response of osteoclast attachment structures and bone resorbing activity in cells in which cytosolic calcium has been augmented by treatment with high extracellular calcium or with K-induced membrane depolarization. In both circumstances the increase in cytosolic calcium was coupled to a decrease in podosome expression and to a concurrent decrease in bone resorption. Thus, our data suggest that cytosolic calcium participates in the regulation of osteoclast activity. These findings have also been confirmed by others (Zaidi et al., 1989).

The Osteoclast as a Polarized Cell

Information recently obtained, using mainly cell culture systems, suggests that resorbing osteoclasts are morphologically and functionally polarized (Baron et al., 1985). Particularly, the osteoclast membrane provides a segregation between the apical (resorbing compartment) and the basolateral (vascular side) spaces. The clear zone has the role of isolating the acidic resorbing compartment. This is comparable to the luminal compartment outlined by a tight epithelium. At the level of the resorbing compartment the plasma membrane specialization of the ruffled border is organized.

The characteristics and distribution of osteoclast plasma membrane ion transport systems confirms this view. As in renal tubular cells and gastric parietal cells, osteoclasts actively acidify the extracellular space. In all these cell types the intracellular source of protons is the carbonic anhydrase-dependent hydration of CO_2 to H_2CO_3. The dissociated H^+ are secreted by the apical proton pump (Baron et al., 1985; Blair et al., 1989), while HCO_3^- effluxes the cell by the basolateral Cl/HCO_3 exchanger (Teti et al., 1989b; Baron, personal communication). Moreover, the basolateral membrane of the osteoclast presents a (Na^+,K^+)ATPase, (Baron et al., 1986; 1988) and a Ca^{2+}ATPase (Akisaka et al., 1988). The maintenance of cell polarization is strictly connected to bone resorption. In fact, clear zone and ruffled border, the most characterizing features of osteoclast polarization, disappear during the resting phase of osteoclast activity in vivo (Miller et al., 1977; 1978). Likely, under this circumstance, the plasma membrane undergoes drastic rearrangements. Thus, it is possible to hypothesize that inhibitory or stimulatory factors could act on osteoclasts, preventing or inducing the onset of a polarized organization.

Acknowledgment

The similarity between osteoclasts and other polarized cells was introduced and discussed by Dr. Roland Baron during the ESCT in 1987.

References

Abbas, S. K., Fox, J. and Care, A. D. (1985) Calcium homeostasis in the chick embryo. *Comp. Biochem. Physiol.* **81B**: 975-979

Akisaka, T., Yamamoto, T. and Gay, C. V. (1988) Ultracytochemical investigation of calcium activated adenosine triphosphatase (Ca^{++}-ATPase) in chick tibia. *J. Bone Min. Res.* **3**: 19-25

Ali, N. N., Boyde, A. and Jones, S. J. (1984a) Motility and resorption: osteoclast activity *in vitro*. *Anat. Embryol.* **170**: 51-56

Ali, N. N., Jones, S. J. and Boyde, A. (1984b) Monocyte-enriched cells on calcified tissues. *Anat. Embryol.* **170**: 169-175

Anderson, R. E., Schraer, H. and Gay, C. V. (1982) Ultrastructural immunocytochemical localization of carbonic anhydrase in normal and calcitonin-treated chick osteoclasts. *Anat. Rec.* **204**: 9-20

Anderson, R. E., Woodbury, D. M. and Jee, W. S. S (1986) Humoral and ionic regulation of osteoclast activity. *Calcif. Tissue Int.* **39**: 252-258

Arnett, T. R. and Dempster, D. W. 91987) A comparative study of disaggregated chick and rat osteoclasts *in vitro*: effect of calcitonin and prostaglandins. *Endocrinology* **120**: 602-608

Arnett, T. R. and Dempster, D. W. (1986) Effect of pH on bone resorption by rat osteoclasts *in vitro*. *Endocrinology* **119** 119-124

Baimbridge, K. G. and Taylor, T. G. (1980) Role of calcitonin in calcium homeostasis in the chick embryo. *J. Endocrinol.* **85**: 171-185

Baron, R., Vignery, A. and Horowitz, M. (1984) Lymphocytes, macrophages and the regulation of bone remodeling. In: *Bone and Mineral Research. Annual 2.* (W. A. Peck, Ed.) pp. 175-243, Elsevier, Amsterdam, New York, Oxford (1984).

Baron, R., Neff, L., Louvard, D. and Courtoy, P. J. (1985) Cell-mediated extracellular acidification and bone resorption: Evidence for a low pH in resorbing lacunae and localization of a 100-kDa lysosomal membrane protein on the osteoclast ruffled border. *J. Cell. Biol.* **101**: 2210-2222

Baron, R., Neff, L., Roy, C., Boisvert, A. and Caplan, M. (1986) Evidence for a high and specific concentration of (Na^{+},K^{+})ATPase in the plasma membrane of osteoclasts. *Cell* **46**: 311-320

Baron, R., Neff, L., Brown, W., Courtoy, P. J., Louvard, D. and Farquhar, M. G. (1988) Polarized secretion of lysosomal enzymes: co-distribution of cation-independent mannose-6-phosphate receptors and lysosomal enzymes along the osteoclast exocytic pathway. *J. Cell. Biol.* **106**: 1863-1872

Blair, H. C. and Ghandur-Mnaymneh, L. (1985) Macrophage-mediate bone resorption in an acidic environment. *Calcif. Tissue. Int.* **37**: 547-550

Blair, H. C., Kahn, A. J., Crouch, E. C., Jeffrey, J. J. and Teitelbaum, S. L. (1986) Isolated osteoclasts resorb the organic and inorganic components of bone. *J. Cell. Biol.* **102**: 1164-1172

Blair, H. C., Teitelbaum, S. L., Schimke, P. A., Konsek, J. D., Koziol, C. M. and Schlesinger, P. H. (1988) Receptor-mediated uptake of a mannose-6-phosphate bearing glycoprotein by isolated osteoclasts. *J. Cell Physiol.* **137** 476-482

Blair, H. C., Teitelbaum, S. L., Ghiselli, R. and Gluck, S. (1989) Osteoclastic bone resorption by a polarized vacuolar proton pump. *Science* **245**: 855-857

Bloom, W., Bloom, H. A. and McLean, F. C. (1941) Calcification and ossification. Medullary bone changes in the reproductive cycle of female pigeon. *Anat. Rec.* **81**: 443-475

Bloom, H. A., Domm, L. V., Nalbandov, A. V. and Bloom, W. (1958) Medullary bone of laying chickens. *Am. J. Anat.* **102**: 411-453

Boyde, A., Ali, N. N. and Jones, S. J. (1984) Resorption of dentine by isolated osteoclasts *in vitro*. *Br. Dent. J.* **156**: 216-220

Bushinsky, D. A., Goldring, J. and Coe, F. L. (1985) Cellular contribution to pH-mediated calcium flux in neonatal mouse calvariae. *Am. J. Physiol.* **248**: F785-F789

Carano, A., Teitelbaum, S., Schlesinger, P. and Blair, H. (1989) Acidosis augments osteoclast-mediated bone resorption *in vitro*. *J. Bone Min. Res.* suppl vol **4**: 521

Chambers, T. J., Athanason, N. A. and Fuller, K. (1984a) Effect of parathyroid hormone and calcitonin on the cytoplasmic spreading of isolated osteoclasts. *J. Endocrinol.* **102**: 281-286

Chambers, T. J., Chambers, J. C., Symonds, J., and Darby, J. A. (1986) The effect of human calcitonin on the cytoplasmic spreading of rat osteoclasts. *J. Clin. Endocrinol. Metab.* **63**: 1080-1085

Chambers, T. J. and Dunn, C. J. (1982) The effect of parathyroid hormone, 1,25dihydroxycholecalciferol and prostaglandins on the cytoplasmic activity of isolated osteoclasts, *J. Pathol.* **137**: 193-203

Chambers, T. J. and Magnus, C. J. (1982) Calcitonin alters the behaviour of isolated osteoclasts. *J. Pathol.* **136**: 27-39

Chambers, T. J., McSheehy, P. M. J., Thomson, B. M. and Fuller, K. (1985) The effect of calcium-regulating hormones and prostaglandins on bone resorption by osteoclasts disaggregated from neonatal rabbit bones. *Endocrinology* **116**: 234-239

Chambers, T. J. and Moore, A. (1983) The sensitivity of isolated osteoclasts to morphological transformation by calcitonin. *J. Clin. Endocrinol. Metab.* **57**: 819-824

Chambers, T. J., Revell, P. A., Fuller, K. and Athanason, N. A. (1984b) Resorption of bone by isolated rabbit osteoclasts. *J. Cell Sci.* **66**: 383-399

Chan, Y. L., Savdie, E., Mason, R. S. and Posen, S. (1985) The effect of metabolic acidosis on vitamin D metabolites and bone histology in uremic rats. *Calcif. Tissue Int.* **37**: 158-164

Chenu, C., Pfeilschifter, J., Mundy, G. R. and Roodman, G. D. (1988) Transforming growth factor β inhibits formation of osteoclast-like cells in long-term human marrow cultures. *Proc. Natl. Acad. Sci. USA* **85**: 5683-5687

Cretin, A. (1951) Contribution histochimique a l'etude de la construction et de la destruction osseuse. *La Presse Medicale* **60**: 1240-1241

Dacke, C. G., Boelkins, J. N., Smith, W. K. and Kenny, A. D. (1972) Plasma calcitonin levels in birds during the ovulation cycle. *J. Endocrinol.* **54**: 369-370

Davies, J., Warwick, J., Totty, N., Philp, R., Helfrich, M. and Horton, M. (1989) The osteoclast functional antigen, implicated in the regulation of bone resorption, is biochemically related to the vitronectin receptor. *J. Cell Biol.* **109**: 1817-1826

de Bernard, B., Stagni, N., Camerotto, R., Vittur, F., Zanetti, M., Zambonin Zallone, A. and Teti, A. (1980) Influence of calcium depletion on medullary bone of laying hens. *Calcif. Tissue Int.* **32**: 221-228

Delaisse', J. M., Boyde, A., Maconnachie, E., Ali, N. N., Sear, C. H. J., Eeckhout, Y., Vaes, G. and Jones, S. J. (1987) The effect of inhibitors of cysteine-proteinases and collagenase on the resorptive activity of isolated osteoclasts. *Bone* **8**: 305-318

de Vernejoul, M.-C., Horowitz, M., Denignon, J., Neff, L. and Baron, R. (1988) Bone resorption by isolated chick osteoclasts in culture is stimulated by murine spleen cell supernatant fluids (osteoclast-activating factor) and inhibited by calcitonin and prostaglandin E_2. *J. Bone Min. Res.* **3**: 69-79

Doty, S. B. and Schofield B.H. (1972) Electron microscopic localization of hydrolytic enzymes in osteoclasts. *Histochem. J.* **4**: 245-258

Dempster, D. W., Murrills, J. R., Horbert, W. R. and Arnett, T. R. (1987) Biological activity of chicken calcitonin: effects on neonatal rat and embryonic chick osteoclasts. *J. Bone Min. Res.* **2**: 443-448

Fallon, M. D., Teitelbaum, S. L. and Kahn, A. J. (1983) Multinucleation enhances macrophage-mediated bone resorption. *Lab. Invest.* **49**: 159-164

Fallon, M. D. (1984) Bone resorbing fluid from osteoclasts is acidic. An *in vitro* micropuncture study. In: *Endocrine Control of Bone and Calcium Metabolism, vol. 4.* (D. V. Cohn, T. Fujita, J. T. Potts Jr., R. V. Talmage, Eds.), pp. 144-146, Elsevier Science Publisher, Amsterdam, (1984).

Ferrier, J., Warda, A., Kanehisa, J. and Heersche, J.N. M. (1986) Electrophysiological responses of osteoclasts to hormones. *J. Cell Physiol.* **128**: 23-26

Fuller, K. and Chambers, T. J. (1989) Effect of arachidonic acid metabolites on bone resorption by isolated rat osteoclasts. *J. Bone Min. Res.* **4**: 209-215

Gay, C. V., Falenski, E. J., Schraer, H. and Schraer, R. (1974a) Localization of carbonic anhydrase in avian gastric mucosa, shell gland and bone by immunohistochemistry. *J. Histochem. Cytol.* **22**: 819-825

Gay, C. V., Ito, M. B. and Schraer, H. (1983a) Carbonic anhydrase activity in isolated osteoclast. *Metab. Bone Dis. Rel. Res.* **5**: 33-39

Gay, C. V., Schraer, H., Anderson, R. E. and Cao, H. (1983b) Current studies on the localization and function of carbonic anhydrase in osteoclasts. *Ann. N.Y. Acad. Sci. Biol. Chem.* **429**: 473-478

Gay, C. V. and Mueller, W. J. 91974b) Carbonic anhydrase and osteoclasts: localization by labeled inhibitor autoradiography. *Science* **183**: 432-434

Gay, C. V. (1988) Avian bone resorption at the cellular level. *Critical Reviews in Poultry Biology* **1**: 197-269

Goldhaber, P. and Rabadjija, L. (1987) H^+ stimulation of cell mediated bone resorption in tissue culture. *Am. J. Physiol.* **253**: E90-E98

Gothlin, G. and Ericsson, J. L. E. (1971) Fine structural localization of acid phosphomonoesterase in the brush border region of osteoclasts. *Histochem.* **28**: 337-344

Gothlin, G. and Ericsson, J. L. E. (1976) The osteoclast. Review of ultrastructure, origin and structure-function relationship. *Clin. Orthop. Rel. Res.* **120**: 201-228

Heersche, J. N. M. (1978) Mechanism of osteoclastic bone resorption: a new hypothesis. *Calcif. Tissue Int.* **26**: 81-84

Hefley, T. J. and Stern, P. H. (1982) Isolation od osteoclasts from fetal rat long bones. *Calcif. Tissue Int.* **34**: 480-487

Holtrop, M. E. and King, G. J. (1977) The ultrastructure of osteoclast and its functional implications. *Clin. Orthop. Rel. Res.* **123**: 177-196

Horton, M. A., Lewis, D., McNulty, K., Pringle, J. A. S. and Chambers, T. J. (1985a) Human fetal osteoclasts fail to express macrophage antigens. *Br. J. Exp. Pathol.* **66**: 103-108

Horton, M. A., Lewis, D., McNulty, K., Pringle, J. A. S. and Chambers, T. J. (1985b) Monoclonal antibodies to osteoclastomas (giant cell tumors): definition of osteoclast-specific cellular antigens. *Cancer Res.* **45**: 5663-5669

Horton, M. A., Pringle, J. A. S. and Chambers, T.J. (1985c) Identification of human osteoclasts with monoclonal antibodies. *New Engl. J. Med.* **312**: 923-924

Hunter, S. J., Schraer, H. and Gay, C. V. (1988) Characterization of isolated and cultured chick osteoclasts: the effect of acetazolamide, calcitonin and parathyroid hormone on acid production as revealed by acridine orange staining. *J. Bone Min. Res.* **3**: 297-303

Ibbotson, K. J., Roodman, G. D., McManus, L. J. and Mundy, G. R. (1984) Identification and characterization of osteoclast-like cells and their progenitors in cultures of felin marrow mononuclear cells. *J. Cell Biol.* **99**: 471-480

Jilka, R. L., Rogers, J. I., Khalifah, R. G. and Vaananen, H. K. (1985) Carbonic anhydrase isoenzyme of osteoclasts and erythrocytes of osteopetrotic microphtalmic mice. *Bone* **6**: 445-449

Jones, S. J., Boyde, A. and Ali, N. N. (1984) The resorption of biological and non-biological substrates by cultured avian and mammalian osteoclasts. *Anat. Embryol.* **170**: 247-256

Jones, S. J., Boyde, A., Ali, A. A. and Maconnachie, E. (1986) Variation of the sizes of resorption lacunae made *in vitro. Scann. Elect. Microsc.* **IV**: 1571-1580

Jotereau, F. V. and Le Douarin, N. M. (1978) The developmental relationship between osteocytes and osteoclasts: A study using the quail-chick nuclear marker in endochondral ossification. *Devel. Biol.* **63**: 253-265

Kahn, A. J. and Simmons, D. J. (1975) Investigation of cell lineage in bone using a chimaera of chick and quail embryonic tissue. *Nature* **258**: 325-327

Kahn, A. J., Simmons, D. J. and Krukowski, M. (1981a) Osteoclast precursor cells are present in the blood of preossification chick embryo. *Devel. Biol.* **84**: 230-234

Kahn, A. J., Steward, C. C. and Teitelbaum, S. L. (1978) Contact-mediated bone resorption by human monocytes *in vitro. Science* **199**: 988-989

Kahn, A. J. and Teitelbaum, S. L. (1981b) Endotoxin inhibition of macrophage-mediated bone resorption. *Calcif. Tissue Int.* **33**: 269-275

King, J. and Holtrop, M. E. (1975) Actin-like filaments in bone cells of cultured mouse calvaria as demonstrated by binding to heavy meromyosin. *J. Cell Biol.* **66**: 445-451

Klein, D. C. and Raisz, L. G. (1970) Prostaglandins: stimulation of bone resorption in tissue culture. *Endocrinology* **85**: 657-665

Kraut, J. A., Mishler, D. R., Singer, F. R. and Goodman, W. G. (1986) The effects of metabolic acidosis on bone formation and bone resorption in the rat. *Kidney Int.* **30**: 694-700

Kukita, T., Chenu, C., McManus, L. M., Mundy, G. R. and Roodman, G. D. (1989a) Abnormal osteoclast-like cells (OCLs) form in Pagetic marrow cultures. *J. Bone Min. Res.* suppl vol. **4**: 320

Kukita, T., McManus, L. M., Miller, M., Civin, C. and Roodman, G. D. (1989b) Osteoclast-like cells formed in long-term bone marrow cultures express a similar surface phenotype as authentic osteoclasts. *Lab. Invest.* **60**: 532-538

Luben, R. A., Wong, G. L. and Cohn, D. V. (1976) Biochemical characterization with parahormone and calcitonin of isolated bone cells: provisional identification of osteoclast and osteoblast. *Endocrinology* **99**: 526-534

Luben, R. A., Wong, G. L. and Cohn, D. V. (1977) Parathormone-stimulated resorption of devitalized bone cultured osteoclast-type bone cells. *Nature* **265**: 629-630

Lucht, V. (1971) Acid phosphatase of osteoclasts demonstrated by electron microscopic histochemistry. *Histochemie* **28**: 103-117

Malgaroli, A., Meldolesi, J., Zambonin Zallone, A. and Teti, A. (1989) Control of cytosolic free calcium in rat and chicken osteoclasts. The role of extracellular calcium and calcitonin. *J. Biol. Chem.* **264**: 14342-14347

Marchisio, P. C., Cirillo, D., Naldini, L., Primavera, M. V, Teti, A. and Zambonin-Zallone, A. (1984) Cell-substratum interaction of cultured avian osteoclasts is mediated by specific adhesion structures. *J. Cell Biol.* **99**: 1696-1705

Marchisio, P. C., Cirillo, D., Teti, A., Zambonin-Zallone, A. and Tarone, G. (1987) Rous sarcoma virus-transformed fibroblasts and cells of monocytic origin display a peculiar dot-like organization of cytoskeletal proteins involved in microfilament-membrane interactions. *Exp. Cell Res.* **169**: 202-214

Marie, P. J. and Hott, M. (1987) Histomorphometric identification of carbonic anhydrase in fetal rat bone embedded in glycolmethacrylate. *J. Histochem. Cytochem.* **35**: 245-250

McDonald, B. R., Takahashi, I., McManus, M., Holahan, J., Mundy, G. R. and Roodman, G. D. (1987) Formation of multinucleated cells that respond to osteotropic hormones in long term human bone marrow cultures. *Endocrinology* **120**: 2326-2333

Marks Jr., S. C. and Walker, D. G. (1981) The hematogenous origin of osteoclasts: experimental evidence from osteopetrotic (microphtalmic) mice treated with spleen cells from beige mouse donors. *Am. J. Physiol.* **161**: 1-10

Martin, T. J., Raisz, L. G. and Rodan, G. A. (1987) Calcium regulation and bone metabolism. **In**: *Clinical Endocrinology of Calcium Metabolism.* (T. J. Martin, L. G. Raisz, Eds), pp. 1-52, Marcel Dekker Inc. New York, Basel

Martin, T. J. and Mundy, G. R. (1987) Hypercalcemia of malignancy. **In**: *Clinical Endocrinology of Calcium Metabolism.* (T. J. Martin, L. G. Raisz, Eds.), pp.171-200, Marcel Dekker Inc., New York, Basel

Mears, D. C. (1971) Effects of parathyroid hormone and thyrocalcitonin on the membrane potential of osteoclasts. *Endocrinology* **88**: 1021-1028

Merke, J., Klaus, G., Hugel, U., Waldherr, R. and Ritz, E. (1986) No 1,25-dihydroxyvitamin D_3 receptors on osteoclasts of calcium-deficient chicken despite demonstrable receptors on circulating monocytes. *J. Clin. Invest.* **77**: 312-314

Miller, S. C. (1977) Osteoclast cell-surface changes during egg-laying cycle in Japanese quail. *J. Cell Biol.* **75**: 104-118

Miller, S. C. (1978) Rapid activation of the medullary bone osteoclast cell surface by parathyroid hormone. *J. Cell Biol.* **76**: 615-618

Mundy, G. R., Altman, A. J., Gonder, M. D. and Bandelin, J. G. (1977) Direct resorption of bone by human monocytes. *Science* **196**: 1109-1111

Miyauchi, A., Hruska, K. A., Greenfield, E. M., Barattolo, R., Colucci, S., Zambonin-Zallone, A., Teitelbaum, S. L. and Teti, A. (1991) Osteoclast cytosolic calcium, regulated by voltage operated calcium channels and extracellular calcium, controls podosome assembly and bone resorption. *J. Cell Biol.* in press.

Mundy, G. R., Varani, J., Orr, W., Gonder, M. D. and Ward, P. A. (1978) Resorbing bone is chemotactic for monocytes. *Nature* **275**: 132-134

Nelson, R. L. and Bauer, G. E. (1977) Isolation of osteoclasts by velocity sedimentation at unit gravity. *Calcif. Tissue Res.* **22**: 303-313

Ng, K.W., Livesey, S. A., Collier, F., Gummer, P. R. and Martin, T. J. (1985) Effect of retinoids on the growth, ultrastructure and cytoskeletal structures of malignant rat osteoblasts. *Cancer Res.* **45**: 5106-5113

Nicholson, G. C., Moseley, J. M. and Martin, T. J. (1987) Chicken osteoclasts do not posses calcitonin receptors. *J. Bone Min. Res.* **2**: 53-55

Nicholson, G. C., Moseley, J. M., Sexton, P. M., Mendelsohn, F. A. O. and Martin, T. J. (1986) Abundant calcitonin receptors in isolated rat osteoclasts. *J. Clin. Invest.* **78**: 355-360

Nijweide, P. J., Vrijheid-Lammers, T., Mulder, R. J. P. and Block, J. (1985) Cell surface antigens on osteoclasts and related cells in the quail studied with monoclonal antibodies. *Histochem.* **83**: 315-324

Okuda, A., Taylor, L. M., Heersche, J. N. M. (1989) Prostaglandin E_2 initially inhibits and then stimulates bone resorption in isolated rabbit osteoclast cultures. *Bone Min.* **7**: 255-266

Oreffo, R. O. C., Francis, M. J. O. and Triffitt, J. T. (1985) Vitamin A effects on UMR 106 osteosarcoma cells are not mediated by specific cytosolic receptors. *Biochem. J.* **232**: 559-603

Oreffo, R. O. C., Triffitt, J. T., Francis, M. J. O., Teti, A., and Zambonin Zallone, A. (1987) Vitamin A action on normal and malignant bone cells. In: *Calcium Regulation and Bone Metabolism. Basic and Clinical Aspects.* (D. V. Cohn, T. J. Martim, P. J. Meunier, Eds). Vol. 9, pp. 349-354, Elsevier Science Publisher, Amsterdam

Oreffo, R. O. C., Teti, A., Triffitt, J. T., Francis, M. J. O, Carano, A. and Zambonin Zallone, A. (1988) Effect of vitamin A on bone resorption: evidence for direct stimulation of isolated chicken osteoclasts by retinol and retinoic acid. *J. Bone Min. Res.* 3: 203-210

Osdoby, P., Martini, M. C. and Caplan, A. I. (1982) Isolated osteoclasts and their presumed progenitor cells, the monocyte, in culture. *J. Exp. Zool.* 244: 331-344

Oursler, M. J., Bell, L. V., Clevinger, B. and Osdoby, P. (1985) Identification of osteoclast-specific monoclonal antibodies. *J. Cell Biol.* 100: 1592-1600

Peck, W. A., Birge Jr., S. J. and Fedak, S. A. (1964) Bone cells: biochemical and biological studies after enzymatic isolation. *Science* 146: 1476-1477

Pfeilschifter, J., Chenu, C., Bird, A., Mundy, G. R. and Roodman, G. D. (1989) Interleukin-1 and tumor necrosis factor stimulate the formation of human osteoclast-like cells *in vitro. J. Bone Min. Res.* 4: 113-117

Pliam, N. B., Nyiredy, K. O. and Arnaud, C. D. (1982) Parathyroid hormone receptors in avian bone cells. *Proc. Natl. Acad. Sci. USA* 79: 2061-2063

Rifkin, B.R., Baker, R. L. and Coleman, S. J. An ultrastructural study of macrophage-mediated resorption of calcified tissue. *Cell Tissue Res.* 202: 125-132

Rifkin, B. R., Baker, R. L., Somerman, M. J., Pointon, S. E., Coleman, S. J. and Wyw, A. U. (1980) Osteoid resorption by mononuclear cells *in vitro. Cell Tissue Res.* 210: 493-500

Rodan, G. A. and Martin, T. J. (1981) Role of osteoblasts in hormonal control of bone resorption. A hypothesis. *Calcif. Tissue Int.* 33: 349-351

Rodan, S. B. and Rodan, G. A. (1974) The effect of parathyroid hormone and calcitonin on the accumulation of cyclic adenosine 3'5'-monophosphate in fresly isolated bone cells. *J. Biol. Chem.* 249: 3068-3074

Roodman, G. D., Ibbotson, K. J., MacDonald, B. R., Kuehl, T. J. and Mundy, G. R. (1985) 1,25-dihydroxyvitamin D_3 causes formation of multinucleated cells with several osteoclast characteristics in culture of primate marrow. *Proc. Natl. Acad. Sci. USA* 82: 8213-8217

Sakamoto, S. and Sakamoto, M., (1982) Biochemical and immunohistochemical studies on collagenase in resorbing bone in tissue culture. *J. Period. Res.* 17: 523-526

Silve, C. M., Hradek, G. T., Jones, A. L. and Arnaud, C. D. (1982) Parathyroid hormone receptor in intact embryonic chicken bone: characterization and cellular localization. *J. Cell Biol.* 94: 379-386

Silver, A., Murrills, R. J. and Etherington, D. J. (1988) Microelectrode studies on the acid microenvironment beneath adherent macrophages and osteoclasts. *Exp. Cell Res.* 175: 266-276

Sundquist, K. T., Leppilampi, M., Jarvelin, K., Kumpulainen, T. and Vaananen, H. K. (1987) Carbonic anhydrase isoenzymes in isolated rat peripheral monocytes, tissue macrophages, and osteoclasts. *Bone* 8: 33-38

Takahashi, N., Yamana, H., Yoshiki, S., Roodman. G. D., Mundy, G. R., Jones, S. J., Boyde, A. and Suda, T. (1988) Osteoclast-like cell formation and its regulation by osteotropic hormones in mouse bone marrow cultures. *Endocrinology* 122: 1373-1382

Takahashi, N., McDonald, B. R., Hon, J., Winkler, E., Derynek, B. R., Mundy, G. R. and Roodman, G. D. (1986) Recombinant human transforming growth-factor α stimulates the formation of osteoclast-like cells in long-term human marrow cultures. *J. Clin. Invest.* 78: 894-898

Teitelbaum, S. L., Malone, D. G. and Kahn, A. J. (1981) Glucocorticoid enhancement of bone resorption by rat peritoneal macrophages *in vitro. Endocrinology* 108: 795-799

Teitelbaum, S.L., Steward, C. C. and Kahn, A. J. (1979) Rodent peritoneal macrophages as bone resorbing cells. *Calcif. Tissue Int.* **27**: 225-261

Testa, N. G., Allen, T. D., Lajtha, L. G. and Onions, D. (1981) Generation of osteoclasts *in vitro*. *J. Cell Sci.* **47**: 127-137

Teti, A., Blair, H. C., Schlesinger, P. H., Grano, M., Zambonin Zallone, A., Kahn, A. J., Teitelbaum, S. L. and Hruska, K. A. (1989a) Extracellular protons acidify osteoclasts, reduce cytosolic calcium and promote expression of cell-matrix attachment structures. *J. Clin. Invest.* **84**: 773-780

Teti, A., Blair, H. C., Teitelbaum, S. L., Kahn, A. J., Koziol, C., Konsek, J., Zambonin Zallone, A. and Schlesinger, P. H. (1989b) Cytoplasmic pH, regulation and chloride/bicarbonate exchange in avian osteoclast. *J. Clin. Invest.* **83**: 227-233

Teti, A., Volleth, G., Carano, A. and Zambonin Zallone, A. (1988) The effects of parathyroid hormone or 1,25-dihydroxyvitamin D_3 on monocyte-osteoclast fusion. *Calcif. Tissue Int.* **42**: 302-308

Vaananen, H. K. and Parvinen, E. K. (1983) High active isoenzyme of carbonic anhydrase in rat calvaria osteoclasts. Immunohistochemical study. *Histochem.* **78**: 481-483

Vaananen, H. K. (1984) Immunohistochemical localization of carbonic anhydrase isoenzyme I and II in human bone, cartilage and giant cell tumor. *Histochem.* **81**: 485-487

Vaananen, H. K., Malmi, R., Tuukkanen, J., Sundquist, K. and Harkonen, P. (1986) Identification of osteoclasts by rhodamine-conjugated peanut agglutinin. *Calcif. Tissue Int.* **39**: 161-165

Vaes, G. (1968) On the mechanism of bone resorption: the action of parathyroid hormone on the excretion and synthesis of lysosomal enzymes and on the extracellular release of acid by bone cells. *J. Cell Biol.* **39**: 676-697

Wakefield, J. St. J., Gale, J. S., Berridge, M. V., Jordan, T. W. and Ford, H. C. (1982) Is Percoll innocuous to cells? *Biochem. J.* **202**: 795-797

Walker, D. G. (1972) Enzymatic and electron microscopic analysis of isolated osteoclasts. *Calcif. Tissue Res.* **9**: 296-309

Walker, D. G. (1973) Osteopetrosis cured by temporary parabiosis. *Science* **180**: 875

Walker, D. G. (1975) Control of bone resorption by hematopoietic tissue. The induction and reversal of congenital osteopetrosis in mice through use of bone marrow and splenic transplant. *J. Exp. Med.* **142**: 651-663

Warshafsky, B., Aubin, J. E. and Heersche, J. N. M. (1985) Cytoskeleton rearrangements during calcitonin-induced changes in osteoclast mobility *in vitro*. *Bone* **6**: 179-185

Wong, G. L. and Cohn, D. V. (1974) Separation of parathyroid hormone and calcitonin-sensitive cells from non-responsive bone cells. *Nature* **252**: 713-715

Yamamoto, T. and Gay, C. V. (1986) Cytochemical detection of adenylate cyclase activity in bone cells. *J. Cell Biol.* **103**: 103a

Zaidi, M., Datta, H. K., Patchell, A., Moonga, B. and MacIntyre, I. (1989) "Calcium-activated" intracellular calcium elevation: a novel mechanism of osteoclast regulation. *Biochem. Biophys. Res. Comm.* **163**: 1461-1465

Zambonin Zallone, A. and Mueller, W. J. (1969) Medullary bone of laying hens during calcium depletion and repletion. *Calcif. Tissue Res.* **4**: 136-146

Zambonin Zallone, A. and Teti, A. (1981) The osteoclasts of hen medullary bone under hypocalcaemic conditions. *Anat. Embryol.* **162**: 379-392

Zambonin Zallone, A., Teti, A. and Primavera, M. V. (1982) Isolated osteoclasts in primary culture: first observation on structure and survival in culture media. *Anat. Embryol.* **165**: 405-413

Zambonin Zallone, A., Teti, A., Primavera, M. V., Naldini, L. and Marchisio, N. C. (1983) Osteoclasts and monocytes have similar cytoskeletal structures and adhesion property *in vitro*. *J. Anat.* **137**: 57-70

Zambonin Zallone, A., Teti, A. and Primavera, M. V. (1984) Resorption of vital and devitalized
    bone by isolated osteoclasts *in vitro*. The role of lining cells. *Cell Tissue Res.* **235**: 561-564
Zambonin Zallone, A., Teti, A., Grano, M., Rubinacci, A., Abbadini, M., Gaboli, M. and
    Marchisio, P. C. (1989) Immunocytochemical distribution of extracellular matrix receptors
    in human osteoclasts: a β3 integrin is colocalized with vinculin and talin in the podosomes
    of osteoclastoma giant cells. *Exp. Cell. Res.8* **182: 645-652**
Zile, M., Bunge, E. C. and De Luca, H. F. (1979) On the physiological basis of vitamin
    A-stimulated growth. *J. Nutr.* **109**: 1787-1796

5

Bone Resorption *In Vivo*

ARNOLD J. KAHN[*] AND NICOLA C. PARTRIDGE[**]
Department of Growth and Development
School of Dentistry
University of California
San Francisco, California

**Departments of Pediatrics and Physiology*
St. Louis University
St. Louis, Missouri

Introduction

Bone resorption is an integral component of skeletal modeling, remodeling and fracture healing. As such, it has been the subject of intensive investigation. However, for reasons related to difficulty in experimental design and interpretation, this effort has focused on *in vitro* models rather than on events within the intact skeleton. As a consequence, little definitive information is available on bone resorption *in vivo*, particularly as it relates to the regulation of resorptive activity. Thus, while a number of agents (hormones, monokines, lymphokines) have been shown to stimulate bone and calcified cartilage resorption in organ or tissue culture, relatively few of these substances have been comprehensively tested for comparable activity in the whole animal and even fewer examined within a physiological context. Consequently, in the present review, we have elected to focus our attention on an analysis of these factors within the context of the major prevailing concepts of skeletal modeling and remodeling. Bone resorption rarely, if ever, occurs outside the context of these two events *in vivo* and, therefore, understanding these processes and what governs them should provide insights into what is both physiologically feasible and biologically relevant. Perhaps more importantly, we hope that by taking this approach, new or alternative frameworks for future experiments will have been established. One such alternative framework is presented below.

Cellular Elements in Bone Resorption

Although the issue has sometimes been disputed, there appears to be little doubt that the osteoclast is the cell principally, if not solely, responsible for resorbing mineralized connective tissue matrix (whether it be bone, calcified cartilage or dentin) (Hancox, 1949). This conclusion follows, in part, from the long established physical association of osteoclasts with focal areas of matrix removal (Howship's lacunae or resorption bays) (Jones *et al.*, 1986) but is most persuasively supported by observations, made *in vitro*, either showing osteoclasts in the act of resorbing mineralized matrix (Hancox and Boothroyd, 1961) or demonstrating (even quantifying) the amount of matrix removed subsequent to osteoclast activity (Chambers *et al.*, 1985; Jones *et al.*, 1986). The primacy of the osteoclast as the principal agent for resorption is also supported, indirectly, by the failure of other cells to express similar resorptive potential when examined by comparable techniques. For example, even the macrophage, which can clearly degrade bone matrix under some circumstances, does so much less efficiently than the authentic osteoclast (Fallon *et al.*, 1983). Precisely how the osteoclast resorbs bone matrix with such efficiency remains uncertain in detail, but the available evidence points to a mechanism that includes the creation of a mineral dissolving acidic environment (probably the result of plasma membrane proton pump activity) (Teti *et al.*, 1989) and the secretion of collagen-degrading proteases (Blair *et al.*, 1986; Vaes, 1988).

Despite the well-documented matrix resorbing capability of osteoclasts, it is equally clear that other cells must also be involved in the resorptive process. Nowhere is this involvement better highlighted than when the apparently related issues of the tissue response to resorption stimulating agents and the osteoblast-lining of bone surfaces are considered. With regard to the former, it now seems certain that most diffusible factors that increase resorptive activity do so *not* by acting directly on the osteoclast but rather by involving one, if not more, local cell types as intermediates in the response mechanism (Rodan and Martin, 1981; McSheehy and Chambers, 1986; Perry *et al.*, 1989). One of these local intermediates appears to be the bone lining cell or osteoblast. This conclusion follows from several lines of evidence and includes, most importantly, the ability of the osteoblast/lining cell to respond to a spectrum of resorption-stimulating agents leading, in some cases, to changes in the morphology of the osteoblast layer (Miller *et al.*, 1976) (thereby providing osteoclast access to the bone matrix) and the production/release of factors that have the potential to stimulate osteoclast precursor proliferation and precursor recruitment (Chambers *et al.*, 1985). In addition, the osteoblast, at least in some species and under some circumstances (perhaps mostly during fetal development; Gershan and Partridge, unpublished observations), is capable of synthesizing neutral collagenase (Sakamoto and Sakamoto, 1982; Heath *et al.*, 1984; Partridge *et al.*, 1987), an enzyme that will degrade the principal organic component of bone matrix, Type I collagen. In fact, one current hypothesis of bone resorption identifies the latter activity as an essential first step in matrix degradation, *viz.*, the removal of a "surface" coat of non- or poorly mineralized matrix ("osteoid") as a consequence of osteoblast-derived collagenolytic activity that permits the osteoclast to resorb the underlying, more fully mineralized matrix (Chambers and Fuller, 1985; Kahn and Partridge, 1987). Finally, as discussed more fully below, the osteoblast/bone lining cell might be the "sensor" detecting those changes in mechanical force that are responsible for initiating remodeling activity.

Bone Resorption in Physiological and Pathological Processes

Although bone resorption occurs under a variety of different circumstances *in vivo*, it is possible to divide these various circumstances into two groups based upon whether or not the removal of matrix is part of a cycle that couples resorption to formation. This distinction is important since it both helps to define the biological context in which resorption is occurring and may aid in the identification of those factors that regulate its occurrence under physiological conditions. In the most widespread circumstance involving cycling, *i.e.*, skeletal remodeling, bone forming cells (osteoblasts) and bone resorbing cells (osteoclasts) co-exist within a mutually interactive framework (BMU; basic multicellular unit) in which the activity of one cell population triggers or represents an essential antecedent for the function of the second (Frost, 1964). Thus, in most current representations of remodeling, the overall process starts with the activation of bone-lining cells (osteoblasts) resulting in the recruitment and resorptive function of osteoclasts (Parfitt, 1984). This latter activity leads, in turn, to the reappearance of matrix-synthesizing osteoblasts and the re-acquisition of bone mass.

In contrast to the "coupling" apparent in remodeling , skeletal modeling (a phenomenon associated with changes in bone shape during growth and development) is characterized by the spatial segregation of the sites of (net) bone formation and resorption (Frost, 1973). This segregation of activity is fundamental to the redistribution of bone mass and is exemplified by the differences seen on endosteal/endocranial surfaces (that show net resorptive activity) as opposed to periosteal/exocranial sites (regions of net matrix synthesis). Under these latter circumstances and, in apparent contrast to remodeling, the steady-state coupling of osteoblast and osteoclast activity is not apparent, suggesting that there are site specific differences in the mechanisms that regulate bone turnover. The nature of these differences is not known, but, as noted again below, site specificity may be an important clue in determining primary signals in the activation of resorption and the triggering of bone remodeling.

Why, then, is remodeling initiated *in vivo*? At present, there is no clear answer to this question but three general possibilities have been identified. These are (1) as a means of recovering mineral from bone in calcium homeostasis, (2) to repair small scale tissue damage (microfractures) and (3) to adjust the structure and mass of the skeleton in response to changes in mechanical force (loading). None of these explanations appears to provide a completely satisfactory answer. With regard to the first, while it is clear that increased calcium demand and/or elevation in calcium mobilizing hormones can lead to changes in remodeling activity (Jaworski, 1981; Miller, 1988; Miller *et al.*, 1989), it is difficult to visualize how such systemic changes, alone, can account for the localized differences in remodeling activity observed as a consequence of changes in loading (*e.g.*, Bouvier and Hylander, 1981) or among the various bones of the skeleton (Atkinson and Woodhead, 1973). With regard to the second, there is little doubt that microfractures and other localized trauma do occur in the skeleton and that these events can trigger remodeling (here seen as a wound healing or tissue repair mechanism) (Bun *et al.*, 1985). However, as with the calcium homeostasis concept, this explanation cannot, by itself, account for the reproducible pattern (distribution) of remodeling found in the skeleton of individual animals of the same species (*e.g.*, Atkinson and Woodhead, 1973) or the differences observed between species (Currey, 1984b). Finally, there is the possibility that mechanical force (loading) or the lack thereof, initiates or regulates remodeling. While such forces do not always account for the apparently non-random distribution of remodeling sites (Marotti, 1961), it is clear that changes in loading can lead to both global and regional differences in remodeling activity. This conclusion follows from a number of highly reproducible observations. First, skeletal mass is always lost, at least initially, whenever mechanical loading is removed or is substantially reduced (Uthoff and Jaworski, 1973). This loss is attributable to increased remodeling (net resorptive) activity and is readily documented in bones that ordinarily function to support weight (*e.g.*, the vertebral column or the bones of the lower extremity; Smith and Gilligan, 1989) or are acted upon by muscle contraction (*e.g.*, bones of the lower jaw; Bouvier and Hylander, 1981). Second, bone adapts to changes in the direction or magnitude of applied force by altering (remodeling) its structure to accommodate to the new loading pattern (Cowin, 1984; Currey, 1984a,b). Finally, the changes in bone mass or structure resulting from the absence of force or changes in force vector are not necessarily accompanied by alterations in bone quality (Frost, 1987a), at least at moderate levels of strain. This implies that mechanical loading effects the activation and, perhaps, the rate of modeling/remodeling but not necessarily the nature of the new matrix produced as part of the process (Burr *et al.*, 1989a). However, it has recently been reported that woven bone may be a normal component of the response if the mechanical challenge is intense enough (Burr *et al.*, 1989b).

The Mechanostat Hypothesis

Recently, Frost (1987a,b) has presented a new hypothesis regarding the control of bone mass during growth, modeling and remodeling that is based upon the primacy of mechanical force in extrinsically controlling bone matrix (mass) accretion or loss. This essential premise follows from numerous observations, summarized briefly above, that indicate a general positive correlation between usage (loading) and mass, and the truism that in healthy skeletons "mass can be overadequate but never inadequate" (Frost, 1987a). These observations suggested to Frost the existence of a homeostatic mechanism within bone (termed a "mechanostat") that monitors usage and sets into motion mechanisms that correct "serious misfits" between mass and mechanical usage. Implicit within this hypothesis are several other essential propositions. First, and foremost, is the concept of minimum effective strain (MES). In modeling, the MES corresponds to that threshold ("setpoint") of load which, when exceeded, will cause an increase in cortical bone mass and appropriate (load resisting) changes in skeletal architecture. In remodeling, the "setpoint" is much lower and, in contrast to modeling MES, is typically activated when the threshold is not reached. Thus, under conditions of diminished load and/or physical activity (*e.g.*, paralysis), remodeling is accelerated and bone mass is lost. The latter result obtains because of the second essential point, *viz.*, that the remodeling process generally results in more matrix being removed than formed, particularly in regions adjacent to bone marrow (Atkinson and Woodhead, 1973; Garn, 1975). It follows, therefore, that *any* circumstance which leads to an increase in remodeling (or, at least, activation of the resorptive component of remodeling) will contribute to a diminution in bone mass.

The final component of the mechanostat hypothesis is the most pertinent to the present review because it attempts to integrate all the various and multiple factors known to influence modeling and remodeling into a single, conceptual framework. Here, the pivotal point is to view these various factors as affecting bone mass and architecture by adjusting the MES setpoints to higher or lower levels. This relationship is depicted by Frost in the following manner (Frost, 1987a):

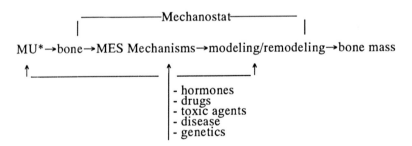

MU = mechanical usage

Fig. 1

Thus, for example, in the presence of glucocorticoids or the absence of estrogens (postmenopausal osteoporosis), the apparent setpoint for remodeling MES might be raised and the mechanostat would "perceive" an excess of bone mass relative to mechanical need. Under these conditions, remodeling would be accelerated and bone lost until the remaining mass matched apparent usage (mechanical loading). At this stage, remodeling activity would diminish and a new steady state would be established. As presented by Frost (1987b), the change in setpoint associated, for example, with osteoporosis is approximately 30%, resulting, if uncorrected, in a corresponding loss of mass of about 30%.

Extrinsic Response Mechanisms

For the present purpose, the term "extrinsic" is used to denote any exogenous chemical or physical factor (or agent) that initiates or modifies skeletal modeling and remodeling activity. The fact that such factors exist and are effective in modifying bone turnover presupposes the existence of a response mechanism sensitive to these various factors. In the case of systemic and locally produced effector substances, the responses can be attributed to binding proteins or receptors located in the plasma membrane or elsewhere in the cell. In the instance of mechanical loading (and, perhaps, resultant changes in electrical potential), the biological or chemical nature of the response mechanism is much less certain and, therefore, much more speculative. However, as discussed again below, it is likely that these responses, too, are receptor mediated and involve the same primary and secondary signalling mechanisms as established for chemical effectors.

1) Signals in Mechanical Force Transduction

Of the various hypotheses that might account for signal generation following the application or removal of mechanical load, only two appear intuitively likely to be involved in the process and these differ substantially in fundamental characteristics. The first hypothesis states that changes in force are detected directly at the cellular level due to presence of mechano- or stretch receptors on osteoblasts, bone lining cells and/or osteocytes. Deformation of these receptors in response to changes in loading could lead to transmembrane ion fluxes (an effect that would be transmitted to electrically-coupled bone cells; also see below) and ion induced alterations in cell function (*e.g.*, the activation of remodeling). At present, there are data showing that the osteoblast and osteoblast-like cells are directly responsive to mechanical stress (at least *in vitro*) (*e.g.*, Hasegawa *et al.*, 1985), but the studies focused on documenting the presence of stretch receptors appear to be relatively limited (see, however, Duncan and Misler, 1989). In any case, one major unknown about this hypothesis is whether the magnitude of shape change associated with mechanical loading at the whole bone level would be adequate to provide the magnitude of physical distortion (stretching) necessary to activate mechanoreceptors. In addition, there is the question of how a reduction in force-induced physical distortion could operate through mechanoreceptors to initiate remodeling or resorptive processes. However, both of these latter these concerns can be addressed by associating stress/strain with (1) changes in forces or flow rate within the fluid compartment of bone where the effect would be amplified and many cells concurrently influenced and (2) controlling an "off-signal" for the synthesis of a remodeling inhibitor. Thus, in the latter situation, the absence or a reduction in force could lead to derepression (*i.e.*, triggering) in modeling/remodeling activity.

The second hypothesis has received much more attention, investigation and debate. Here, as opposed to the circumstance described above, bone cells are not activated directly by changes in force but are postulated to respond to either endogenous bioelectrical potential (Brighton and McCluskey, 1986) or alterations in electrical potential produced by the piezoelectric properties of bone matrix (Pollack, 1984) and/or streaming potentials resulting from an ionic exchange between the bone matrix and the bone fluid/blood vascular compartment (Eriksson, 1974). These stress generated potentials (SGP) would, therefore, constitute the signal event in initiating resorption/remodeling. The nature of the response mechanism to potential changes is not known. However, one attractive possibility that would integrate SGP with hormone action is to postulate that the ionic or potential differences produced by SGP alter the structure/function relationship of receptors associated with local or systemic osteotropic agents (Ferrier, 1989). If such activities did occur and were to include up or down regulation of receptors or alterations in receptor activity, it might be sufficient to initiate or suppress the onset of resorption/remodeling. In this regard, it is of interest to consider the findings of Luben and his co-workers (Cain *et al.*, 1987) and Brighton and McClusky (1988) who have examined the PTH response of osteoblastic cells in pulsed electromagnetic and electrical fields, respectively. Their observations not only indicate a shift in the dose-response curve (as measured by cAMP levels), but also a diminished amplitude in response to hormone. With this in mind, among the compelling features of a control mechanism based upon electrical/ionic potentials are (1) its ability to account for the site and regional specificity of remodeling activated by applied force, (2) its transmission (*via* ion flow) to adjacent cells by gap junctions (the latter structures apparently link subsets of osteoblasts and osteocytes) (Doty, 1981) and (3) the sensitivity of the modeling and remodeling processes to experimental and clinical alterations in electrical potential (Becker, 1979; Brighton and McCluskey, 1986).

2) Target Cells in Initiating Resorption/Remodeling

Although, conceptually, almost any cell type associated with the bone surface might be the target of the initiating signal in resorption/remodeling, the bone lining cell/osteoblast (and perhaps contiguous osteocytes) seems best suited to fulfill this role. (However, for an alternative view, see section [5] below on Immune System Regulation of Resorption.) This tentative conclusion follows from the proximity of lining cells/osteoblasts/osteocytes to both blood borne and matrix derived regulatory factors, including ionic changes resulting from streaming potentials, their involvement in mediating ionic exchange between the blood vascular compartment and the mineral component of the bone matrix (Talmage, 1967; Parfitt, 1979), and their probable role in controlling the recruitment and activity of osteoclasts (*Supra vidae*), the cells ultimately responsible for bone resorption. As noted above, this postulated intermediate function for osteoblasts/bone lining cell/osteocyte derives, in part, from observations indicating that these cells and not osteoclasts have receptors for and/or exhibit responses to resorption stimulating factors, *e.g.*, PTH. Thus, to link two important elements together; osteoblast/bone lining cell/osteocyte would respond to ionic changes resulting from mechanical stress by altering receptor binding or activity to systemic or local effector substances.

3) Effector Interaction in Mechanostat Function: An Extended Hypothesis

The mechanostat is a homeostatic device of a special type; sensitive to mechanical force, self-regulating with regard to force/structure relationships and containing two feed-back loops. One of these loops operates at the upper limit of the strain threshold such that when this "set point" is exceeded, new bone formation is triggered. The other loop functions at the lower limit of the strain threshold and is activated when the force acting on bone falls below certain minimal levels (the MES). In this instance, it is remodeling that is triggered and with it, over time, the loss of bone mass. Although we still lack definitive information on the nature of the primary signal resulting from mechanical force and on the identity of the cell responsive to this signal for reasons stated previously, it seems reasonable to postulate that the former is represented by local differences in ionic or electrical potential and the latter by the bone lining cell. If such be the case, what, then, is the nature of the interaction that might lead to alterations in remodeling activity? Note that the bone lining cell (osteoblast/osteocyte) is responsive to a variety of systemic and local effector substances, and that many of these substances act *via* receptors located in the cell membrane (Raisz, 1988; Canalis *et al.*, 1989). Note also that many (all?) of these substances appear to show dose-dependent, biphasic effects on bone and bone cells such that at low concentrations they enhance "anabolic" activity while at high concentrations they are "catabolic". Thus, to cite one example, low levels of PTH stimulate osteoblast proliferation and growth (MacDonald *et al.*, 1986; Majeska and Rodan, 1981; Hock *et al.*, 1988) and high levels of growth inhibition (Partridge *et al.*, 1985) and a cessation of matrix synthesis (Kream *et al.*, 1980; Lian *et al.*, 1984). Within such a spectrum, it might be expected that physiological concentrations of PTH would favor a phenotypic "steady-state" for the osteoblast or bone lining cell; a state in which the primary activity would be the maintenance of the tissue (bone) fluid compartment located between the bone matrix and the lining cells. In fact, in humans, on average, 80% of the cells lining the endosteum have a morphology consistent with this interpretation (Parfitt, 1982).

Previously, we noted the possibility that stress-induced electrical or ionic changes might operate by altering receptor binding and/or activity. If, as one example, such changes were manifest in the PTH receptor, then alterations in cell function associated with mechanical loads (*e.g.*, remodeling) could be attributed, at least in part, to a shift in the dose-activity relationship of this hormone (Fig. 2).

It is important to emphasize that the present example, based upon PTH, is meant to be representative of a general class of interactions involving ligands, receptors and stress-induced changes in the milieux of the lining cells. Thus, the ligands could include matrix proteins and cytokines as well as steroids and prostanoids, the receptors might be located intracellularly as well as in the plasma membrane and the stress induced changes could act *via* stretch or mechanoreceptors rather than ionic/electrical potential signals. What is essential here is the recognition (1) that the bone lining cell, like other cells, integrates extrinsic information (signals) from a wide range of sources, (2)

Hormone-Mechanical Load Relationships on Osteoblasts

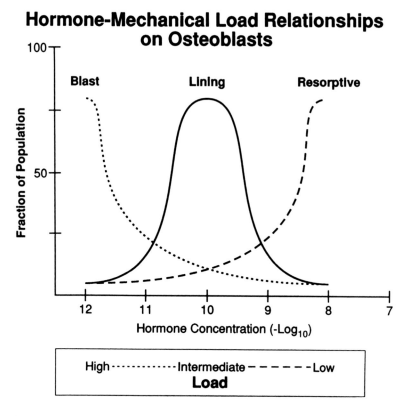

Fig. 2 In this depiction, the fraction of the osteoblast population displaying a particular phenotype is shown as a function of hormone concentration and mechanical force. Under normal circumstances of loading and hormone concentration, most (~ 80%) osteoblasts function as lining cells (designated lining, solid line), while smaller fractions (~ 10%) are involved in proliferation and matrix synthesis (blast, dotted line) or resorption-related activities (resorptive, dashed line). When loading is increased beyond threshold levels or hormone levels are substantially diminished, the hormone-activity relationship is shifted such that the majority of cells (~ 80% or greater) become sensitive to lower concentrations of hormone and respond by functioning in a blast-like manner. On the other hand, when loading drops beneath threshold levels and/or hormone concentration is significantly increased, the activity curve shifts in the opposite direction resulting in lower concentrations of hormone stimulating resorption related activity in a vast majority of the cells.

that such integration occurs in a manner that both stabilizes phenotype and permits functional adaptation in accord with changing need and (3) that the response to alterations in stress or load is based upon shifting the activity relationships of the cell to other effectors in the environment (including hormones and cytokines). Whether the reciprocal of the last postulate is also true, *viz.*, that marked changes in the level of effector results in modifications in the response to stress, is interesting to contemplate and theoretically possible. Fortunately, both this and the original formulation are amenable to testing.

4) Systemic Factors in Resorptive/Remodeling Activity

There are a number of systemic factors that have been associated with the regulation of resorptive/remodeling activity including the classic calcitropic hormones, sex steroids, and growth hormone and functionally related insulin-like growth factors (IGFs). Of these, the best explored because of their established relationship to calcium homeostasis are parathyroid hormone, vitamin D and, somewhat more problematically, calcitonin.

Parathyroid hormone (PTH) is released from the parathyroid gland in response to low circulating levels of Ca^{++} and acts to elevate the serum levels of this divalent cation by increasing tubular reabsorption of Ca^{++} in the kidney (Klahr and Hruska, 1983), promoting calcium absorption in the gut (*via* hydroxylation of vitamin D_3) (Drezner and Harrelson, 1979) and stimulating bone resorption in the skeleton (Wong, 1986). The latter action of the hormone, however, must be indirect (since the osteoclast lacks PTH receptors) therefore necessitating the presence of an intermediate, PTH-responsive meditating cell(s). In this instance, one, not necessarily exclusive hormone target, appears to be the osteoblast which clearly has receptors for and responds to PTH in a manner consistent with a resorption mediator (Wong, 1986; Rodan and Martin, 1981). This response may include the synthesis and/or release from matrix of proteins that have the potential to augment osteoclast precursor proliferation (*e.g.*, GM-CSF) (Horowitz *et al.*, 1989) and recruitment (bone *gla* protein, alpha$_2$ HS-glycoprotein, collagen peptides) (Malone *et al.*, 1982), indirectly stimulate the activity of extant osteoclasts (Holtrop *et al.*, 1974; Miller *et al.*, 1984) and, perhaps, prepare the bone surface for osteoclast degradative function (Chambers and Fuller, 1985). In addition, PTH can curtail osteoblast biosynthetic activity (particularly of Type I collagen) (Kream *et al.*, 1980); an inhibition that could contribute to a net loss in bone mass. Finally, as a consequence of chronic exposure to PTH *in vivo*, an endosteal fibrosis occurs that is characteristic of hyperparathyroidism and that may reflect the participation of one or more local mediators in the accelerated remodeling process including interleukin-1 (Il-1) and transforming grwoth factor-Beta (TFG-B). Both of these substances have the potential of increasing bone cell number and collagen synthesis (Canalis *et al.*, 1989; Centrella *et al.*, 1988).

The situation with vitamin D3 and resorptive activity *in vivo* is, if anything, more complex than that of PTH. This complexity follows, in part, because the production of the most active metabolite of vitamin D3, 1,25 $(OH)_2D_3$ (hereafter 1,25 D3) is stimulated by PTH (Drezner *et al.*, 1979) and, in part, because the action of the vitamin/hormone on osteoclast-mediated resorption appears indirect, *i.e.*, not on mature osteoclasts. In this instance, 1,25 D3 appears capable of stimulating osteoclast differentiation (*e.g.*, Hattersley and Chambers, 1989; Takahashi *et al.*, 1988) as well as of promoting the maturation and, perhaps, function of other bone and bone marrow cells potentially involved in the resorptive process. These cells include lymphocytes as a possible source of tumor necrosis factor-beta (TNF-beta) and interferon-gamma, monocytes as a potential source of Il-1, TNF-alpha and prostaglandin, and osteoblasts as a possible source of prostaglandin and osteoinductive and osteoclast-activating factors (Canalis *et al.*, 1989; Huffer, 1988; and Suda *et al.*, 1986;). In addition, because 1,25 D3 increases circulating calcium levels *via* augmentation of calcium uptake in the gut (Bikle, 1981; Drezner *et al.*, 1979), cartilage mineralization is promoted providing, ultimately, for the orderly removal of such mineralized tissue by osteo(chondro)clastic activity.

Of the several, intensively studied calcitropic agents, only calcitonin appears to act directly on mature osteoclasts to inhibit resorption, (Arnett and Dempster, 1987; Murrills *et al.*, 1989). In this instance, the principle effect of the hormone, as assessed *in situ*, appears to be detachment of osteoclasts from the bone surface and a diminution in the extent of cell specialization associated with resorptive activity, notably in the clear zone (the site of attachment to the bone matrix) and the ruffled membrane (the site of resorptive activity) (Holtrop *et al.*, 1974; Singer *et al.*, 1976). However, it must be emphasized that the physiological role of calcitonin in calcium homeostasis has not been clearly established.

There are, of course, a number of other systemic effector substances that have been implicated in the regulation of remodeling (resorption) *in vivo* but, for the most part, firm conclusions about underlying mechanism are difficult to establish. This list of putative regulators include, but is not limited to, glucocorticoids, thyroid hormone, growth hormone and physiologically associated insulin-like growth factors and the sex steroids.

5) Local Factors in Resorption/Remodeling

In recent years, there has accrued a very large and complex body of information related to the possible action and interaction of local factors in regulating bone resorption and remodeling. These paracrine factors are produced by a number of different cell types found in bone and bone marrow, and variously influence the proliferation, maturation and/or function of osteoblasts and osteoclasts (Raisz, 1988; Canalis *et al.*, 1989). What is clearly important about the existence of such effectors is their ability to modulate events within focally-defined regions of bone and to link systemic regulatory substances (*e.g.*, hormones) to local, site-specific activities (Huffer, 1988; Raisz, 1988). Thus, while circulating PTH may directly enhance osteoclast precursor maturation (Wong, 1986), much of its influence on the latter and more mature osteoclasts seems to occur by stimulating cytokine production by vicinal, mediating cells (also see Section [6] below). In the instance of PTH acting on osteoblasts, for example, intermediary activity might include the synthesis and release of prostaglandins which can affect both bone formation and resorption (Raisz and Martin, 1984) and the generation of an OAF-like substance capable of stimulating osteoclast formation and resorptive activity (*e.g.*, Perry *et al.*, 1989). Systemic 1,25 $(OH)_2D_3$ has similar direct effects on osteoblasts (including dose-dependent, biphasic activity (Huffer, 1988) but can act on mature osteoclasts only indirectly; either by stimulating immature osteoclast development or the production of paracrine, osteoclast-effecting substances synthesized by mononuclear cells and osteoblasts (Elford *et al.*, 1987; Huffer, 1988; Suda *et al.*, 1986).

One of the more important insights into the local control of remodeling relates to the possible role of bone matrix-associated molecules on osteoblast and osteoclast activity. These effectors become active (*i.e.*, acquire cytokine-like functions) either as a consequence of direct secretion by matrix synthesizing cells (osteoblasts) or through release from the bone matrix subsequent to resorption. Historically, the best known example of the latter circumstance is bone morphogenetic protein (BMP), a substance (substances?) which, when isolated from bone matrix, is capable of inducing ectopic bone formation (Urist, 1979). Molecules with BMP-like activity have recently been purified and characterized (*e.g.*, Bentz *et al.*, 1989) and, in one instance, cloned (Wozney *et al.*, 1988). Among the most interesting findings to emerge from these and similar studies are the augmenting activity of TGF-beta in inducing bone formation (*e.g.*, Bentz *et al.*, 1989) and the TGF-beta-like structure of some of the cloned BMPs (Wozney *et al.*, 1988). TGF-beta, itself localized in bone matrix, has multiple and complex effects on bone cells (Centrella *et al.*, 1988).

While local factors can serve as intermediates to regionalize and amplify the activity of systemic effectors, they cannot, alone, dictate the specific sites of resorptive or remodeling activity. This must come from some other site-determining, initiating event; perhaps, as discussed above, from a local change in mechanical loading. Under these particular circumstances, one could again postulate that such changes would alter receptor function leading to a diminished or enhanced response to systemic, paracrine or matrix-associated effector substances.

6) Immune System Regulation of Resorption and Remodeling

There is little doubt that immune cells and immune effector substances can stimulate bone resorption *in vitro* and probably *in vivo*, at least in some pathological situations. The pivotal question is whether such cells and effectors are also active in regulating these events under normal physiological circumstances, including for the sake of the present discussion, osteoporotic changes associated with aging. While a comprehensive review of this question goes well beyond the scope of this chapter, there are two aspects of it that merit at least brief consideration. First, there are the observations suggestive of possible physiological role for the immune system in remodeling. These include:

(1) observed immune (or mononuclear cell) deficiencies that accompany the skeletal lesions seen in some forms of inherited and diphosphonate and virally-induced osteopetrosis (Labat and Milhaud, 1986).

(2) the modeling/remodeling deficits described in some naturally occurring and induced immune deficiency states. The former is exemplified by data accumulated in the *nude* (athymic) mouse (McCauley *et al.*, 1989) and the latter by *in vivo* (Moskowitz *et al.*, 1988)and *in vitro* (Stewart *et al.*, 1986) observations on the immunosuppressive agent Cyclosporin A.

(3) the *in vitro* resorption enhancing effects of the monokines interleukin-1 (Gowan *et al.*, 1983; Heath *et al.*, 1985) and tumor necrosis factor (Bertolini *et al.*, 1986; Pfeilschifter *et al.*, 1989), and the modulatory affects of several lymphokines, including interferon-

gamma (Gowan *et al.*, 1986; Hoffman *et al.*, 1987; Takahashi *et al.*, 1986) and the colony stimulating factors on osteoclast differentiation. With regard to the latter interleukin-3 (Il-3) seems to be of particular importance (Barton and Mayer, 1989; Sheven *et al.*, 1986).

While none of these observations, even considered collectively, is sufficient to establish a causal relationship between immune system function and physiological remodeling, they are clearly consistent with such a possibility. If the immune system is involved in regulating remodeling, it raises a second and, perhaps more fundamental issue, namely whether the osteoblast/bone lining cell is the sole (or principal) intermediate controlling remodeling/resorptive activity. An augmented version of the concept developed above (Section 2 above), could include a role for mononuclear or dendritic cells in surveying the lining cell population for stress-induced changes in ligand/receptor properties. Upon detecting such changes, these surveying cells would alter remodeling activity by (locally) releasing monokines (*e.g.*, Il-1) or triggering the synthesis and secretion of lymphokines. Among the attractive features of this modified concept is the linkage provided between the immune system and mechanical force, and the alternative manner of viewing the action of hormones that affect remodeling.

Intrinsic Factors in Resorption

While it is not possible to directly identify intrinsic factors that likely contribute to the regulation of resorptive activity, there can be little doubt that such factors do exist. Predictable and consistent architectural differences between homologous bones of different species and of different bones within the same species indicate the presence and differential activity of genes that regulate skeletal morphology. Such genes must act, at least in part, by regulating resorptive activity, perhaps by establishing MES thresholds. Such a conclusion is consistent with the findings of several recent studies of bone mass in adult human twins (Pocock, 1987; Smith *et al.*, 1973). These data clearly demonstrate a genetic contribution to determining bone mass and, indirectly, relative remodeling (resorptive) activity. In this regard, it is also of interest to recall that there are site and region specific differences in remodeling activity that are not readily accounted for by variations in mechanical loading or circulating systemic factors. Thus, for example, Atkinson and Woodhead (1973) found in each of three bones studied (2nd lumbar vertebra, femur and mandible) that the pattern (distribution) of porosity (remodeling) remained constant during aging. From this finding, they concluded that while "bone remodeling may be influenced superficially by stress", "bone structure is genetically inbuilt and that its basic pattern (of remodeling) is established during development". This pattern of remodeling persists throughout life. Similarly, Currey (1984) and Marotti (1961) have shown that there is a marked similarity in the regional distribution of cortical remodeling in paired bones of the same animal. Such persistent patterns of remodeling, evident both developmentally and bilaterally, imply the existence of relatively stable, but as yet undefined, epigenetic factors that contribute to the activation of the remodeling cycle and the initiation of resorptive function.

Summary and Conclusions

It is clear from the present, brief review of the literature, that much remains to be learned about the *in vivo* control of bone resorption and, by extension, the modeling and remodeling processes. One persistent major difficulty that has and continues to limit progress in understanding is the small data base derived from whole animal or human studies. This is a problem that arises, in large measure, from the difficulty in both executing and interpreting *in vivo* experiments; a problem that will not readily disappear, although some of the newer cell transplant and transgenic technologies may help. On the other hand, a closer examination of the several different concepts that have been developed to explain modeling and remodeling, does suggest testable hypotheses that can be initially explored *in vitro* and that may provide better insight into comparable events occurring under physiological conditions. For example, if mechanical forces, directly or indirectly, change the cellular response to hormone (*e.g.*, PTH, 1,25 $(OH)_2D_3$), then such changes should be manifest either in receptor binding kinetics and/or second messenger generation in cells deformed by stress. Alternatively, one might predict that osteoblasts or bone lining cells obtained from bones with inherently different remodeling activity or "set points" would express differences in receptor binding or second messenger generation. In any case, the challenge to understanding the *in vivo* regulation of resorption looms as large as ever, but is amenable, we believe, to experimental analysis and resolution.

References

Arnett, T. R. and Dempster, D. W. (1987) A comparative study of disaggregated chick and rat osteoclasts *in vitro*:Effects of calcitonin and prostaglandins. *Endocrinol.* 120:602-608.

Atkinson, P. J., and Woodhead, C. (1973) The development of osteoporosis. A hypothesis based on a study of human bone structure. *Clin. Orthop. Rel. Res.* 90:217-228.

Barton, B. E., and Mayer, R. (1989) Il-3 induces differentiation of bone marrow precursor cells to osteoclast-like cells. *J. Immunol.* **143**:3211-3216.

Becker, R. O. (1979) The significance of electrically stimulated osteogenesis. More questions than answers. *Clin. Orthop. Rel. Res.* **141**:266-274.

Bentz, H., Nathan, R. M., Rosen, D. M., Armstrong, R. M., Thompson, A. Y., Segarini, P. R., Mathews, M. C., Dasch, J. R., Piez, K. A., and Seyedin, S. M. (1989) Purification and characterization of a unique osteoinductive factor from bovine bone. *J. Biol. Chem.* **264**:20805-20810.

Bertolini, D. R., Nedwin, G. E., Bringman, T. S., Smith, D. D., and Mundy, G. R. (1986) Stimulation of bone resorption and inhibition of bone formation *in vitro* by human tumor necrosis factors. *Nature* **319**:516-518.

Bikle, D. D., Morrisey, R. L., Zolock, D. T., and Rasmussen, H. (1981) The intestinal response to vitamin D. *Rev. Physiol. Biochem. Pharmacol.* **89**:63-142.

Blair, H. C., Kahn, A. J., Crouch, E. C., Jeffrey, J. J., and Teitelbaum, S. L. (1986) Isolated osteoclasts resorb the organic and inorganic components of bone. *J. Cell Biol.* **102**:1164-1172.

Bouvier, M., and Hylander, W. L. (1981). Effect of bone strain on cortical bone structure in macaques (*Macaca mulatta*). *J. Morph.* **167**:1-12.

Brighton, C. T., and McCluskey, W. P. (1986) Cellular response and mechanisms of action of electrically induced osteogenesis. In: *Bone and Mineral Research/4*. (W. A. Peck, Ed.). Elsevier Science Publishers BV, Amsterdam, pp. 213-254.

Brighton, C. T., and McCluskey, W. P. (1988) Response of cultured bone cells to a capacitively coupled electric field: inhibition of cAMP response to parathyroid hormone. *J. Orthop. Res.* **6**:567-571.

Bun, D. B., Martin, R. B., Schaffler, M. B., and Raden, E. L. (1985) Bone remodeling in response to *in vivo* fatigue microdamage. *J. Biochem.* **18**:189-200.

Burr, D. B., Schaffler, M. B., Yang, K. H., Wu, D. D., Lukoschek, M., Kandzasi, D., Sivaneri, N., Blaha, J. D., and Rodan, E. L. (1989a) The effects of altered strain environments on bone tissue kinetics. *Bone* **10**:215-221.

Burr, D. B., Schaffler, M. B., Yang, K. H., Lukoschek, M., Sivaneri, N., Blaha, J. D., and Rodan, E. L. (1989b) Skeletal change in response to altered strain environments: Is woven bone a response to elevated strain? *Bone* **10**:223-233.

Cain, C. D., Adey, W. R., and Luben, R. A. (1987) Evidence that pulsed electromagnetic fields inhibit coupling of adenylate cyclase by parathyroid hormone in bone cells. *J. Bone Min. Res.* **2**(5):437-441.

Canalis, E., McCarthy, T., and Centrella, M. (1989) The regulation of bone formation by local growth factors. In: *Bone and Mineral Research/6* (Peck, W. A., Ed.). Elsevier Science Publishers BV, Amsterdam, pp. 27-56.

Centrella, M., McCarthy, T. L., and Canalis, E. (1988) Skeletal tissue and transforming growth factor B. *The FASEB Journal* **2**:3066-3073.

Chambers, T. J., McSheehy, P. M., Thompson, B. M., and Fuller, K. (1985) The effect of calcium regulating hormones and prostaglandins on bone resorption by isolated rabbit osteoclasts disaggregated from neonatal rabbit bones. *Endocrinol.* **116**:234-239.

Chambers, T. J., and Fuller, K. (1985) Bone cells predispose bone surface to resorption by exposure of mineral to osteoclastic contact. *J. Cell Sci.* **76**:155-165.

Cowin, S. C. (1984) Mechanical modeling of the stress adaptation process in bone. *Calcif. Tiss. Int.* **36**:S98-S103.

Currey, J. D. (1984a) Can strains give adequate information for adaptive bone remodeling? *Calcif. Tiss. Int.* **36**:S118-S122.

Currey, J. D. (1984b) *The Mechanical Adaptations of Bones*. Princeton University Press. pp. 294.

Doty, S. B. (1981) Morphological evidence of intercellular junctions between bone cells. *Calcif. Tiss. Int.* **33**:509-512.

Drezner, M. K. and Harrelson, J. M. (1979) Newer knowledge of vitamin D and its metabolites in health and disease. *Clin. Orthop. Rel. Res.* **139**:206-230.

Duncan, R. and Misler, S. (1989) Voltage-activated and stretch-activated Ba^{2+} conducting channels in an osteoblast-like cell line (UMR 106). *FEBS. Lett.* **251**:17-21.

Elford, P. R., Felix, R., Cecchini, M., Trechsel, U., and Fleisch, H. (1987) Murine osteoblast-like cells and the osteogenic cell MC3T3-E1 release a macrophage colony-stimulating activity in culture. *Calcif. Tiss. Int.* **41**:151-156.

Eriksson, C. (1974) Streaming potentials and other water-dependent effects in mineralized tissues. *Ann. N.Y. Acad. Sci.* **38**:321-338.

Fallon, M. D., Teitelbaum, S. L., and Kahn, A. J. (1983) Multinucleation enhances macrophage-mediated bone resorption. *Lab. Invest.* **49**:159-164.

Ferrier, J. (1989) Electrical modulation of bone cell behavior. In: *Metabolic Bone Disease: Cellular and Tissue Mechanisms.* (C. S. Tam, J. N. M. Heersche, and T. M. Murray, Eds.). CRC Press, Boca Raton, Fl. pp. 269.

Frost, H. M. (1964) Dynamics of bone remodeling. In:*Bone Biodynamics.* (Frost, H. M., Ed.). Little, Brown and Co., Boston. pp. 315-333.

Frost, H. M. (1973) *Bone modeling and skeletal modeling errors.* C. C. Thomas, Pub., Springfield, 214 pp.

Frost, H. M. (1987a) Bone "mass" and the "mechanostat": A proposal. *Anat. Rec.* **219**:1-9.

Frost, H. M. (1987b) The mechanostat: a proposed pathogenic mechanism of osteoporoses and the bone mass effects of mechanical and nonmechanical agents. *Bone and Min.* **2**:73-85.

Garn, S. M. (1975) *Bone loss and aging in physiology and pathology of aging.* Academic Press, New York, pp. 39-57.

Gowen, M., Nedwin, G., and Mundy, G. R. (1986) Preferential inhibition of cytokine-stimulated bone resorption by recombinant interferon-gamma. *J. Bone Min. Res.* **1**:469-474.

Gowen, M., Wood, D. D., Ihire, E. J., McGuire, M. K. B., and Russell, R. G. G. (1983) An interleukin I like factor stimulates bone resorption *in vitro*. *Nature* **306**:378-380.

Hancox, N. M. (1949) The osteoclast. *Biol. Rev.* **24**:448-469.

Hancox, N. M., and Boothroyd, B. (1961) Motion picture and electron microscope studies on the embryonic avian osteoclast. *J. Biophy. Biochem. Cytol.* **11**:651-661.

Hasegawa, S., Sato, S., Saito, S., Suzuki, Y., and Brunette, D. M. (1985) Mechanical stretching increases the number of cultured bone cells synthesizing DNA and alters their pattern of protein synthesis. *Calcif. Tiss. Int.* **37**:431-436.

Hattersley, G. and Chambers, T. J. (1989) Generation of osteoclastic function in mouse bone marrow cultures: Multinuclearity and tartrate-resistant acid phosphatase are unreliable markers of osteoclast differentiation. *Endocrinol.* **124**:1689-1696.

Heath, J. K., Atkinson, S. J., Meikle, M. C., and Reynolds, J. J. (1984) Mouse osteoblasts synthesize collagenase in response to bone resorbing agents. *Biochem. Biophys. Acta* **802**:251-254.

Heath, J. K., Saklatvala, J., Meikle, M. D., Atkinson, S. T., and Reynolds, J. J. (1985) Pig interleukin-1 (catabolin) is a potent stimular of bone resorption *in vitro*. *Calcif. Tiss. Int.* **37**:95-97.

Hock, J. K., Gera, I., Fonseca, J., and Raisz, L. G. (1988) Human parathyroid hormone-(1-34) increases bone mass in ovariectomized and orchidectomized rats. *Endocrinol.* **122**:2899-2904.

Hoffman, O., Klaushofer, K., Gleispach, H., Leis, H. J., Luger, T., Koller, K., and Peterlik, M. (1987) Gamma interferon inhibits basal and interleukin-1-induced prostaglandin production and bone resorption in neonatal mouse calvaria. *Biochem. Biophys. Res. Commun.* 143:38-43.

Holtrop, M. E., Raisz, L. G., and Simmons, H. A. (1974) The effects of parathyroid hormone, colchicine and calcitonin on the ultrastructure and the activity of osteoclasts in organ culture. *J. Cell Biol.* 60:346-355.

Horowitz, M. C., Coleman, D. L., Ryaby, J. T., and Einhorn, T. A. (1989) Osteotropic agents induce the differential secretion of granulocyte-macrophage colony-stimulating factor by the osteoblast cell line MC3T3-E1. *J. Bone Min. Res.* 4:911-921.

Huffer, W. E. (1988) Biology of Disease. Morphology and biochemistry of bone remodeling: possible control by vitamin D, parathyroid hormone and other substances. *Lab. Invest.* 59:418-442.

Jaworski, Z. F. G. (1981) Physiology and pathology of bone remodeling. *Orthop. Clinics of North America* 12:485-512.

Jones, S. J., Boyde, A., and Ali, N. N. (1986) The interface of cells and their matrices in mineralized tissues: a review. *Scanning Electron Microscopy* IV:1555-1569.

Jones, S. J., Boyde, A., Ali, N. N., and Maconnachie, E. (1986) Variation in the sizes of resorption lucunae made *in vitro*. *Scanning Electron Microscopy* IV:1571-1580.

Kahn, A. J. and Partridge, N. C. (1987) New concepts in bone remodeling: An expanding role for the osteoblast. *Am. J. Otolaryngol.* 8:258-264.

Klahr, S., and Hruska, K. (1983) Effects of parathyroid hormone on the renal reabsorption of phosphorous and divalent cations. **In:** *Bone and Mineral Research/2.* (Peck, W. A., Ed.). Elsevier Science Publishers BV., Amsterdam, pp. 65-124.

Kream, B. E., Rowe, D. W., Gworek, S. C., and Raisz, L. G. (1980) Parathyroid hormone alters collagen synthesis and procollagen mRNA in fetal rat calvaria. *Proc. Nat. Acad. Sci. USA* 77:5654-5658.

Labat, M. L., and Milhaud, G. (1986) Osteopetrosis and the immune deficiency syndrome. **In:** *Bone and Mineral Research/4.* (Peck, W. A., Ed.). Elsevier Science Publishers BV, Amsterdam, pp. 131-212.

Lian, J. B., Coults, M., and Canalis, E. (1984) Regulation of osteocalcin synthesis in cultured fetal rat calvariae. *Calcif. Tiss. Int.* 36:518.

MacDonald, B. R., Gallagher, J. A., and Russell, R. G. (1986) Parathyroid hormone stimulates proliferation of cells derived from human bone. *Endocrinol.* 118:2445.

Majeska, R. J., and Rodan, G. A. (1981) Low concentrations of parathyroid hormone enhance growth of clonal osteoblast-like cells *in vitro*. *Calcif. Tiss. Int.* 33:323.

Malone, J. D., Teitelbaum, S. L., Griffin, G. L., Senior, R. M., and Kahn, A. J. (1982) Recruitment of osteoclast precursors by purified bone matrix constituents. *J. Cell Biol.* 92:227-230.

Marotti, G. (1961) Physiology, number and arrangement of osteons in corresponding regions of homotypic long bones. *Nature* 191:1400-1401.

McCauley, L. K., Rosol, T. J., Capen, C. C., and Horton, J. E. (1989) A comparison of bone turnover in athymic (nude) and euthymic mice: biochemical, histomorphometric, bone ash and *in vitro* studies. *Bone* 10:29-34.

McSheehy, P. M. J., and Chambers, T. J. (1986) Osteoblastic cells mediate osteoclastic responsiveness to parathyroid hormone. *Endocrinol.* 118:824-828.

Miller, M. A., Omura, T. H., and S. C. Miller. (1989) Increased cancellous bone remodeling during lactation in beagles. *Bone* 10:279-285.

Miller, S. C., Bowman, B. M., and Meyers, R. C. (1984) Morphological and ultrastructural aspects of the activation of avian medullary bone osteoclasts by parathyroid hormone. *Anat. Rec.* 208:223-231.

Miller, S. C. (1988) Hormonal regulation of osteogenesis. In: *The Biological Mechanisms of Tooth Eruption and Root Resorption*. (Davidovitch, Z., Ed.). EBSCO Media, Birmingham, pp. 71-79.

Miller, S. S., Wolf, A. M., and Arnaud, C. D. (1976) Bone cells in culture: morphologic transformation by hormones. *Science* 192:1340-1343.

Moskowitz, C., Epstein, S., Fallon, M., Ismail, F., and Thomas, S. (1988) Cyclosporin-A *in vivo* produces severe osteopenia in the rat: Effect of dose and duration of administration. *Endocrinol.* 123:2571-2577.

Murrills, R. J., Shane, E., Lindsay, R., and Dempster, D. W. (1989) Bone resorption by isolated human osteoclasts *in vitro*: Effects of calcitonin. *J. Bone Min. Res.* 4:259-268.

Parfitt, A. M. (1979) Equilibrium and disequilibrium hypercalcemia. New light on an old concept. *Metab. Bone Dis. Rel. Res.* 1:279-293.

Parfitt, A. M. (1982) The coupling of bone formation to bone resorption: a critical analysis of the concept and of its relevance to the pathogenesis of osteoporosis. *Metab. Bone Dis. Rel. Res.* 4:1-6.

Parfitt, A. M. (1984) The cellular basis of bone remodeling: The quantum concept reexamined in light of recent advances in the cell biology of bone. *Calcif. Tiss. Int.* 36:S37-S45.

Parfitt, A.M. (1989) Plasma calcium control at quiescent bone surfaces: a new approach to the homeostatic function of bone lining cells. *Bone* 10:87-88.

Partridge, N. C., Opie, A. L., Opie, R. T., and Martin, T. J. (1985) Inhibitory effects of parathyroid hormone on growth of osteogenic sarcoma cells. *Calcif. Tiss. Int.* 37: 519-525.

Partridge, N. C., Jeffrey, J. J., Ehlich, L. S., Teitelbaum, S. L., Fliszar, C., Welgus, H. G., and Kahn, A. J. (1987) Hormonal regulation of the production of collagenase and collagenase inhibitor activity by rat osteogenic sarcoma cells. *Endocrinol.* 120:1956-1962.

Perry, H. M., Skogen, W., Chappel, J., Kahn, A. J., Wilner, G., and Teitelbaum, S. L. (1989) Partial characterization of a parathyroid hormone-stimulated resorption factor(s) from osteoblast-like cells. *Endocrinol.* 125:2075-2082.

Pfeilschifter, J., Chenu, C., Bird, A., Mundy, G. R., and Roodman, G. D. (1989) Interleukin-1 and tumor necrosis factor stimulate the formation of human osteoclast-like cells *in vitro. J. Bone Min. Res.* 4:113-118.

Pocock, N. A., Eisman, J. A., Hopper, J. L., Yeates, M. G., Sambrook, P. N., and Ebert, S. (1987) Genetic determinants of bone mass in adults. A twin study. *J. Clin. Invest.* 80:706-710.

Pollack, S. R. (1984) Bioelectrical properties of bone: endogenous electrical signals. *Orthop. Clinics of North America* 15:3-14.

Raisz, L. G. and Martin, T. J. (1984) Prostaglandins in Bone and Mineral Metabolism. In: *Bone and Mineral Research/2*. (Peck, W. A., Ed.). Elsevier Science Publishers BV, Amsterdam. pp. 286-310.

Raisz, L. G. (1988) Local and systemic factors in the pathogenesis of osteoporosis. *New Eng. J. Med.* 318:818-828.

Rodan, G. A., and Martin, T. J. (1981) Role of osteoblasts in hormonal control of bone resorption. *Calcif. Tiss. Int.* 33:349-351.

Sakamoto, S., and M. Sakamoto. (1982) Biochemical and immunohistochemical studies on collagenase in resorbing bone tissue. *J. Periodont. Res.* 17:523-526.

Scheven, B. A. A., Visser, J. W. M., and Nijweide, P. J. (1986) *In vitro* osteoclast generation from different marrow fractions, including a highly enriched hematopoietic stem cell population. *Nature* 321:79-81.

Singer, F. R., Melvin, K. E. W., and Mills, B. G. (1976) Acute effects of calcitonin in man. *Clin. Endocrinol.* 5 (Suppl.):3335-3405.

Smith, D. M., Nance, W. E., Kang, K. W., Christian, J. C., and Johnson, C. C., Jr. (1973) Genetic factors in determining bone mass. *J. Clin. Invest.* 52:2800-2808.

Smith, E. L., and Gilligan, C. (1989) Mechanical forces and bone. In: *Bone and Mineral Research/6*. (W. A. Peck, Ed.). Elsevier Science Publishers BV, Amsterdam, pp. 139-173.

Stewart, P. J., Green, O. L., and Stern, P. H. (1986) Cyclosporin-A inhibits calcemic hormone-induced bone resorption *in vitro*. *J. Bone Min. Res.* 1:285-291.

Suda, T., Miyaura, C., Abe, E., and Kuroki, T. (1986) Modulation of cell differentiation, immune responses and tumor promotion by vitamin D compounds. *Bone and Mineral Research/4*. (Peck, W. A., Ed.). Elsevier Science Publishers BV, Amsterdam, pp. 1-48.

Takahashi, N., Mundy, G. R., and Roodman, G. D. (1986) Recombinant human interferon-gamma inhibits formation of human osteoclast-like cells. *J. Immunol.* 137:3544-3549.

Takahashi, N., Yamaua, H., Yoshiki, S., Roodman, G. D., Mundy, G. R., Jones, S. J., Boyde, A., and Suda, T. (1988) Osteoclast-like cell formation and its regulation by osteotropic hormones in mouse bone marrow cultures. *Endocrinol.* 122:1373-1382.

Talmage, R. V. (1967) A study of the effect of parathyroid hormone on bone remodeling and on calcium homeostasis. *Clin. Orthop. Rel. Res.* 54:163-173.

Teti, A., Blair, H. C., Schlessinger, P., Grano, M., Zambonin-Zallone, Kahn, A. J., Teitelbaum, S. L., and Hruska, K. A. (1989) Extracellular protons acidify osteoclasts, reduce cytosolic calcium and promote expression of cell-matrix attachment structures. *J. Clin. Invest.* 84:773-780.

Urist, M. R. (1979) Bone morphodifferentiation and tumorigeneses. *Persp. Biol. Med.* 22:S89-S113.

Uthoff, H. K., and Jaworski, Z. F. G. (1978) Bone loss in response to long-term immobilization. *J. Bone Joint. Surg.* 60-B(3):420-429.

Vaes, G. (1988) Cellular biology and biochemical mechanism of bone resorption. A review of recent developments on the formation, activation, and mode of action of osteoclasts. *Clin. Orthop. Rel. Res.* 231:239-271.

Wong, G. L. (1986) Skeletal effects of parathyroid hormone. In: *Bone and Mineral Research/4*. (W. A. Peck, Ed.). Elsevier Science Publishers BV, Amsterdam, pp. 103-129.

Wozney, J. M., Rosen, V., Celeste, A. J., Mitsock, L. M., Whitters, M. J., Kriz, R. W., Hewick, R. M., and Wong, E. A. (1988) Novel regulators of bone formation: molecular clones and activities. *Science* 242:1528-1534.

6

Regulation of Osteoclastic Bone Resorption *In Vitro*

T. J. CHAMBERS
Department Of Histopathology
St George's Hospital Medical School
London SW17 ORE
England

Introduction
Mechanisms of resorption
The effects of calcitonin on osteoclasts
Regulation of osteoclastic resorption by osteoblasts
Prostaglandins and bone resorption
Regulation of osteoclast production
Concluding remarks
References

Introduction

For more than a century osteoclasts have been identified as multinucleate cells in bone. From the first they were strongly implicated by association as the cells of resorption, a function directly confirmed more recently by observation of bone resorption by osteoclasts incubated on bone, and by *in vivo* experiments in which transplanted hemopoietic cells are both incorporated into osteoclasts and cure the resorptive defect in osteopetrosis (Ash *et al.*, 1980; Coccia *et al.*, 1980; Marks and Walker, 1981). Other cells in bone, particularly macrophages and cells of the osteoblastic lineage (osteoblasts, osteocytes, bone lining cells) also possess and secrete proteolytic enzymes, and this, together with the lack of demonstrable collagenase in osteoclasts, has led to suggestions that such cells may act as alternative or accessory bone resorptive cells (Heersche, 1978; Sakamoto, 1987). However, it has not been possible to demonstrate that these cells are capable of the excavation of bone, and enzyme release by osteoblastic cells may have other roles (see later). Excavation of bone seems to be a function unique to the osteoclast, and the osteoclast effects this without assistance from other cell types (Chambers *et al.*, 1984).

Mechanisms of Resorption

Bone resorption is accomplished through the formation, by osteoclasts, of a sealing zone of close adhesion between osteoclast and bone, which extends around the circumpherence of the bond-apposed surface of the osteoclast (Miller *et al.*, 1984). Special adhesive structures are probably involved in this process (Marchisio *et al.*, 1989) and subjacent cytoplasm contains concentrations of cytoskeletal elements that exclude other organelles ('clear zone'). Within this circumpherential sealing zone the osteoclastic plasma membrane is thrown into complex folds ('ruffled border'), the elaboration and size of which is proportional to bone resorbing activity (Holtrop *et al.*, 1974; Doman and Wakita, 1986). The ruffled border probably represents a means whereby the membrane-associated activities required for bone resorption are concentrated. There is now considerable evidence that osteoclasts resorb bone through secretion of protons and enzymes into the confined space between bone and the ruffled border, within the circumpherential sealing zone. In this specialised extracellular microenvironment bone is degraded by acid hydrolase activity. The resorptive hemivacuole is the functional equivalent of an extracellular phagolysosome, the specialisation of the osteoclast.

Although it was suggested two decades ago (Vaes, 1968) that osteoclasts resorb bone through the formation of an extracellular acid compartment, direct evidence of a low pH in the resorptive hemivacuole has been presented only recently. Baron *et al.* (1985) used the fluorescent weak base acridine orange, which accumulates in acidic compartments, to show that the osteoclast actively acidifies the zone beneath the ruffled border. Osteoclast acidification has been shown to be predictably modulated by regulators of osteoclastic bone resorption (Anderson *et al.*, 1986). Etherington *et al.* (1987) placed pH electrodes beneath osteoclasts on plastic substrates and found that the pH in the contact zone fell to a value of pH 3 or less within a few minutes.

The mechanism by which protons are transported into the hemivacuole remains to be identified. An antiserum raised against a 100 kDa polypeptide in lysosomal membranes, that cross-reacts with a 100kDa H^+,K^+ proton pump ATPase of hog gastric mucosa, binds to the ruffled border of osteoclasts (Baron *et al.*, 1986). Antibody-reactivity suggests that the osteoclastic antigen, may also be a proton pump component, but the study enabled no distinction between whether osteoclasts transport protons through a H^+,K^+

type ATPase or electrogenic H^+ATPase of the vacuolar apparatus. In preliminary communications, Parvinen *et al.*, (1987) report immunogold labelling of ruffled border with antibody to H^+,K^+ATPase, while Ghiselli *et al.* (1987) found the ruffled border bound antibody to H^+ATPase. Akisaka and Gay (1986a) used ultracytochemical techniques to attempt to identify proton pumps in osteoclasts. They found strong inhibition by duramycin, a potent inhibitor of the H^+ATPase. However, other inhibitors gave unexpected results - for example, inhibitors of mitochondrial proton pumps actually increased the amount of reaction product in mitochondria. Anderson *et al.* (1986) incubated bone in organ culture and found that acridine orange fluorescence of osteoclasts was increased by parathyroid hormone and inhibited by calcitonin. A H^+,K^+ATPase was implicated in this acidification by the observation that omeprazole, a potent inhibitor of the gastric parietal cell H^+,K^+ATPase, reduced fluorescence. However, omeprazole abolished proton pumping in the stomach, while even the highest concentration used in these experiments (10^{-4}M) reduced fluorescence by only 20 per cent. A H^+,K^+ATPase seems inherently less likely than a H^+ATPase, since the former required the continuous presence of K^+ions within the hemivacuole for its activity.

Acidification of the hemivacuole may occur through H^+Na^+ exchange, rather than through proton pumping: the energy from a sodium electrochemical gradient provided by a Na^+,K^+ATPase could be used to transport protons against a concentration gradient (Diamond and Machen, 1983; Paradiso *et al.*, 1984). Such a model, although like the K^+,H^+ ATPase dependent upon K^+ availability in the hemivacuole, would be consistent with the finding by Anderson *et al.* (1986) that amiloride, which blocks channels involved in Na^+,H^+ exchange, strongly inhibits PTH-stimulated acidification in organ cultured bone. Baron *et al.* (1986), and Akisaka and Gay (1986b) have shown that Na^+,K^+ ATPase is present in osteoclasts in considerably greater quantities that in other bone cells. However, the membrane pump is present in greatest density in the basolateral membrane, rather than the ruffled border (Baron *et al.*, 1986, 1988), suggesting that the energy of the Na^+,K^+ATPase may not be primarily involved with supporting the coupled transport of protons. Even in the ruffled border, the Na^+ electrochemical gradient may be utilised not for H^+,Na^+ exchange but for co-transport of amino acids and other degradation products of bone resorption.

Sensitivity of osteoclastic acidifications to inhibition by amiloride may be due to inhibition of Na^+,H^+ exchange processes not primarily involved in hemivacuole acidification. The exchange plays a role in the maintenance of cytoplasmic pH levels. Moreover, the effect on PTH-induced bone resorption and acidification in organ culture may be due to an effect by amiloride on the osteoblastic cells that mediate PTH-stimulation of osteoclasts (see later). Osteoblasts respond to PTH with perturbation of their ion-equilibrium mechanisms (DeLuise and Harker, 1986) and their physiology or responsiveness, which is involved in osteoclast-stimulation in response to PTH (Mc-Sheehy and Chambers, 1986a), may depend upon a Na^+,H^+ exchange system.

An alternative, or additional role for the Na^+,K^+ ATPase may be in coupled transport of Ca^{2+}. The low pH in the hemivacuole is sufficient to dissolve the mineral phase of bone matrix. Although Ca^{2+} transport from the hemivacuole to the basolateral extracellular space may be vesicular, Ca^{2+} ions may, alternatively, passively diffuse across the ruffled border into the osteoclastic cytoplasm, followed by transcellular movement similar to that in cells of renal distal tubules and small intestine (Schatzmann, 1985). If the latter occurs, the osteoclast would be expected to possess powerful mechanisms for Ca^{2+} extrusion in the face of surges of Ca^{2+} ingress from bone resorptive activity. The basolateral Na^+,K^+ATPase may provide an electrochemical gradient for Na^+,Ca^{2+} exchange. Such a mechanism may supplement the Ca^{2+} ATPase recently demonstrated in the basolateral membrane of the osteoclast (Akisaka *et al.*, 1988): the burden of calcium efflux is shared by a calcium pump and a Na^+,Ca^{2+} exchange system in many cells (Penniston, 1982).

Protons are made available for transport through the action of carbonic anhydrase, isoenzyme II, which provides protons by catalysing the conversion of carbon dioxide and water to bicarbonate and hydrogen ions. Carbonic anhydrase plays a key role in bone resorption: bone resorption is inhibited by carbonic anhydrase inhibitors (Minkin and Jennings, 1972), and congenital absence of carbonic anhydrase isoenzyme II is associated with deficient bone resorption (osteopetrosis) (Sly *et al.*, 1983), The enzyme is localised on the plasma membrane in active osteoclasts (Anderson *et al.*, 1982; Gay *et al.*, 1984). It is likely that the excess bicarbonate remaining after proton extrusion is exchanged through a plasma membrane Cl^-,HCO_3^- exchanger (Anderson *et al.*, 1982; Titi *et al.*, 1987). A model for osteoclastic ion and nutrient transport based on the available evidence is shown in Fig. 1.

Histochemical studies have demonstrated the presence of a variety of acid hydrolases in osteoclasts in the area beneath the ruffled border of the osteoclast (Doty and Schofield, 1972, 1976; Lucht, 1971 1973a,b; Miller, 1985) which increase in amount in the hemivacuole in response to parathyroid

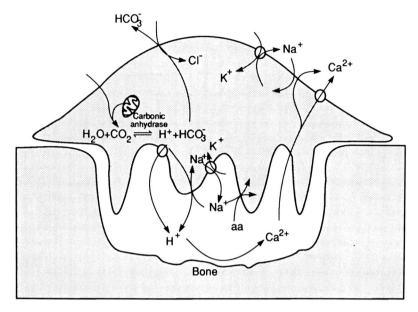

Fig. 1 Diagrammatic representation of possible ion transport mechanisms involved in bone resorption by osteoclasts. The Na^+ exchange systems at the ruffled border are shown as possible explanations for the presence of $Na^+,K^+ATPase$ which, although predominantly basolateral, is also present at this site. Membrane ATPases represented by circles. Coupled arrows represent passive co-transport.

hormone (Miller, 1985), Lysosomal enzyme release into culture medium from bone organ cultures changes in response to CT and PTH and correlates with, and precedes, changes in bone resorptive activity (Vaes, 1972; Eilon and Raisz, 1978). Enzymes are secreted by isolated osteoclasts in a hormone-responsive manner (Chambers *et al.*, 1987). These enzymes can be demonstrated in Golgi cisternae, that are often close to the deep invaginations of the ruffled border, and enzymes are also observed in small vesicles surrounding the Golgi stacks, which appear to fuse with the membrane of numerous closed profiles close to the ruffled border where acid hydrolase reaction product can also be observed. Unlike secondary lysosomes, these small vesicles do not contain the 100kDa antigen that cross-reacts with parietal cell membranes (Baron *et al.*, 1985). This suggests that the vesicles are primarily destined for secretion.

Although many histochemical activities have been described, the natural substrates, biochemical characteristics and role in bone resorption of the majority of the osteoclastic acid hydrolases is unknown. Collagen is the major substrate in bone. Native collagen can only be enzymatically cleaved by collagenase, but under the acidic conditions of the hemivacuole collagen is likely to become denatured, and once partially uncoiled becomes accessible to hydrolysis by lysosomal cysteine proteases (cathepsins). By using cysteine protease inhibitors, Vaes and collaborators (Delaisse *et al.*, 1980, 1984) have provided evidence for the involvement of cathepsins in the degradation of bone collagen. A cathepsin has recently been purified from chicken osteoclasts (Blair *et al.*, 1986).

The current state of ignorance concerning enzymes that are central to bone biology is attributable to the scarcity of osteoclasts in bone, and their heavy contamination by other cells. It seems likely that osteoclastic acid hydrolases will be found to differ quantitatively and qualitatively from those of other cells. The lysosomes of most cells have a relatively diverse macromolecular digestive burden. Because the osteoclast is a cell specialised for digestion of a particular substrate of unique composition, it may have developed specialised acid hydrolases that differ significantly from the lysosomal hydrolases of other cells. This appears to be the case for at least one enzyme, tartrate-residant acid phosphatase (TRAP). TRAP is relatively specific for osteoclasts, although other cells, particularly mononuclear phagocytes, either contain (Chambers *et al.*, 1987; Efstratiadis and Moss, 1985) or develop in culture (Snipes *et al.*, 1986) a similar enzyme. We have found, however, that the TRAP extracted from tumors consisting largely of normal osteoclasts show major differences from TRAPs characterised from other sources (submitted).

The Effects of Calcitonin on Osteoclasts

The osteoclast is a major target for the action of calcitonin (CT), a hormone which inhibits osteoclastic resorption at extremely low concentrations. There is convincing evidence that the hormone inhibits bone resorption through a direct effect on the osteoclast. Although there is some evidence that the behaviour of other bone cells changes after administration of pharmacological quantities of CT *in vivo* (Norimatsu *et al.*, 1978; Salmon *et al.*, 1983), responsiveness has not been demonstrated in isolated cell populations, and CT receptors are absent from cells of the osteoblastic lineage (Martin and Partridge, 1981) (except in a later passage clone of osteosarcoma cells

(Gutierrez *et al.*, 1984; Forrest *et al.*, 1985)): the response of bone cells *in vivo* is thus likely to be secondary to hormonal or ionic changes induced by the hormone. Osteoclastic responsiveness is seen at sufficiently low concentrations, and is sufficiently rapid and dramatic that it seems likely to be able to account for the inhibition of calcium efflux from bone (Grubb *et al.*, 1977) after systemic administration.

Pharmacologic does of CT completely inhibit osteoclastic bone resorption (Holtrop *et al.*, 1974). This is accompanied by loss of the ruffled borders of osteoclasts within 30 minutes (Kallio *et al.*, 1972; Singer *et al.*, 1976) together with loss of the cytoplasmic coating of the ruffled border plasmalemma, and a physical separation from the underlying bone (Kallio *et al.*, 1972). CT induces a rapid decrease in osteoclast numbers (Baron and Vignery, 1981; Hedland *et al.*, 1983). Loss of ruffed borders by osteoclasts in response to CT correlates with inhibition of ^{45}Ca release in organ culture (Holtrop *et al.*, 1974). CT treatment inhibits osteoclastic $Na^+,K^+ATPase$ activity (Akisaka and Gay, 1986a) and alters carbonic anhydrase II localisation. In untreated osteoclasts the enzyme is detected along the ruffled border; after CT-administration the enzyme appears in the adjacent cytosol (Anderson *et al.*, 1982). These enzymes are believed to play an important role in acidification of the digestive hemivacoule, and inhibition of their activity may represent a mechanism whereby CT inhibits bone resorption.

Techniques have recently become available whereby osteoclasts can be isolated from mammalian bone. The hormonal responsiveness of such isolated cells can be assessed *in vitro*, free from the influence of other bone cells (Chambers *et al.*, 1984). Studies with such preparations have demonstrated that osteoclasts respond directly to CT, and have also emphasised the rapidity and sensitivity with which they respond to the hormone. In these preparations, osteoclasts represent about 40 per cent of nuclei, widely dispersed at low cell density over plastic or bone substrates. Addition of salmon CT, in picogramme/ml concentrations, to isolated populations of rat osteoclasts is rapidly followed by a dramatic change in behavior and a characteristic morphological transformation (Chambers and Magnus, 1982; Chambers and Moore, 1983). Untreated osteoclasts demonstrate continuous cytoplasmic motility, ceaselessly protruding and retracting broad, smoothly lobulated cytoplasmic processes, from whose periphery membrane ruffles move back over the dorsal cell surface. The cell body frequently shows rhythmic contractions. Within a minute of CT-addition pseudopodial motility and membrane ruffling activity abruptly cease: the cell appears paralysed. Over the ensuing hours the peripheral cytoplasm gradually retracts. Some areas retract before others, so that the cytoplasmic outline of the cell loses its smoothly lobulated contour and becomes irregular, as cytoplasm retracts between peripheral adhesion sites (Fig. 1). Ultimately, in the rat, cytoplasmic retraction becomes so extensive that the cell takes on a neurone-like appearance. Osteoclasts from human and rabbit bone show a similar but less dramatic, complete or sustained behavorial change in response to CT. This quiescence response of isolated osteoclasts to CT is quite different from the cytoplasmic contraction that follows exposure of osteoclasts to injurious agents or circumstances. Osteoclastic injury causes rapid contraction to an even, smooth circular outline. The quiescence response is reversed on removed CT, and is abrogated by prior treatment of osteoclasts with trypsin, which support a receptor-mediated process (Chambers and Magnus, 1982).

The rapidity with which osteoclasts respond, in cultures where they are widely separated from other cells, suggest that CT acts directly on osteoclasts. The predictability of the response, its specificity for osteoclasts, and the low, new physiological concentrations of CT required, suggest that the phenomenon is of physiological significance, a morphological expression of their inhibited ability to resorb bone. The nature of the behavioral change supports this: bone resorption is likely to require motile processes for activities such as enzyme extrusion. One mechanism through which CT may inhibit resorption is through inhibition of motility-dependent processes in the resorbing cell.

Cyclic AMP (cAMP) generation seems to be involved in the inhibition of osteoclasts by CT. CT increases the cAMP content of bone (Murad *et al.*, 1970); CT-receptor localisation studies have demonstrated CT receptors only in osteoclasts, in sections of bone and in disaggregated bone cell preparations (Warshawsky *et al.*, 1980; Rao *et al.*, 1981; Nicholson *et al.*, 1986a). Purified populations of primary cultures of osteoblastic cells lack an adenyl cyclase response to CT (Martin and Partridge, 1981). cAMP generation has been demonstrated directly in rat osteoclasts in response to CT, by immunocytochemistry (Nicholson *et al.*, 1986b). cAMP itself, and analogues of cAMP, induce in rat osteoclasts a state of sustained immotility identical to that caused by CT (Chambers and Ali, 1983). Theophylline, an intracellular inhibitor of cAMP degradation, which by itself has no effect on osteoclastic motility *in vitro*, potentiates CT-induced osteoclastic quiescence, while imidazole, which increases cAMP degradation, reduces osteoclastic sensitivity to CT (Chambers and Ali, 1983).

The mechanism by which cAMP inhibits cytoplasmic motility is unknown. cAMP is known to cause phosphorylation of cytoskeletal elements (*e.g.* Wallach *et al.*, 1978; Glenn, Kerrick and Hoar, 1981). Warshafsky *et al.*, (1985) studied cytoskeletal rearrangement during calcitonin-induced changes in osteoclast motility, and found that specific cytoskeletal components were altered in response to CT, and that actomyosin interactions may be involved in the early stages of cytoplasmic retraction.

The morphologic response of osteoclasts to CT is sufficiently reproducible that it can be used as a bioassay for the hormone (Chambers and Moore, 1982). Since the immotile state is accompanied by a shape-change, the response of large numbers of osteoclasts can be assessed simultaneously after incubation with CT. We have found, using this approach, that osteoclasts respond to CT as a very uniform population, with a narrow dose-response range. The cytoplasmic retraction that accompanies the immotile state has also been developed as a more objective and readily quantifiable parameter of osteoclastic responsiveness (Chambers *et al.*, 1986). Cytoplasmic spreading is significantly impaired by 2pg/ml of human CT.

When osteoclasts, mechanically disaggregated from bone, are sedimented onto slices of devitalised cortical bone, they form excavations in the bone surface within a few hours. This process is inhibited by very low concentrations of CT (Chambers *et al.*, 1985; Zaidi *et al.*, 1987): salmon CT (1pg/ml) abolishes bone resorption for at least 18 hrs; resorption is reduced to half by 0.1pg/ml of salmon CT. Porcine and human CT have the same effects at concentrations approximately 30 times higher, a ratio that correlates with the relative effects as hypocalcaemic agents. Calcitonin gene-related peptide is also inhibitory, but only at concentrations three orders of magnitude greater (Zaidi *et al.*, 1979).

Osteoclasts are more sensitive to resorption-inhibition that motility-inhibition. Presumably the motile potential required for bone resorption is greater than that required for pseudopodial movement - just as an athlete may feel disinclined from competitive activity by a sedative, but will continue to undertake more routine activities (which will themselves be prevented by higher doses of the same sedative). In fact, with the caveat that higher concentrations of CT are required to abolish pseudopodial motility than to inhibit bone resorption, effects on motility and resorption correlate well: the relative potencies of salmon, human, porcine CT, and CGRP are very similar as inhibitors of motility to their relative potencies as inhibitors of resorption (Chambers and Ali, 1983; Chambers *et al.*, 1986; Chambers and Moore, 1983;

Zaidi *et al.*, 1987). The same applies to prostaglandins (PGs) E_1 and E_2 (Chambers and Ali, 1983; Chambers *et al.*, 1985). All the agents so far found to inhibit motility also inhibit resorption (PGs, cAMP, CT, CGRP), and agents that have no effect on motility generally do not influence bone resorption (PTH, $1,25(OH)_2D_3,IL1$). The relationship between motility and resorption has been questioned on the dubious basis of experiments in which CT was said to inhibit the motility of 'most' osteoclasts on plastic, but did not 'completely prevent' resorption of dentine (Ali *et al.*, 1984). These results seem, if anything, to support a correlation. No quantification of hormone effects was attempted.

Two exceptions to the correlation between changes in motility and resorption have been found: macrophage colony stimulating factor (M-CSF) in rodent osteoclasts, and PGs in the chick. We have found (submitted) that M-CSF directly inhibits bone resorption, but has no discernable effect on osteoclastic motility. This suggests that M-CSF may inhibit osteoclastic resorption through a pathway that does not involve cAMP or changes in motility. In the macrophage, M-CSF receptors may act through stimulation of tyrosine kinase activity (Rettenmeir *et al.*, 1986), and may thus utilise a transduction mechanism distinct from that of CT and PGs, which appear to involve adenyl cyclase. It is likely that there are multiple pathways through which osteoclasts can be inhibited from resorption of bone.

The second possible exception is the effect of PGs on isolated chick osteoclasts. As in the rat, PGs inhibit osteoclastic resorption (Arnett and Dempster, 1987) and induce cAMP generation (Nicholson *et al.* ,1986a) but unlike the rat, there was no detectable change in cytoplasmic motility (Arnett and Dempster, 1984). This may imply that resorption is inhibited by PGs in the chick through a mechanism other than motility, or it may be that PGs cause a reduction in motile potential below that necessary for bone resorption, but to a level still sufficient for pseudopodial movement.

The responsiveness of chicken osteoclasts to CT is unclear. While rat osteoclasts possess large numbers of CT receptors (approx 10^6 per cell), and show cAMP generation, motility-inhibition and cessation of bone resorption in response to CT, several authors have found these phenomena to be undemonstrable in osteoclasts isolated from chick and chicken bones, even using chicken CT (Arnett and Dempster, 1986; Ito, Schraer and Gay, 1985; Dempster *et al.*, 1987; Nicholson *et al.*, 1986a). Others, however, have found inhibition of bone resorption at similar concentrations (de Vernejoul *et al.*, 1988), CT receptors (Rifkin *et al.*, 1988) and morphological evidence for CT effects on chicken osteoclasts (Cao and Gay, 1985). This discrepancy may be at least partially explained by the very high level of circulating CT in chickens (Kenny, 1971), which may cause down-regulation of osteoclastic CT-responsiveness. The experiments which failed to identify CT-responsiveness used normal chickens, while those experiments that showed CT-responsiveness in isolated osteoclasts used calcium-deficient animals (in which circulating CT would be expected to be depressed). This suggestion is supported by a recent preliminary report (Eliam *et al.*, 1987) in which chicken osteoclasts were shown to possess a small number of CT receptors which can be demonstrated only in animals maintained hypocalcaemic for several weeks.

The physiological role of CT is unknown. Several functions have been proposed, but none has been universally accepted. The action on osteoclasts is probably the only action of physiological significance. Changes in osteoclastic morphology occur sufficiently rapidly to account for the time course of the hypocalcaemic effect, and osteoclasts are the only cell type in bone shown to possess CT receptors or responsiveness. The primary function of CT does not seem to be that of a hypocalcaemic hormone since it causes hypocalcaemia, and then transiently, only in growing animals and in adults with Paget's disease, both situations associated with high levels of osteoclastic activity. In normal adults and in older animals CT has little or no hypocalcaemic effect (see MacIntyre, 1983). These observations suggest that the primary role of CT is as an inhibitor of osteoclastic bone resorption. This inhibition may temporarily disturb calcium homeostasis if sufficient numbers of osteoclasts are simultaneously inhibited from resorption. The hormone also acts on the kidney to inhibit normal calcium excretion, and to increase $1,25(OH)_2$ vitamin D_3 production (See Borle, 1983; Doepfner, 1983). Neither of these actions would be expected if CT were primarily a hypocalcaemic agent. CT seems to have an overall action, through osteoclasts and perhaps the kidney, to conserve total body calcium. The extreme sensitivity of osteoclasts to inhibition by CT suggest that osteoclasts are the major cell target for this role.

Regulation of Osteoclastic Resorption by Osteoblasts

The osteoclast takes ultimate origin from a mononuclear precursor that reaches bone surfaces through the circulation (see below). Despite this hematogenous origin osteoclasts localise in intricate and dynamic patterns appropriate for skeletal morphogenesis and restructuring. It is difficult to envisage a mechanism by which an essentially wandering cell could achieve such patterns without direction from local tissue. Cells of the osteoblastic lineage (osteoblasts, osteocytes and bone lining cells) appear *a priori* well equipped to provide the morphogenetic information required for osteoclastic localisation. The cells of this (osteoblastic) lineage form a extensive network in which osteocytes, interred in bone, communicate with each other and with osteoblasts and bone lining cells on the bone surface through long and numerous cytoplasmic processes. This network of cells may generate positional information during morphogenesis, and may transduce mechanical stimuli (Rodan *et al.*, 1975; Rubin and Lanyon, 1984), to the bone surface, where formation or resorption may be induced in appropriate sites. Thus, osteoblastic cells may be able to recruit, localise, activate, regulate and terminate osteoclastic bone resorption (Chambers, 1980).

Similar reasoning can be applied to systemic stimulators of osteoclastic bone resorption such as parathyroid hormone (PTH). PTH increases both the activity of pre-existing osteoclasts and the number of osteoclasts in bone (Binhham, Brazell and Owen, 1969; Roberts, 1975; Miller, 1978; Miller *et al.*, 1984). We would expect newly recruited osteoclasts to localise in areas most appropriate for bone resorption. This implies (except in the physiologically unlikely circumstance that there is normally a deficit between osteoblastic demand for resorptive cells, and osteoclastic supply, which could be reduced by a direct action on osteoclastic precursors) that osteoblastic cells are, by the argument above, involved in mediating the PTH responsiveness of bone resorption: the increased number and activity of osteoclasts induced by parathyroid hormone could be effected without disturbance to the overall pattern of osteoclastic resorption if PTH were to act primarily on osteoblastic cells, which are able to take local structure into account in determining where increased bone resorption is more appropriate (Chambers, 1980). The model is consistent with the presence of PTH receptors on osteoblastic calls (see Rodan and Martin, 1981) and their absence from osteoclasts reported by most (O'Grady and Cameron, 1971; Silve *et al.*, 1982; Rouleau *et al.*, 1986), but not all (Rao *et al.*, 1983) investigators.

We have tested the extent to which osteoblastic cells mediate the environmental response of osteoclasts, and have found that, with the sole exception of CT, the ultimate response of osteoclasts in intact bone to all the calcium regulating hormones, cytokines and other local hormones so far tested is mediated by osteoblastic cells. This demonstrates a central role for osteoblastic cells in the regulation of bone resorption.

PTH stimulates bone resorption *in vivo* and in organ culture, but we have found no effect on either the bone resorption or motility of isolated osteoclasts (Chambers and Ali, 1983; Chambers *et al.*, 1985). This suggests that the populations of cells we use are deficient in some cell type that mediates the PTH-responsiveness of bone. This deficiency can be restored by incubation of osteoclasts with osteosarcoma cells, or osteoblastic cells from neonatal rat calvariae (McSheehy and Chambers, 1986a). Such co-cultures respond to concentrations as low as 10^{-4} IU/ml PTH, with increases in bone resorption to 2-4 fold those seen in cultures of osteoclasts alone, or in co-cultures incubated without PTH.

Stimulation of bone resorption in osteoblast-osteoclast co-cultures can be accounted for by the release, by PTH-incubated osteoblastic cells, of osteoclast resorption stimulating activity (ORSA) into culture supernatants (McSheehy and Chambers, 1986b): addition to osteoclasts of supernatants from osteosarcoma cells or rat calvarial cells previously incubated for 24 hours with PTH increases osteoclastic resorption to a similar extent to that seen in co-cultures.

The bone slice assay is poorly productive and makes identification of ORSA by analysis of osteoblastic supernatants impracticable. An alternative approach is to screen agents known to stimulate bone resorption in organ culture for a direct effect on osteoclasts. The factor seems not to be a prostaglandin (PG): despite the undoubted ability of PGs to stimulate resorption in intact bone (Klein and Raisz, 1970; Tashjian *et al.*, 1973) they act as direct inhibitors of osteoclasts (see later) (Chambers and Ali, 1983; Chambers *et al.*, 1985); and indomethacin does not impair ORSA-production by osteoblasts (McSheehy and Chambers, 1986b). Leukotrienes A_4, B_4, C_4 and D_4 do not stimulate resorption by isolated osteoclasts (unpublished observations). Interleukin 1, tumour necrosis factor and lymphotoxin, which are all potential local messengers for stimulation of osteoclasts by osteoblasts, are all without direct effect, but stimulate resorption in co-cultures (Thomson *et al.*, 1986; Thomson *et al.*, 1987). Although these agents do not represent the mechanism through which osteoblasts stimulate osteoclasts, the sensitivity of co-cultures to their presence is sufficiently great to suggest that these cytokines may play a role, either as agents of systemic catabolism during the systemic response to injury (and non-adaptive, pathological bone resorption if produced inappropriately or locally by neoplastic or inflammatory tissue) or as messengers between bone cells (for example, if produced by osteocytes to act on the bone surface cells).

A third approach to identification of ORSA is to use the (more productive) organ culture assay as a detection system. Perry *et al.* (1987) have found that osteoblastic cells are stimulated by PTH to produce a macromolecular agent that stimulates ^{45}Ca release from rat long bones. Unfortunately, the assay cannot be used to identify direct osteoclastic stimulators: for example IL1 itself stimulates resorption in the assay, but does not directly stimulate osteoclasts (Thomson and Chambers, 1986). Bone cells are known to produce agents *in vitro*, such as IL1 (Heath *et al.*, 1984; Hanazawa *et al.*, 1985), that stimulate resorption in organ culture but activate osteoclasts indirectly, through osteoblastic cells. Some osteoblast-derived products (PGs) stimulate organ culture resorption but paradoxically inhibit osteoclasts directly (see later). Even those cytokines whose production by osteoblasts can be shown to be increased by agents which, like PTH, stimulate organ culture resorption do not necessarily represent the osteoblast-derived osteoclast stimulator. For example, macrophage colony stimulating factor (M-CSF) is produced by osteoblastic cells in response to lipopolysaccharide and 1,25 dihydroxyvitamin D$_3$ (Elford *et al.*, 1987) and tumour necrosis factor a (Sato *et al.*, 1987, but we have found that M-CSF inhibits osteoclastic resorption in the isolated osteoclast bone slice assay (submitted).

Osteoblastic cells seem to be able to regulate osteoclastic resorption by a second, distinct mechanism, through mineral exposure. Implantation of inorganic materials such as hydroxyapatite crystals into tissues evokes a macrophage foreign body response, that results in sequestration or dissolution of the implanted material (see Chambers, 1978). Presumably, therefore, bone has evolved some means of protecting bone mineral from phagocytic attack, This protective mechanism is unlikely to be cellular for when bone lining cells die (as in osteonecrosis) bone does not evoke a foreign body response (Ham and Harris, 1972; Glimcher and Kenzora, 1979) but may well be the unmineralised layer of organic material that is regularly observed lining bone surfaces (Raina, 1972; Fornasier, 1980; Vanderwiel, 1980). Then, when bone resorption is required, bone lining cells may remove the organic protective material, and induce exposure of mineral to contact with the specialised digestive cells of bone, the osteoclasts (Chambers, 1980).

We tested this hypothesis by using devitalised slices of cortical bone. Because these slices are sections of bone, mineral is exposed on the cut surface. Such slices, lacking the unmineralised organic covering present on native surfaces, are spontaneously resorbed by osteoclasts *in vitro*. If, however, bone mineral is removed, resorption does not occur (Chambers, Thomson and Fuller, 1984).

The hypothesis was also tested using native bone surfaces. Pre-existing cells were removed from calvariae of adult rats, and osteoclasts were incubated on the endocranial surface. We found that osteoclasts did not excavate this (unmineralised) surface, but did so if the unmineralised organic surface was first removed by collagenase (Chambers *et al.*, 1984; Chambers, Darby and Fuller, 1985). Since osteoclasts are clearly capable of destruction of both inorganic and organic components of bone (Chambers *et al.*, 1984) this indicates that contact with bone mineral induces osteoclasts to resorptive activity, while unmineralised organic material does not. We also found, consistent with the hypothesis, that osteoblasts are able to remove the surface layer of unmineralised organic material *in vitro*, in response to PTH, and expose underlying bone mineral; and that bone so modified has an increased susceptibility to osteoclastic resorption, and that this susceptibility is abrogated by demineralisation (Chambers and Fuller, 1985).

Do these experimental results reflect physiological processes? Removal of organic material by osteoblasts took the unphysiological time of several days. For practical reasons we used a bone surface on which the unmineralised layer was approximately 10μm deep (osteoid). It is likely that bone resorption *in vivo* is generally initiated on bone surfaces upon which bone formation has long since ceased. On such (resting) surfaces, the unmineralised organic layer is only a few hundred nanometers thick, and if bone lining cells remove this at a similar rat to that we observed *in vitro*, mineral exposure could be effected in a relatively short time. The results are consistent with the events observed preceding resorption *in vivo*, where previously-covered mineral becomes exposed onto the bone surface just before osteoclasts appear at the same site (Tran Van *et al.*, 1982).

The model (that mineral is protected from contact with osteoclasts (and mononuclear phagocytes) by unmineralised organic material, and that bone lining cells initiate and localise osteoclastic resorption by localised neutral protease activity, which exposes mineral onto the bone surface and activates resorptive behaviour in osteoclasts) enables a reinterpretation of the significance of neutral protease release by osteoblastic cells. Osteoblastic cells produce collagenase and tissue plasminogen activator *in vitro*, and secrete increased amounts of these proteases, and decreased amounts of protease inhibitor in the presence of PTH and other bone resorbing hormones (Hamilton *et al.*, 1984; Heath *et al.*, 1984; Sakamoto and Sakamoto, 1984; Thomson *et al.*, 1987). Collagenase has been identified in bone lining cells in situ in circumstances of increased bone resorption, and synthesis in bone is increased by exposure to a resorptive stimulus (Sakamoto and Sakamoto, 1985; Eeckhout *et al.*, 1986). This has been interpreted as evidence for a role for collagenase secreting cells as accessory cells in bone resorption (viz, accessory cells remove collagen, osteoclasts digest mineral). However, even if, as is likely, collagenase is absent from osteoclasts, it is not required by them for collagen digestion; since osteoclasts resorb both organic and inorganic components of bone. Acid protease (cathepsin) release correlates with ^{45}Ca release in organ culture, and cysteine protease (including cathepsin) inhibitors inhibit bone resorption (Delaisse *et al.*, 1980, 1984): osteoclasts are likely to digest organic matrix through acid hydrolase secretion (see earlier).

A second possible explanation for osteoblastic collagenase secretion is that these cells act as alternative bone resorptive cells. However, we found osteoblasts removed only the organic surface layer, and exposed but did not detectably resorb the underlying mineral. Also, there is neither ^{45}Ca release nor bone resorption in response to PTH in osteopetrotic mice with normal osteoblasts but defective osteoclasts (Jilka and Hamilton, 1985).

Several recent observations support a role for osteoblastic collagenase as the mechanism by which osteoclasts are induced to resorptive activity. According to this model, there are two distinct processes: osteoblastic collagenase digestion of the organic layer, preceding and enabling acid hydrolytic resorption of bone. Inhibition or incompetence of the latter process, due to acetazolamide, CT or in osteopetrosis, does not affect collagenase release and uncalcified collagen digestion in response to PTH (Jilka and Cohn, 1983; Jilka and Hamilton, 1985; Eeckhout *et al.*, 1986), but there is failure to degrade mineralised tissue. On the other hand, digestion of unmineralised collagen is inhibited by a synthetic collagenase inhibitor (Delaisse *et al.*, 1985; Delaisse *et al.*, 1988). Thus, collagenase secretion accounts for digestion of unmineralised collagen, occurs when osteoclasts are inactive, but cannot by itself account for one resorption. Nevertheless, osteoclastic resorption seems dependent on this neutral protease secretion: collagenase and products of collagen digestion are detected before ^{45}Ca release (Sakamoto and Sakamoto, 1985); inhibition of collagenase by anticollagenase antibody (Sakamoto *et al.*, 1984), cartilage derived anti-collagenase factor (Horton *et al.*, 1978) or a synthetic collagenase inhibitor (Vaes, 1985) inhibits PTH-stimulation of ^{45}Ca release in organ culture. Inhibition is not complete, but increases with time (Horton *et al.*, 1978); presumably osteoclasts already in contact with mineral continue to resorb, but there is inhibition of induction of osteoclasts to new resorptive sites in response to the hormone.

Prostaglandins and Bone Resorption

Prostaglandins (PGs) are known from many experiments to stimulate resorption of bone in organ culture (*e.g.* Klein and Raisz, 1970; Tashjian *et al.*, 1973; Dietrich *et al.*, 1975). We have found, however, that the same PGs (PGE$_1$ PGE$_2$ and PGI$_2$) that stimulate organ culture resorption strongly inhibit bone resorption at low concentrations in the isolated osteoclast bone slice assay (Chambers *et al.*, 1985). Inhibition is not transient, but is maintained for at least 6 hours, and recovery is to control, not supranormal levels (Fuller and Chambers, in preparation). Inhibition of bone resorption by isolated osteoclasts has been confirmed by others using isolated osteoclasts (Arnett and Dempster, 1987; de Vernejoule *et al.*, 1988). Time-lapse video observations of osteoclastic responsiveness to PGs strongly suggest that this is a direct effect on osteoclasts: osteoclasts, widely separated from other cell types, respond within a minute, with cessation of motility and subsequent cytoplasmic retraction, a behavioral change identical to that observed using CT, and with an indistinguishable time-course (Chambers and Ali, 1983; Arnett and Dempster, 1987). Like CT, PGs inhibit enzyme release by isolated osteoclasts (Chambers *et al.*, 1987). Also, like CT, PGs cause cyclic AMP production in osteoclasts (Nicholson *et al.*, 1986a) and their effect on motility is potentiated by phosphodiesterase inhibitors (Chambers and Ali, 1983). It is difficult to escape the conclusion that PGs act as strong and direct inhibitors of osteoclasts, and that this is their sole demonstrable direct effect.

This inhibitory effect is also observed in organ cultures and lasts up to 9 hours (Conaway *et al.*, 1986; Lerner *et al.*, 1987). However, by 24-48 hours stimulation of bone resorption is regularly demonstrated. We see a similar sequence in osteoblast-osteoclast co-cultures (Chambers and Fuller, 1984). Thus, PGs act as direct inhibitors, with tachyphylaxis, but also induce osteoblastic cells to stimulate osteoclasts, through a effect on osteoblasts that, to account for the delayed net stimulation, suffers less tachyphylaxis. This may explain the phenomenology, but does not elucidate the role of PGs in the regulation of bone resorption.

PGs directly inhibit osteoclastic resorption (Chambers *et al.*, 1985), and are produced by osteoblastic cells (Feyen *et al.*, 1984; Partridge *et al.*, 1985; Rodan *et al.*, 1986). This makes it likely that at least some osteoblastic cells produce PGs as local inhibitors of osteoclastic resorption: PG's may be the means by which osteoblasts oppose ORSA-stimulation, and inhibit or terminate osteoclastic resorption. Osteoblastic cells thus have the potential for both direct inhibition and direct stimulation of osteoclastic activity. The explanation for the apparently paradoxical effects of PGs on one resorption may be that the balance between osteoblastic PG and ORSA production is homeostatically regulated. This balance may be maintained through the PTH-like effect of PGs on osteoblastic adenyl cyclase (Yu et al., 1976; Heersche et al., 1978; Partridge et al., 1981), an effect that may, like PTH, increase ORSA production, or may sensitise osteoblastic cells to stimulators of ORSA production, as compensation for what is perceived by osteoblasts as excessive PG production. Addition of PGs from an external source (for example, by addition to bone on organ culture, or by inflammatory cells in vivo) would be perceived by osteoblasts as excessive PG production, and the appropriate homeostatic response would be to produce increased amounts of ORSA. Whatever the explanation for PG stimulation of bone resorption in organ culture, PGs are such powerful direct inhibitors of osteoclastic resorption that they seem unlikely to have a physiological role as stimulators in intact bone. If this is so, agents that stimulate bone resorption in organ culture through PG production (Stern et al., 1985; Tashjian et al., 1985) probably act physiologically as inhibitors, rather than stimulators, or osteoclastic resorption in vivo (where tissue perfusion, absent in organ culture, is likely to prevent accumulation of PGs sufficient to cause osteoclastic tachyphylaxis or disrupt osteoblastic homeostasis). Such agents may nevertheless, like PGs themselves, act as stimulators under pathological circumstances of excessive production by inflammatory or neoplastic cells in bone. In this model, PGs are essentially anabolic (and agents that stimulate bone resorption in organ culture through PG production may be essentially anabolic in vivo). This role is in keeping with many in vivo observations in which PG administration is associated with increased bone formation (Baron et al., 1978; Sone et al., 1980; Veda et al., 1980; Ringel et al., 1982; Jee et al., 1985).

A second possibility is that a subpopulation of bone cells exploits the above system and produces PGs as (indirect) stimulators of osteoclastic resorption. It is of interest that there is an inverse relationship in the rank order of osteoclastic and osteoblastic sensitivity to PGE_2 and PGI_2, such that while osteoclasts seem to be approximately 100 times more sensitive to inhibition by PGI_2 than PGE_2 (Chambers and Ali, 1983), the reverse is true for osteoblasts (Partridge et al., 1981a,b). Thus, a cell such as an osteocyte, by producing PGE$_2$ in response to mechanical or morphogenetic information, could perturb the homeostasis of bone lining cells in the direction of resorption-stimulation at a concentration too low to cause significant osteoclastic inhibition: a PG-mediated resorptive stimulus. Similarly, a bone lining cell determined to inhibit osteoclastic resorption could produce PGI$_2$ sufficient for osteoclast-inhibition without significantly disturbing the adenyl cyclase activity of bone lining cells. Resolution of this issue awaits the localisation of PG production, and identification of environmental responsiveness, intact bone.

Regulation of Osteoclast Production

We have identified several points at which bone resorption by mature osteoclasts can be regulated: non-resorptive osteoclasts can be induced to resorptive activity through mineral exposure; osteoclasts already undertaking resorption can be stimulated to increased activity; and resorptive cells can be inhibited by PGs or CT. Apart from CT, which acts directly on osteoclasts, the remainder of the environmental responsiveness of osteoclastic regulation seems to be mediated by the cells of the osteoblastic lineage, which are capable of induction, stimulation and inhibition of bone resorption by mature osteoclasts. Regulation of osteoclast production is likely to be an additional mechanism through which bone resorption is regulated. *in vivo*, local and systemic levels of osteoclastic activity correlate with osteoclast number: PTH increases, and CT decreases, the number of osteoclasts in bone (Bingham *et al.*, 1969; Roberts, 1975; Miller, 1978; Baron and Vignery, 1981; Hedland *et al.*, 1983; Miller *et al.*, 1984).Virtually nothing is known of the mechanism underlying these changes in osteoclast numbers. The increased number of osteoclasts that appears under circumstances of increased bone resorption may be mediated either through a PTH action on osteoblastic cells, to produce a signal for increased osteoclast production, or through a direct action of PTH on osteoclast precursors (which then lose receptors on maturation). It may be that both mechanisms contribute, but at least an element of osteoblastic mediation is likely, to facilitate co-ordination between osteoclast production and osteoblastic demand. The same considerations apply to other agents that stimulate bone resorption through an effect on cells of the osteoblastic lineage.

Parabiosis experiments, quail-chick chimeras and bone marrow and spleen cell transplantation experiments have established that osteoclasts take origin from hemopoietic tissue (see Marks, 1983; Chambers, 1985). In all three systems local osteoclasts and potential precursors are, by nature or artifice, deficient. Under such circumstances osteoclasts are supplied through the circulatory system, ultimately from hemopoietic tissue. In physiology such circumstances may only hold in the embryo: Hemopoietic tissue may supply a (radiosensitive) stem call through the circulation to bone surfaces, that is dedicated to osteoclast production and sustains osteoclast number independent of both hemopoiesis and continued vascular supply. Alternatively there may be continuous recruitment of precursors, incapable of self-maintenance, through the vascular system.

Amongst the progeny of hemopoietic tissue, from which osteoclasts derive, the mononuclear phagocyte system was immediately the most likely contender for the role of osteoclast precursor (see Loutit and Nisbet, 1979). While the other major circulating descendants of the hemopoietic system are quite unlike osteoclasts, monocytes superficially have much in common morphologically, enzymatically, functionally (both are specialised for degradation) and in the ability to form multinucleate cells. Osteoclasts demonstrate several antigens otherwise specific for or typical of mononuclear phagocytes (Burmester et al., 1983; Nijweide et al., 1985; Ousler et al., 1985; Athanasou et al., 1986). However, despite these similarities, osteoclasts differ from mononuclear phagocytes in several important ways. Mononuclear and multinucleate macrophages are unable to excavate bone (Chambers and Horton, 1984); they do not show the behavorial and morphological transformation induced in osteoclasts by CT (Chambers and Magnus, 1982); osteoclasts lack many antigens typical of mononuclear phagocytes, and possess several antigens that are absent from these cells (Horton et al., 1985a, 1985b, 1985c).

These dissimilarities do not exclude an ontogenetic relationship. What is required, to show that mononuclear phagocytes can act on osteoclastic precursors, is to induce in mononuclear phagocytes phenotypic markers characteristic of osteoclasts. Osdoby et al., (1986) have attempted this. Chick monocytes were induced by osteoblastic cells to express osteoclast-specific antigen. The extent to which antigen-induction, which may well represent osteoclast differentiation, also represents differentiation of monocytes to osteoclasts cannot be assessed from this preliminary communication, since no information was given concerning either the purity of the monocyte preparation or the proportion of monocytes that responded: the responders may have been a non-monocytic subpopulation. We have found that osteoclast-specific antigens can be induced in cultures of hemopoietic tissue, but only in a very small proportion of cells, in a population that seems quite distinct from the mononuclear phagocytes also present in the cultures (Fuller and Chambers, 1987).

In another experimental system, osteoclast development in bone rudiments (themselves lacking demonstrable osteoclast precursors) is detected as bone-resorbing multinucleate cells that form in the rudiment during culture with putative osteoclast precursors (Burger *et al.*, 1982, 1984). Bone rudiments alone did not form multinucleate cells, but when co-cultured with long-term liquid marrow cultures consisting largely of immature mononuclear phagocytes, osteoclasts appeared. It is presumed because no osteoclasts developed when dead rudiments were used, that the rudiment provided signals that induced osteoclastic differentiation in the co-cultured cells. The main problem in applying this technique for lineage analysis is the small number of osteoclasts that develop before the detection system is saturated: a very minor contaminant, rather than the major cell type, could be providing the osteoclasts. Indeed, subsequent experiments using the same system found that the precursor did not fractionate with mononuclear phagocytes, but with pluripotent stem cells (Scheven *et al.*, 1986). This conclusion is supported by bone marrow transplantation experiments in which, while mononuclear phagocytes cannot cure the resorptive defect in osteopetrosis (Loutit and Nisbet, 1982; Schneider and Byrnes, 1983), granulocyte and granulocyte-macrophage colony forming cells, but not macrophage colony forming cells can (Schneider and Relfson, 1988). These results suggest that osteoclastic precursors diverge from the ancestors of the mononuclear phagocyte lineage before the latter becomes established. The results imply that osteoclasts develop from a derivative of the hemopoietic stem cell that can become committed specifically to osteoclast-generation, equivalent to the cells that supply other hemopoietic lineages, and do not derive from cells of the mononuclear phagocyte series. Analysis of osteoclast lineage-relationships should soon be resolved through identification of osteoclasts, and the cells that develop with them, in the colonies formed in semi-solid cultures of bone marrow cells.

Little is known of osteoclast ancestry, and even less is known of the regulation of its differentiation, largely due to lack, until recently, of reliable markers for osteoclast-identification. The development of multinuclear cells in culture has been widely used as evidence of osteoclast formation (Testa *et al.*, 1981; Ibbotson *et al.*, 1984; Pharoah and Heersch, 1985; Roodman *et al.*, 1985; MacDonald *et al.*, 1986; Takahashi *et al.*, 1986). However, mononuclear phagocytes are present in large numbers in the culture systems utilised, and mononuclear phagocytes are known to readily fuse to form multinucleated giant cells *in vitro*.

Although multinuclearity is a reliable criterion for osteoclasts in bone, it cannot be used as the major criterion for osteoclast *in vitro*. Allen *et al.* (1981) found that the giant cells that formed in feline bone marrow cultures were incapable of excavation of mineralised tissue, and we (Horton *et al.*, 1986) found that the giant cells that arise in long-term cultures of rabbit bone marrow cells were similarly unable to excavate the surface of bone slices. Moreover, the giant cells did not bind osteoclast-specific monoclonal antibodies, but were positive for macrophage markers. Thus, the multinucleate cells remain macrophage-like, and are not rendered discernably more osteoclast-like by multinuclearity.

Tartrate-resistant acid phosphates (TRAP) positivity and calcitonin-responsiveness have been construed as additional support for an osteoclastic nature for these nultinucleate giant cells. However, macrophages contain (Efstratiadis and Moss, 1985) and develop TRAP *in vivo* (Chambers *et al.*, 1987), and in culture (Snipes *et al.*, 1986). No convincing evidence has been published that the multinucleate giant cells identified as osteoclasts show an osteoclast-like response to CT. Nor does bone resorption (Takahashi *et al.*, 1988) in such cultures identify the giant cells as the cells responsible. We have found that the cells developing in bone marrow cultures that express osteoclastic characteristics (bone resorption, osteoclast-specific antigen positivity) are mononuclear cells and cells of low multinuclearity, and appear morphologically distinctively different from the (non-resorptive, antigen negative) multinucleate giant cells that also develop in these cultures (Fuller and Chambers, 1987). These problems make interpretation of experiments in which osteoclasts are counted as the number of multinucleate cells that arise in bone marrow cultures difficult to interpret in terms of the regulation of osteoclastic differentiation. However, more reliable criteria (excavation of bone, osteoclast-specific monoclonal antibodies, CT receptors) are now being applied to identification of osteoclast production from hemopoietic tissue by several groups, and much new information on both lineage and regulation is likely to become available in the next few years.

Concluding Remarks

The available evidence suggests a central role for osteoblastic cells in the regulation of osteoclastic resorption. This intercommunicating network of cells seems well suited to generate morphogenetic information and to assess the mechanical performance of bone, and to identify those sites in bone where resorption is appropriate. There are at least three mechanisms by which regulation may be effected. Osteoblastic cells may initiate osteoclastic resorption by neutral protease digestion of the unmineralised surface of bone, thus exposing resorption-stimulating mineral to osteoclastic contact; once resorption is under way osteoclasts are able to stimulate the process through ORSA production; and may reduce or terminate resorption through PG production. It seems likely that these mechanisms regulate resorption during bone morphogenesis and restructuring, in response to unknown signals generated by osteocytes or bone lining cells, independent of calcium regulating hormones. If calcium homeostasis requires increased bone resorption, the stimulus (PTH, $1,23(OH)_2D_3$) is directed at osteoblastic cells. This alters the threshold of osteoblastic cells in favour of resorption throughout the skeleton: resorption will be stimulated in places where this is already underway, and may be initiated in new areas by osteoblasts that were previously nearest the threshold for resorption-stimulation: by acting on osteoblastic cells, the increased resorption occurs in those sites more appropriate for the maintenance of the structure of bone.

This simple model is clearly incomplete. It is likely that osteoblastic cells also play a role in the regulation of osteoclastic development, recruitment to bone surfaces, and chemotaxis to appropriate areas. Also, nothing is known of the signals produced by osteocytes or bone lining cells that transmit the requirement for increased resorption to osteoblastic cells in the appropriate area. Osteoblastic cells are clearly heterogenous, but it is not know whether there are distinct phenotypes on the bone surface separately responsible for, for example, osteoclastic induction, stimulation and inhibition. Osteoblastic cell lines differ in functions such as PG production (See Raisz and Martin, 1984) but the extent to which this reflects the state of affairs in bone is unknown. It may be that osteoclasts themselves produce, or release from bone matrix during resorption, substances that either provide feedback information to osteoblastic cells, or even stimulate subsequent bone formation. But bone formation does not regularly follow resorption, even in the adult, and if osteoblastic cells have the capacity to decide where bone resorption is appropriate, the same capacity should enable them to decide when resorption is sufficient, and whether subsequent bone formation should occur.

Bone resorption is also clearly affected by other cells and tissues. Resorption occurs in inflammation, and around tumours, and in myeloid hyperplasia. Do these pathological circumstances reflect mechanisms of significance to the physiology of bone? Certainly cells of the immune system produce cytokines that stimulate bone resorption *in vitro*. However, production of these cytokines is not limited to cells of the immune system, and immunological cells produce cytokines whether bone is present or not. If the same cytokines cause bone resorption, this implies that bone cells use similar paracrine systems, not that immune cells make a contribution (difficult for wandering cells) to skeletal morphogenesis and restructuring. Similarities between the paracrine systems of bone and lymphoid cells may explain how excessive (pathological) accumulations of lymphoid or other cells cause osteolysis in disease, but this is a pathological, not a physiological mechanism. What bone does learn from the immune system is that cytokines are important in cell-cell interactions, and that the source and environmental responsiveness of production of cytokines in bone will need to be identified before we can reach an adequate understanding of the cellular physiology of bone formation and resorption.

References

Akisaka, T. and Gay, C. V. (1986a) Ultracytochemical evidence for a proton pump adenosine triphosphate in chick osteoclasts. *Cell Tiss. Res.* **245**: 507-512

Akisaka, T. and Gay, C. V. (1986b) An ultracytochemical investigation of ouabain-sensitive p-nitrophenylphosphatase in chick osteoclasts. *Cell Tiss. Res.* **244**: 57

Akisaka, T., Yamamoto T. and Gay, C. V. (1938) Ultracytochemical investigation of calcium-activated adenosine triphosphatase (Ca^{2+}-ATPase) in chick tibia. *J. Bone and Min. Res.* **3**: 19-25

Ali, M. N., Boyde A. and Jones, S. J. (1984) Motility and resorption: osteoclastic activity *in vitro*. *Anat. Embryol.* **170**: 51-56

Allen, T. D., Testa, N. G., Suda, T., Schor, S. L., Onions, D., Jarrett O. and Boyde, A. (1981) The production of putative osteoclasts in tissue culture - ultrastructure, formation and behaviour. *Scanning Electron Microscopy* **III**: 347-354

Anderson, R. E., Schraer H. and Gay, C. V. (1982) Ultrastructural immunocytochemical localisation of carbonic anhydrase in normal and calcitonin-treated chick osteoclasts. *Anat. Rec.* **204**: 9

Anderson, R. E., Woodbury D. M. and Jee, W. S. S. (1986) Humoral and ionic regulation of osteoclast acidity. *Calc. Tiss. Int.* **39**: 252-258

Arnett T. R. and Dempster, D. W. (1987) A comparative study of disaggregated chick and rat osteoclasts *in vitro*: effects of calcitonin and prostaglandins. *Endocrinology* **120**: 602-608

Ash, P., Loutit J. F. and Townsend, K. M. S. (1980) Osteoclasts derive from haemopoietic stem cells. *Nature* **283**: 669-670

Athanasou, N. A., Heryet, A., Quinn, J., Gatter, K. C., Mason D. Y. and McGee, J. O'D. (1986) Osteoclasts contain macrophage and ?? antigens. *J. Pathol.* **150**: 239-246

Baron, R., Kellokumpu, S., Neff, L., Jamsa-Kellokumpu, S., Emanuel, J., Sweadner K. and Levenson, R. (1988) Sodium pumps and bone resorption: presence of basolateral kidney type alpha subunits in osteoclasts, effects of ouabain on bone resorption and interaction with calcitonin in MDCK cells. *Calc. Tiss. Int.* Suppl. vol **42**: abs. 54

Baron, R., Neff, L., Louvard D. and Courtoy, P. J. (1985) Cell-mediated extracellular acidification and bone resorption: evidence for a low pH in resorbing lacunae and localisation of a 100kDa lysosomal membrane protein on the osteoclast ruffled border. *J. Cell Biol.* **101**: 2210-2222

Baron, R., Neff, L., Roy, C., Boisvert A. and Caplan, M. (1986) Evidence for a high and specific concentration of $(Na^+, K^+)ATPase$ in the plasma membrane of the osteoclast. *Cell* **46**: 311-320

Baron, R., Nefussi, J. R., Duflot-Vignery, A., Lasfargues, J. J., Cohen F. and Puzas, E. (1978) Failure of prostaglandin E to induce local bone resorption *in vivo*. In: Proc. mechanisms of localised bone loss. (J. E. Horton, T. M. Tarpley and W. R. Davis Eds). Suppl. to *Calc. Tiss. Res.* pp 433-434

Barmon R., and Vignery, A. (1981) Behaviour of osteoclasts during a rapid change in their number induces by high doses of parathyroid hormone or calcitonin in intact rats. *Met. Bone Dis. and Rel. Res.* **2**: 339-346

Bingham, P. J., Brazell, I. A. and Owen, M. (1969) The effect of parathyroid extract on cellular activity and plasma calcium levels *in vivo*. *J. Endoc.* **45**: 387-400

Blair, H. C., Kahn, A. J., Crouch, E. C., Jeffrey J. J. and Teitelbaum, S. L. (1986) Isolated osteoclasts resorb the organic and inorganic components of bone. *J. Cell Biol.* **102**: 1164-1172

Borle, A. B. (1983) Calcitonin and the regulation of calcium transport and of cellular calcium metabolism. *Triangle* **22**: 75-80

Burger, E. H., Van der Meer, J. V. M., Van de Gevel, J. S., Gribnan, J. C., Thesingh C. W. and Van Furth, R. (1982) *In vitro* formation of osteoclasts from long-term cultures of bone marrow mononuclear phagocytes. *J. Exp. Med.* **156**: 1604-1614

Burger, E. H., Van der Meer, J. W. M. and Nijweide, P. J. (1984) Osteoclast formation from mononuclear phagocytes: role of bone-forming cells. *J. Cell Biol.* **99**: 1901-1906

Burmester, G. R., Winchester, R. J., Dimitriu-Bona, A., Klein, M., Steiner, G. and Sissons, H. A. (1983) Delineation of four cell types comprising the giant cell tumor of bone. *J. Clin. Invest.* **71**: 1966-1645

Cao, H. and Gay, C.V. (1985) Effects of parathyroid hormone and calcitonin on carbonic anhydrase location in osteoclasts of cultured embryonic chick bone. *Experimentation* **41**: 1472-1474

Chambers, J. P., Peters, S. P., Glew, R. H., Lee, R. E., McCafferty, L. R., Mercer, D. W. and Wenger, D. A. (1978) Multiple forms of acid phosphatase activity in Gaucher's disease. *Metabolism* **27**: 801-814

Chambers, T. J. (1978) Multinucleated giant cells. *J. Pathol.* **126**: 125-146

Chambers, T. J. (1980) The cellular basis of bone resorption. *Clin. Orthop. Rel Res.* **151**: 283-293

Chambers, T. J. (1985) The pathobiology of the osteoclast. *J. Clin. Pathol.* **38**: 241-252

Chambers, T. J. and Ali, N. N. (1983) Inhibition of osteoclastic motility by prostaglandins I_2, E_1, E_2 and 6-oxo-E_1. *J. Pathol.* **139**: 383-398

Chambers, T. J., Chambers, J. C., Symonds J. and Darby, J. A. (1986) The effect of human calcitonin on the cytoplasmic spreading of rat osteoclasts. *J. Clin. Endoc. Metab.* **63**: 1080-1085

Chambers, T. J., Darby J. A and Fuller, K. (1985) Mammalian collagenase predisposes bone surfaces to osteoclastic resorption. *Cell Tiss. Res.* **241**: 671-675

Chambers, T. J. and Fuller, K. (1985) Bone cells predispose endosteal surfaces to resorption by exposure of bone mineral to osteoclastic contact. *J. Cell Science* **76**: 155-165

Chambers, T. J., Fuller, K. and Athanasou, N. A. (1984) The effect of prostaglandins I_2, E_1 and E_2 and dibutryl cyclic AMP on the cytoplasmic spreading of rat osteoclasts. *Brit J. Exp. Pathol.* **65**: 557-566

Chambers, T. J., Fuller K. and Darby, J. A. (1987) Hormonal regulation of acid phosphatase release by osteoclasts disaggregated from neonatal rat bone. *J. Cell Physiol.* **132**: 90-97

Chambers, T. J. and Horton, M. A. (1984) Failure of cells of the mononuclear phagocyte series to resorb bone. *Calc. Tiss. Int.* **36**: 556-558

Chambers, T. J., McSheehy, P. M. J., Thomson, B. M. and Fuller, K. (1985) The effect of calcium-regulating hormones and prostaglandins on bone resorption by osteoclasts disaggregated from neonatal rabbit bones. *Endocrinology* **116**: 234-239

Chambers, T.J. and Magnus, C.J. Calcitonin alters behaviour of isolated osteoclasts. *J. Pathol.* **136**: 27-39

Chambers, T. J. and Moore, A. (1983) The sensitivity of isolated osteoclasts to morphological transformation by calcitonin. *J. Clin. Endoc. Metabolism* **57**: 819-824

Chambers, T. J., Revell, P. A., Fuller, K. and Athanasou, N. A. (1984) Resorption of bone by isolated rabbit osteoclasts. J. Cell *Science* **66**: 383-399

Chambers, T. J., Thomson, B. M. and Fuller, K. (1984) The effect of substrate composition on bone resorption by isolated rabbit osteoclasts. *J. Cell Science* **70**: 61-71

Coccia, P. F., Krivit, W., Cervenka, J., Clawson, C., Kersey, J. H., Kim, T. H., Nesbit, M. E., Ramsay, N. K. C., Warkentin, P. I., Teitelbaum, S. L., Kahn, A. J. and Brown, D. M. (1980) Successful bone marrow transplantation for infantile osteopetrosis. *New Eng. J. Med.* **302**: 701-708

Conaway, H. H., Diez, L. F. and Raisz, L. G. (1986) Effects of prostacyclin and prostaglandin E_1 (PGE_1) on bone resorption in the presence and absence of parathyroid hormone. *Calc. Tiss. Int.* **38**: 130-134

Delaisse, J.-M., Eeckhout, Y., Sear, C., Galloway, A., McCullagh, K. and Vaes, G. (1985) A new synthetic inhibitor of mammalian tissue collagenase inhibits bone resorption in culture. *Biochem Biophys. Res Commun.* **133**: 483-490

Delaisse, J-M., Eeckhout, Y. and Vaes, G. (1984) *In vivo* and *in vitro* evidence for the involvement of cysteine proteinases in bone resorption. *Biochem. Biophys. Res Commun.* **125**: 441-447

Delaisse, J-M., Eeckhout, Y. and Vaes, G. (1988) Possible role of collagenase in bone resorption. *Calc. Tissue. Int.* suppl. to Vol. **42**: abs. 59

De Luise, M. and Harker, M. (1986) Parathyroid hormone stimulation of the Na^+,K^+ pump in rat clonal osteosarcoma cells. *J. Endoc.* **111**: 61-66

Dempster, D. W., Nurills, R. J., Horbert, W. and Arnett, T. R. (1987) Biological activity of chicken calcitonin: Effects on neonatal rat and embryonic chick osteoclasts. *J. Bone Min. Res.* **2**: 443-448

de Vernejoul, M-C., Horowitz, M., Demignon, J., Neff,·L. and Baron, R. (1988) Bone resorption by isolated chick osteoclasts in culture is stimulated by murine spleen cell supernatant fluids (osteoclast activating factor) and inhibited by calcitonin and prostaglandin E_2. *J. Bone & Min. Res.* **3**: 69-80

Diamond, J. M. and Machen, T. E. (1983) Impedance analysis in epithelia and the problem of gastric acid secretion. *J. Memb. Biol.* **72**: 17-41

Dietrich, J. W., Goodson, J.M. and Raisz, L. G. (1975) Stimulation of bone resorption by various prostaglandins in organ culture. *Prostaglandins* **10**: 231-240

Doepfner, W. E. H. (1983) Pharmacological effects of calcitonin. *Triangle* **22**: 57-68

Domon, T. and Wakita, M. (1986) Electron microscope study of osteoclasts with special reference to the three-dimensional structure of the ruffled border. *Arch. Histol. Jap.* **49**: 593

Doty, S. B. and Schofield, B. H. (1972) Electron microscopic localisation of hydrolytic enzymes in osteoclasts. *Histochem. J.* **4**: 245-258

Eeckhout, Y., Delaisse, J-M. and Vaes, G. (1986) Direct extraction and assay of bone tissue collagenase and its relation to parathyroid-hormone-induced bone resorption. *Biochem. J.* **239**: 793-796

Efstratiadis, T. and Moss, D. W. (1985) Tartrate-resistant acid phosphatase of human lung: apparent identity with osteoclastic acid phosphatase. *Enzyme* **33**: 340-40

Eilon, G. and Raisz, L. G. (1978) Comparison of the effects of stimulator and inhibitors or resorption on the release of lysosomal enzymes and radioactive calcium from fetal bone in organ culture. *Endocrinology* **103**: 1969-1978

Elford, P. R., Felix, R., Cecchini, M., Treschel, U. and Fleisch, H. (1987) Murine osteoblast-like cells and the osteogenic cell MC3T3-E$_1$ release a macrophage colony-stimulating activity in culture. *Calc. Tiss. Int.* **41**: 151-156

Eliam, M. C., De Vernejoul, M. C., Bonizar, Z. and Monkhtar, M. S. (1987) Calcitonin receptors in chicken osteoclasts. *J. Bone Min. Res.* **2**: (suppl. 1), abs 261

Etherington, D. J., Maciewicz, R. A., Taylor, M. A. J. and Wardale, R. D. (1987) The role of collagen-degrading cysteine proteinases in connective tissue metabolism. In: *Cysteine Proteinases and their Inhibitors*. (V. Turb, Ed.) Walter de Gruyter, Berlin

Feyen, J. H. M., vander Wilt, G., Moonen, P., Did Bon A. and Nijweide, P. J. (1984) Stimulation of arachidonic acid metabolism in primary cultures of osteoblast-like cells by hormones and drugs. *Prostaglandins* **28**: 769-781

Fornoisier, V. L. (1980) Transmission electron microscopy studies of osteoid maturation. *Met. Bone Dis. & Rel. Res.* **25**: 103-108

Forrest, S. M., Ng, K. W., Findlay, D. M., Micelangeli, V. P., Livesey, S. A., Partridge, N. C., Zajac, J.D. and Martin, T. J. (1985) Characterization of an osteoblast-like clonal cell line which responds to both parathyroid hormone and calcitonin. *Calc. Tiss. Int.* **37**: 51-56

Fuller, K. and Chambers, T. J. (1987) Generation of osteoclasts in cultures of rabbis bone marrow and spleen cells. *J. Cell Physiol.* **132**: 441-452

Gay, C. V., Schraer, H., Anderson, R. E. and Cao, H. (1984) Current studies on the location and function of carbonic anhydrase in osteoclasts. Annals New York Acad. *Science* **429**: 473-478

Ghiselli, R., Blair, H., Teitelbaum S. L. and Gluck, S. (1987) Identification of the osteoclast proton pump. *J. Bone & Min. Res.* **2**: (suppl. 1), abs 275

Glenn, W., Kerrick L. and Hoar, P. E. (1981) Inhibition of smooth muscle tension by cyclic AMP-dependent protein kinase. *Nature* **292**: 253-255

Glimcher, M. J. and Kenzora, J. E. (1979) The biology of osteonecrosis of the human femoral head and its clinical implications. *Clin Orthop.* **138**: 284

Grubb, S. A., Markham, T. C. and Talmage, R. V. (1977) Effect of salmon calcitonin infusion on plasma concentrations of recently administered ^{45}Ca. *Calc. Tiss. Res.* **24**: 201-208

Gutierrez, G. E., Mundy, G. R. and Katz, M. S. (1984) Adenylate cyclase of osteoblast-like cells from rat osteosarcoma is stimulated by calcitonin as well as parathyroid hormone. *Endocrinology* **115**: 2342-2346

Hamiton, J. A., Lingelbach, S. R., Partridge, N. C. and Martin, T. J. (1984) Stimulation of plasminogen activator in osteoblast-like cells by bone-resorbing hormones. *Biochem. Biophys. Res. Commun.* **122**: 230-236

Ham, A. W. and Harris, W. R. (1982) In: *The Biochemistry and Physiology of Bone*. (G. H. Bourne, Ed.). 2nd ed, vol. 1 p 337. Academic Press, New York

Hanazawa, S., Ohmori, Y., Amana, S., Miyoshi, T., Kumegawa, M. and Kitano, S. (1985) Spontaneous production of interleukin-1-like cytokine from mouse osteoblastic cell line (MC3T3-E$_1$). *Biochem. Biophys. Res. Comm.* **131**: 774-779

Heath, J. K., Atkinson, S. J., Miekle, M. C. and Reynolds, J. J. (1984a) Mouse osteoblasts synthesis collagenase in response to bone resorbing agents. *Biochem. Biophys Acta* **802**: 151-154

Heath, J. K., Meikle, M. C., Atkinson, S. J. and Reynolds, J J. (1984b) A factor synthesised by rabbit periosteal fibroblasts stimulates bone resorption and collagenase production by connective tissue cells *in vitro. Biochem. Biophys Acta* **800**: 301-305

Hedlund, T. Hulth, A. and Johnell, O. (1983) Early effect of parathormone and calcitonin on the number of osteoclasts and on serum calcium in rats. *Acta Orthop. Scand.* **54**: 802

Heersche, J. N. M. (1978) Mechanism of osteoclastic bone resorption: a new hypothesis. *Calc. Tiss. Res.* **26**: 81-84

Heersche, J. N. M., Heyboer, M. P. M. and Ng, B. (1978) Hormone specific suppression of adenosine 3151-monophosphate responses in bone *in vitro* during prolonged incubation with parathyroid hormone, prostaglandin E1 and calcitonin. *Endocrinology* **103**: 333

Holtrop, M. E., Raisz, L. G. and Simmons, H. A. (1974) The effects of parathyroid hormone, colchicine and calcitonin on the ultrastructure and the activity of osteoclasts in organ culture. *J. Cell Biol.* **60**: 346-365

Horton, M. A., Lewis, D., McNulty, K., Pringle, J. A. S. and Chambers, T. J. (1985a) Human foetal osteoclasts fail to express macrophage antigens. *Brit. J. Exp. Pathol.* **66**: 103-108

Horton, M. A., Lewis, D., McNulty, K., Pringle, J. A. S. and Chambers, T. J. (1985b) Monoclonal antibodies to osteoclastomas: definition of osteoclast-specific cellular antigens. *Cancer Research* **45**: 5663-5669

Horton, M. A., Rimmer, E. F. and Chambers, T. J. (1986) Giant cell formation in rabbit long-term bone marrow cultures: immunocytological and functional studies. *J. Bone & Min. Res.* **1**: 5-14

Horton, M. A., Rimmer, E. F., Moore, A. and Chambers, T. J. (1985c) On the origin of the osteoclast: the cell surface phenotype of rodent osteoclasts. *Calc. Tiss. Int.* **37**: 46-50

Horton, J. E., Wezeman, F. H. and Kuettner, K. E. (1978) Inhibition of bone resorption *in vitro* by a cartilage-derived anticollagenase factor. *Science* **199**: 1342-1344

Ibbotson, K. J., Roodman, G. D., McManus, L. M. and Mundy, G. R. (1984) Identification and characterization of osteoclast-like cells and their progenitors in culture of feline marrow mononuclear cells. *J. Cell Biol.* **99**: 471-480

Ito, M. B., Schraer, H. and Gay, C. V. (1985) The effects of calcitonin, parathyroid hormone and prostaglandin E2 on cyclic AMP levels of isolated osteoclasts. *Comp. Biochem. Physiol.* **81A**: 653-657

Jee, W. S. S., Veno, K., Deng, Y. P. and Woodbury, D. M. (1985) The effects of prostaglandin E2 in growing rats: increased metaphysical hard tissue and cortico-endosteal bone formation. *Calc. Tiss. Int.* **37**: 145-157

Jilka, R. L. and Cohn, D. V. (1983) A collagenolytic response to parathormone, 1,25 dihydroxy-cholecalciferol D3 and prostaglandin E2 in bone of osteoporotic (mi/mi) mice. *Endocrinology* **112**: 945-950

Jilka, R. L. and Hamilton, J. W. (1985) Evidence for two pathways for stimulation of collagenolysis in bone. *Calc. Tiss. Int.* **37**: 300-306

Kallio, D. M., Garant, P. R. and Minkin, C. (1972) Untrastructural effects of calcitonin on osteoclasts in tissue culture. *J. Ultrastruct. Res.* **39**: 205-216

Kenny, A. D. (1971) Determination of calcitonin in plasma by bioassay. *Endocrinology* **89**: 1005-1013

Klein, D. C. and Raisz, L. G. (1970) Prostaglandins: stimulation of bone resorption in tissue culture. *Endocrinology* **86**: 1436-1440

Lerner, U. H., Ransjo, M. and Ljunggren, O. (1987) Prostaglandin E_2 causes a transient inhibition of mineral mobilisation, matrix degradation, and lysosomal enzyme release from mouse calvarial bones *in vitro*. *Calc. Tiss. Int.* **40**: 323-331

Loutit, J. F. and Nisbet, N. W. (1979) Resorption of bone. *Lancet* ii: 26-28

Loutit, J. F. and Nisbet, N. W. (1982) The origin of the osteoclast. *Immunology* **161**: 193-203

Lucht, U. (1971) Acid phosphatase of osteoclasts demonstrated by electron microscopic histochemistry. *Histochemie* **28**: 103-117

Lucht, U. (1973) Effects of calcitonin on osteoclasts *in vivo*: An untrastructural and histochemical study. *Zeitschrift fuer Zellforschung und Mikroskopische Anatomie* **145**: 75-82

Lucht, U. and Maunsbach, A. B. (1973) Effects of parathyroid hormone on osteoclasts *in vivo*: an ultrastructural and histochemical study. *Zeitschrift fuer Zellforschund und Mikroskopische Anatomie* **145**: 75-82

MacDonald, B. R., Mundy, G. R., Clark, S., Wang, E. A., Kuehl, T. J., Stanley, E. R. and Roodman, G. D. (1986) Effect of human recombinant CSF-GM and highly purified CSF-1 on the formation of multinucleated cells with osteoclast characteristics in long-term bone marrow cultures. *J. Bone & Min. Res.* **1**: 227-232

MacIntyre, I. (1983) The physiological actions of calcitonin. *Triangle* **22**: 69-74

McSheehy, P. M. J. and Chambers, T. J. (1986a) Osteoblastic cells mediate osteoclastic responsiveness to PTH. *Endocrinology* **118**: 824-828

McSheehy, P. M. J. and Chambers, T. J. (1986b) Osteoblast-like cells in the presence of parathyroid hormone release soluble factor that stimulates osteoclastic bone resorption. *Endocrinology* **119**: 1654-1659

Marchisio, P. C., Cirillo, D., Laldini, L., Primavera, M. V., Tei, A. and Zambonin-Zallone, A. (1984) Cell-substratum interaction of cultured avian osteoclasts is mediated by specific adhesion structures. *J. Cell Biol.* **99**: 1696-1705

Marks, S. C. (1984) The origin of osteoclasts. *J. Oral Pathol.* **12**: 226-256

Marks, S. C. and Walker, D. G. (1981) The haematogenous origin of osteoclasts: experimental evidence from osteopetrotic (microphthalmic) mice treated with spleen cells from beige mouse donors. *Amer. J. Anat.* **161**: 1-10

Martin, J. T. and Partridge, N. C. (1981) Initial events in the activation of bone cells by parathyroid hormone, prostaglandins and calcitonin. In: *Hormonal Control of Calcium Metabolism*. (D. V. Cohn, R. V. Talmage, J. C. Matthews, Eds.). Excepta Medica Int. Congress Series, no. 511, pp 147-156

Miller, S. C. (1978) Rapid activation of the medullary bone osteoclast cell surface by parathyroid hormone. *J. Cell Biol.* **76**: 615-618

Miller, S. C. (1985) The rapid appearance of acid phosphatase activity at the developing ruffled border of parathyroid activated medullary bone osteoclasts. *Calc. Tiss. Int.* **37**: 526-529

Miller, S. C., Bowman, B. M and Myers, R. L. (1984) Morphological and ultrastructural aspects of the activation of avian medullary osteoclasts by parathyroid hormone. *Anatomical Record* **208**: 223-231

Minkin, C. and Jennings, J. M. (1972) Carbonic anhydrase and bone remodeling: sulphonamide inhibition of bone resorption in organ culture. *Science* **176**: 1031

Murad, F., Brewer, H. B. and Vaughan, M. (1970) Effect of thyrocalcitonin on adenosine 3'5' cyclic monophosphate formation in rat kidney and bone. *Proc. Natl. Acad. Sci. USA* **65**: 446-453

Nicholson, G. C., Livesey, S. A., Moseley, J. M. and Martin, T. J. (1986a) Actions of calcitonin, parathyroid hormone, and prostaglandin E_2 on cyclic AMP formation in chicken and rat osteoclasts. *J. Cell Biochem.* **31**: 229-241

Nicholson, G. C., Moseley, J. M., Sexton, P. M., Mendelsohn, F. A. O. and Martin, T. J. (1986b) Abundant calcitonin receptors in isolated rat osteoclasts. *J. Clin. Invest.* **78**: 355-360

Nijweidge, P. J., Vrijheid-Lammers, T., Mulder, R. J. P. and Blok, J. (1985) Cell surface antigens on osteoclasts and related cells in the quail studied with monoclonal antibodies. *Histochemistry* **83**: 315-324

Norimatsu, H., Vander Wiel, C. J. and Talmage, C. V. (1978) Electron microscope study of the effects of calcitonin on bone cells and their extracellular milieu. *Clin. Orthop. Rel. Res.* **139**: 250-258

O'Grady, R. L. and Camerson, D. A. (1971) Demonstration of binding sites of parathyroid hormone in bone cells. In: *Endocrinology 1971: Proceedings of the 3rd Int. Symposium.* pp 374-379. Heinemann, London

Osdoby, P., Oursler, M. J. and Anderson, F. (1986) The osteoblast and osteoclast cytodifferentiation. In: *Progress in Developmental Biology.* Part B, pp 409-414. Alan Liss Inc. New York

Oursler, M. J., Bell, L. V., Clevinger, B. and Osdoby, P. (1985) Identification of osteoclast-specific monoclonal antibodies. *J. Cell Biol.* **100**: 1592-1600

Paradiso, A. M., Tsien, R. Y. and Machen, T. E. (1985) Na^+,H^+ exchange in gastric glands as measured with a cytoplasmic-trapped fluorescent pH indicator. *Proc. Natl. Acad. Sci. USA.* **81**: 7436-7440

Partridge, N. C., Hillyard, C. J., Nolan, R. D. and Martin, T. J. (1985) Regulation of prostaglandin production by osteoblast-rich calvarial cells. *Prostaglandins* **30**: 527-539

Partridge, N. C., Alcorn, D., Michelangeli, V. P., Kemp, B. E., Ryan, G. B and Martin, T. J. (1981a) Functional properties of hormonally responsive cultured normal and malignant rat osteoblastic cells. *Endocrinology* **108**: 213-219

Partridge, N. C., Kemp, B. E., Veroni, M. C. and Martin, T. J. (1981b) Activation of adenosine 3′,5′-monophosphate-dependent protein kinase in normal and malignant bone cells by parathyroid hormone, prostaglandin E_2 and prostacyclin. *Endocrinology* **108**: 220-225

Parvinen, E-K., Slot, J. W. and Vaarianen, H. K. (1987) Osteoclast acidifying enzymes, carbonic anhydrase II and H^+,K^+ATPase immunogold localisation on ultracryosections. *Calc. Tiss. Int.* Suppl. 2, Vol. **41**: p 20, abs. OP35

Pharoah, M. J. and Heersche, J. N. M. (1985) 1,25 dihydroxyvitamin D_3 causes an increase in the number of osteoclast-like cells in cat bone marrow cultures. *Calc. Tiss. Int.* **37**: 276-281

Penniston, J. T. (1982) Plasma membrane Ca^{2+}-pumping ATPases. *Ann. New York Acad. Sci.* **402**: 296

Perry, H. M., Skogen, W., Chappel, J. C., Wilner, G. D., Kahn, A. J. and Teitelbaum, S. L. (1987) Conditioned medium from osteoblast-like cells mediate parathyroid hormone-induced bone resorption. *Calc. Tiss. Int.* **40**: 298-300

Raina, V. (1972) Normal osteoid tissue. *J. Clin. Path.* **25**: 229-232

Raisz, L. G. and Martin, T. J. (1984) Prostaglandins in bone and mineral metabolism. In: *Bone & Min Res Ann.* **2**: 286-310.(W. A. Peck, Ed.) Elsevier Science Pubs, Amsterdam. (1984).

Rao, L. G., Heersche, J. N. M., Marchu, L. L. and Sturtridge, W. (1981) Immunohistochemical demonstration of calcitonin binding to specific cell types in fixed rat bone tissue. *Endocrinology* **108**: 1982-1992

Rao, L. G., Murray, T. M. and Heersche, J. N. M. (1983) Immunohistochemical demonstration of parathyroid hormone binding to specific cell types in fixed rat bone tissue. *Endocrinology* **112**: 805-810

Rettenmier, C. W., Sacca, R., Furman, W. L., Roussel, M. F., Holt, J. T., Nienhuis, A. W., Stanley, E. R. and Sherr, C. J. (1986) Expression of the human c-fms protoncogene product (colony-stimulating factor-1 receptor) on peripheral blood mononuclear cells and choricarcinoma cells. *J. Clin. Invest.* **77**: 1740-1746

Rifkin, B. R., Auszmann, J. M., Kleckner, A. P., Vernillo, A. T. and Fine, A. S. (1988) Calcitonin stimulates cAMP accumulation in chicken osteoclasts. *Life Sciences* **42**: 779-804

Ringel, R. E., Brenner, J. I., Haney, P. J., Burns, J. E., Moulton, A. L. and Berman, M. A. (1982) Prostaglandin-induced periostitis: a complication of long-term PGE$_1$ infusion in an infant with congenital heart disease. *Radiology* 142: 657-658

Roberts, W. E. (1975) Cell population dynamics of periodontal ligament stimulated with parathyroid extract. *Amer. J. Anat.* 143: 363-370

Rodan, G. A., Bourret, L. A., Harvey, A. and Mervi, T. (1975) 3',5' cyclic GMP: Mediators of the mechanical effects on bone modelling. *Science* 189: 467-469

Rodan, B., Wesolowski, G. and Rodan, G. A. (1986) Clonal differences in prostaglandin synthesis among osteosarcoma cell lines. *J. Bone & Min. Res.* 1: 213-220

Roodman, G. D., Ibbotson, K. J., MacDonald, B. R., Kuehl, T. J. and Mundy, G. R. (1985) 1,25 dihydroxyvitamin D$_3$ causes formation of multinucleated cells with several osteoclastic characteristics in cultures of primate marrow. *Proc. Natl. Acad. Sci. USA.* 82: 8213-8217

Rouleau, M. F., Warshawsky, H. and Goltzman, D. (1986) Parathyroid hormone binding *in vivo* to renal, hepatic and skeletal tissues of the rat using a radioautographic technique. *Endocrinology* 118: 919-931

Rubin, C. T. and Lanyon, L. E. (1984) Regulation of bone formation by applied dynamic loads. *J. Bone Joint Surg.* 66A: 397-402

Sakamoto, S. and Sakamoto, M. (1984) Osteoblast collagenase: collagenase synthesis by clonally-derived mouse osteogenic cells. *Biochem. Int.* 9: 51-59

Sakamoto, S. and Sakamoto, M. (1985) On the possibility that bone matrix collagen is removed prior to bone mineral during cell-mediated bone resorption. **In:** *Current Advances in Skeletogenesis.* (A. Ornoy, A. Harell and J. Sela, Eds.). pp 65-70. Elsevier Science Pubs.

Sakamoto, S. and Sakamoto, M. (1986) Bone collagenase, osteoblasts, and cell mediated bone resorption. **In:** *Bone & Min. Res. Ann.* 4: pp 49-102. (W. A. Peck, Ed.). Pub. Elsevier Science Pubs, Amsterdam

Sakamoto, S., Sakamoto, M. and Horton, J. E. (1984) Evidence that collagenase is involved in the mechanism of bone resorption stimulated with parathyroid hormone: a study in two difference culture systems. **In:** *Endocrine Control of Bone and Calcium Metabolism.* (D. V. Cohn, F. Fujita, J. T. Potts and R. Va. Talmage, Eds.). pp 140-143. Elsevier Science Pubs. (1984).

Salmon, D. M., Azria, M. and Zanelli, J. M. (1983) Quantitative cytochemical responses to exogenously administered calcitonins in rat kidney and bone cells. *Molecular & Cell. Endocrinology* 33: 293-304

Sato, K., Kasono, K., Fujii, Y., Kawakami, M., Tsushima, T. and Shizume, K. (1987) Tumour necrosis factor a stimulates mouse osteoblast-like cells (MC3T3-E$_1$) to produce macrophage-colony stimulating activity and prostaglandin E$_2$. *Biochem. Biophys. Res. Commun.* 145: 323-329

Schatzmann, H. J. (1985) Calcium extrusion across the plasma membrane by the calcium pump and the Ca^{2+}Na$^+$ exchange system. **In:** *Calcium and Cell Physiology.* (D. Marme, Ed.). pp 19-52. Springer-Verlag, Berlin

Scheven, B. A. A., Visser, J. W. M. and Nijweide, P. J. (1986) *In vitro* osteoclast generation from different bone marrow fractions, including a highly-enriches haemopoietic stem cell population. *Nature* 321: 79-81

Schneider, G. B. and Byrnes, J. E. (1983) The cellular specificity of the cure for neonatal osteopetrosis in the rat. *Exp. Cell Biol.* 51: 44-50

Schneider, G. B. and Relfson, M. (1988) The effects of transplantation of granulocyte-macrophage progenitors on bone resorption in osteopetrotic rats. *J. Bone & Min. Res.* 3: 225-232

Silve, C. M., Hradek, G. T., Jones, A. L. and Arnand, C. D. (1982) Parathyroid hormone receptor in intact embryonic chicken bone: characterization and cellular localisation. *J. Cell Biol.* 94: 379-386

Singer, F. R., Melvin, K. E. W. and Mills, B. G. (1976) Acute effects of calcitonin on osteoclasts in man. Clin. Endrinology 5: Suppl. 333s-3340s

Sly, W. S., Hewett-Emmett, D., Whyte, M. P., Lu, Y-S. L. and Tashian, R. E. (1983) Carbonic anhydrase II deficiency identified as the primary defect in the autosomal recessive syndrome of osteopetrosis with renal tubular acidosis and cerebral calcification. Proc. Natl. Acad. Sci. USA. 80: 2725

Snipes, R. G., Lam, K. W., Dodd, R. C., Gray, T. K. and Cohen, M. S. (1986) Acid phosphatase in mononuclear phagocytes and the U937 cell line: monocyte-derived macrophages express tartrate-resistant acid phosphatase. Blood 67: 729-734

Sone, K., Tashiro, M., Fujinaga, T., Romomasa, T., Tokuyama, K. and Kuirome, T. (1980) Long-term does prostaglandin E_1 administration. J. Paediatrics 97: 866-867

Stern, P. H., Krieger, N. S., Nissenson, R. A., Williams, R. D., Winkler, M. E., Derynck, G. and Strewler, G. J. (1985) Human transforming growth factor-alpha stimulates bone resorption in vitro. J. Clin. Invest. 76: 2016-2019

Takahasi, N., MacDonald, B. R., Hon, J., Winkler, M. E., Derynck, R., Mundy, G. R. and Roodman, G. D. (1986) Recombinant human transforming growth factor-alpha stimulates the formation of osteoclast-like cells in long-term human marrow cultures. J. Clin. Invest. 78: 894-898

Takahashi, N., Yamama, H., Yoshiki, S., Roodman, D. G., Mundy, G. R., Jones, S. J., Boyde, A. and Suda, T. (1988) Osteoclast-like cell formation and its regulation by osteotropic hormones in mouse marrow cultures. Endocrinology 122: 1373-1382

Tashjian, A. H., Vaelkels, E. F., Goldhaber, P. and Levine, L. (1973) Prostaglandins, bone resorption and hypercalcaemia. Prostaglandins 3: 515-524

Tashjian, A. H., Voelkel, E. F., Lazzaro, M., Goad, D., Bosma, T. and Levine, L. (1987) Tumour necrosis factor-a (cachectin) stimulates bone resorption in mouse calvaria by a prostaglandin-mediated mechanism. Endocrinology 120: 2029-2036

Testa, N. G., Allen, T. D., Lajtha, L. G., Onions, D. and Jarret, O. (1981) Generation of osteoclasts in vitro. J. Cell Sci. 47: 127-137

Tei, A., Blair, H., Kahn, A., Knosek, J., Koziol, C., Zambonin-Zallone, A., Teitelbaum, S. and Schlesinger, P. (1987) Intracellular pH regulation of isolated osteoclasts by chloride/bicarbonate exchange. J. Bone & Min. Res. 2: Suppl. 1, abs. 276

Thomson, B. M., Atkinson, S. J., Reynolds, J. J. and Meickle, M. C. (1987) Degradation of type I collagen fibres by mouse osteoblasts is stimulated by 1,25 dihydroxyvitamin D_3 and inhibited by human recombinant TIMP. Biochem. Biophys. Res. Commun. 148: 596-602

Thomson, B. M., Saklatvala, J. and Chambers, T. J. (1986) Osteoblasts mediate interleukin 1 responsiveness of bone resorption by rat osteoclasts. J. Exp. Med. 104: 104-112

Thomson, B. M., Mundy, G. R. and Chambers, T. J. (1987) Tumor necrosis factors a and b induce osteoblastic cells to stimulate osteoclastic bone resorption. J. Immunol. 138: 775-779

Van Tran, P., Vignery, A. and Baron, R. (1982) Cellular kinetics of the bone remodelling sequence in the rat. Anat. Rec. 202: 445-451

Veda, K., Saito, A., Nakano, K., Aoshima, M., Yokoto, M., Muraoka, R. and Iwaya, T. (1980) Cortical hyperosteosis following long-term administration of prostaglandin E_1 in infants with cyanotic congenital heart disease. J. Paediatrics 97: 834-836

Vaes, G. (1968) On the mechanism of bone resorption. The action of parathyroid hormone on the excretion and synthesis of lysosomal enzymes and on the extracellular release of acid by bone cells. J. Cell Biol. 39: 676-684

Vaes, G. (1972) Inhibitory actions of calcitonin on resorbing bone explants and on their release of lysosomal hydrolases. J. Dent. Res. Suppl. to No. 2, 51, 363-366

Vanderwiel, C. J. (1980) An ultrastructural study of the components which make up the resting surface of bone. Metab. Bone Dis. & Rel. Res. 25: 109-116

Wallach, D., Davies, P., Bechtel, P., Willingham, M. and Paston, I. In: *Advances in Cyclic Nucleotide Research*, vol 9. (W. J. George and L. J. Ignarro, Eds.). pp 371-380. Raven Press, New York

Warshafsky, B., Aubin, J. E. and Heersche, J. N. M. (1985) Cytoskeleton rearrangements during calcitonin-induced changes in osteoclast motility *in vitro. Bone* 6: 179-185

Warshawsky, H., Goltzman, D., Rouleau, M. F. and Bergeron, J. J. M. (1980) Direct in-vivo demonstration by autoradiography of specific binding sites for calcitonin in skeletal and renal tissues of the rat. *J. Cell Biol.* 85: 682-694

Zaidi, M., Fuller, K., Bevis, P. J. R., Gaines, R. E., Das, Chambers, T. J. and MacIntyre, I. (1987) Calcitonin gene-related peptide inhibits osteoclastic bone resorption - a comparative study. *Calc. Tiss. Int.* 40: 149-154

Yu, H., Wells, H., Ryan, W. J. and Lloyd, W. (1976) Effect of prostaglandins and other drugs on the cyclic AMP content of cultured bone cells. *Prostaglandins* 12: 501-513

7

Bone Resorbing Cells and Human Clinical Conditions

BARBARA G. MILLS
University of Southern California
Orthopaedic Hospital
Bone Physiology Laboratory
University Park
Los Angeles, California

Postmenopausal and Senile Osteoporosis
Osteoporosis and Osteopenia
Idiopathic Osteoporosis
Rheumatoid Arthritis
Osteoarthritis
Functional Failure
Metabolic Bone Disease
Circulatory Disturbances
Avascular Necrosis
Blood Dyscrasias
Sickle Cell Disease
Hemophilia
Gastrointestinal Disorders
Malabsorption of Vitamins and Minerals
Chronic Liver Disease
Hormonal Disorders
Diabetes Mellitus
Estrogen
Testosterone
Adrenal Hormones
Thyroid Excess and Deficiency
Hyperthyroidism
Hypothyroidism
Calcitonin
Parathyroid Function
Primary Hyperparathyroidism
Hypoparathyroidism
Chronic Renal Failure, with Uremia
Renal Osteodystrophy
Nephrotic Syndrome
Treatment by Chronic Dialysis
Renal Transplants
Hypophosphatemic Rickets and Osteomalacia
Results of Therapeutic Intervention
Immobilization or Disuse
Heparin Therapy
Prostheses and Implants
Chronic Drug Intake

> Fluorides
> Anticonvulsants
> Diphosphonates
> Corticoids
> Cytotoxic Drugs

Idiopathic
> Genetic
> Osteogenesis Imperfecta Congenita and Tarda
> Osteopetrosis
> Pycnodysostosis
> Lower Motor Neuron Degeneration with Skeletal Manifestations
> Skeletal Dysgenesis
> Klinefelter's Syndrome
> Storage Diseases
> Hypophosphatemia
> Hyperphosphatasia
> Systemic Mastocytosis
> Hyperoxaluria
> Osteitis Deformans
> Fibrogenesis Imperfecta Ossium
> Ectopic Bone Resorption

Bone Cysts
> Simple
> Aneurysmal Bone Cysts
> Florid Osseous Dysplasia

Neoplasms
Benign
> Fibrous Dysplasia
> Osteochondroma
> Benign Osteoblastoma
> Giant Cell Tumor

Malignant
> Medullary Thyroid Cancer
> Fibrosarcoma
> Osteosarcoma
> Malignant Giant Cell Tumor
> Multinucleated Giant Cells in the Stroma of Malignant Tumors
> Malignant Giant Cell Tumors of Soft Tissues

Introduction

The study of man and his ailments has preoccupied scholars and healers since earliest times. The marks of disease are engraved on bone to survive through the ages (Wellesley, 1964). This chapter will concentrate on bone resorbing cells that play a part in the pathophysiology of human skeletal disease.

Bone resorbing cells and their functional characteristics have been described in preceding chapters in this volume and in recent reviews (Bonucci, 1981; Chambers, 1985, 1988). In order to discuss bone resorbing cells observed in clinical conditions, we shall adhere to definitions of resorbing cells based on morphologic cell characteristics, and not attempt to resolve controversies that are beyond the scope of this chapter and are included in the recently published pathologic discussions of Teitelbaum (1985) and others. In this chapter we will employ the following descriptive criteria to define resorbing cells, as found in human tissues.

Osteoclast

Osteoclasts in normal humans of various ages and osteoclasts from animals have many of the same well known morphologic characteristics described in many publications since that of Kolliker in 1873. Osteoclasts, by definition, are large multinucleated cells with a ruffled border (Hall, 1975) and sealing zone (Holtrop, 1977) that resorb bone (Fig. 1). [Mononuclear cells that have these characteristics are found by electron microscopy on bone surfaces that have the frayed appearance or "brush border" of osteoclastic bone resorption (Ham et al., 1979). They may represent a mononuclear osteoclast or only part of a larger osteoclast. These cells will not be referred

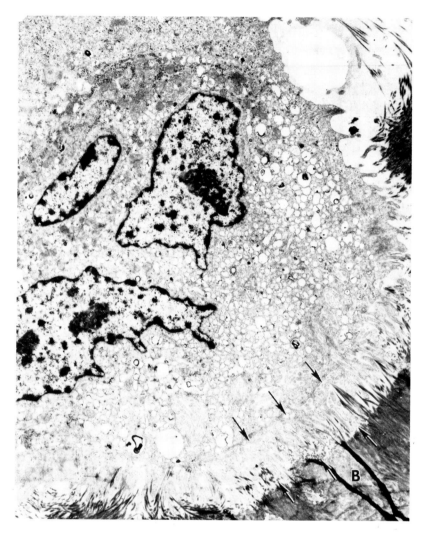

Fig. 1 Brush border of decalcified bone matrix (B) with interdigitating cytoplasmic components of ruffled border of osteoclast from a patient with fibrous dysplasia. Note cross striations of collagen fibrils as well as cellular components in cytoplasmic extensions (arrows). Collagen fibrils appear to be tapered toward the osteoclast. Magn. × 13,000

to as osteoclasts]. Using a strict definition, cells removed from the surface by one or two cell diameters cannot be called osteoclasts, even though in most circumstances the giant cells probably are functional non-resorbing os-

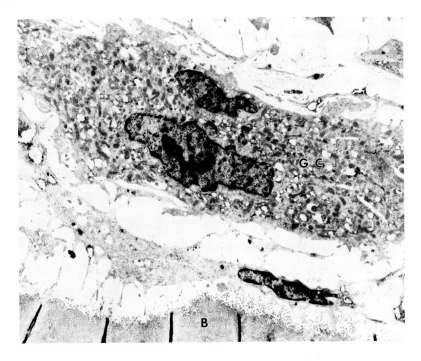

Fig. 2 Multinucleated cell (GC) with appearance of osteoclast but not interdigitated with bone surface from normal human adult bone (B). Magn. × 10,000

teoclasts in transit (Fig. 2). Osteoclasts have receptors for calcitonin, unique surface antigens, (Chambers, 1988) characteristic enzymes and respond to certain humoral factors (Minkin *et al.*, 1986). Fetal osteoclasts are capable of resorbing bone but may not respond to calcitonin with the same changes in motility or morphology as rat osteoclasts (Murrills *et al.*, 1989). Osteoclasts are not "born" and do not "die" in any well described way according to Young (1962) and Bonucci (1981). There are different morphologic forms of osteoclasts in pathologic bone which may represent different stages in the life cycle of osteoclasts, with differing potential for resorption of bone. Increased or decreased overall numbers of osteoclasts, changes in the number of multinucleated cells which show a ruffled border, changes in the extent of the ruffled border and sealing zone, increased or decreased numbers of nuclei, changes in mitochondria, endoplasmic reticulum, golgi apparatus and vacuolization are the most common ultrastructural observations in pathologic material. A disorganized arrangement of cells (Burkhardt *et al.*, 1984) and the appearance of inclusions in the nucleus or cytoplasm of osteoclasts in certain diseases are less common (Yabe *et al.*, 1986; Beneton *et al.*, 1987).

Histomorphometry is a method of evaluating the effects of osteoclastic action on the trabecular bone volume, the total bone density and the cortical thickness in clinical specimens (Meunier *et al.*, 1985). Iliac crest biopsy is a good predictor of the amount of trabecular bone, but not of cortical bone (Sedlin *et al.*, 1963; Podenphant *et al.*, 1986). Biopsies and surgical specimens have been used to evaluate the intersample variations either for a group or for one single patient. For each parameter the intersample variation differs according to the diagnosis but is much lower for groups of 10 and 20 patients (Chavassieux *et al.*, 1985).

Chondroclasts

These cells are morphologically identical to osteoclasts except that the matrix they resorb is calcified cartilage.

Odontoclasts

Odontoclasts are multinucleated giant cells much like osteoclasts except that they are found resorbing human primary teeth. These multinucleated cells exhibit varying numbers of nuclei and it is believed that there is an optimum size for resorption of teeth related to the development of an efficient ruffled border during periods of active resorption (Addison, 1978).

Giant Cells

Giant cells are multinucleate cells containing from two, to more than two hundred, nuclei which exist in two forms, as discussed by Mariano and Spector (1974). Foreign body giant cells form and participate in the phagocytosis of alien indigestible particulate matter, including dead bone. Their nuclei are dispersed throughout the cytoplasm. Neoplasms may contain multinucleated cells which may be clustered in an area adjacent to, but not necessarily against, bone (Fig. 3). Pathological bone resorption may be induced locally by neoplastic or inflammatory tissues that produce factors such as interleukin I, tumour necrosis factor and lymphotoxin (Chambers, 1988).

Langhans giant cells differ from foreign body giant cells in that the nuclei are distributed around the periphery of the cell. This configuration is maintained by a critical equilibrium between contractile cytoskeletal components with opposing actions. Loss of this equilibrium results in reversion to the arrangement of nuclei typical for "foreign body" multinucleate giant cells (Rigby, 1984). Langhans cells are rarely found in bone except in

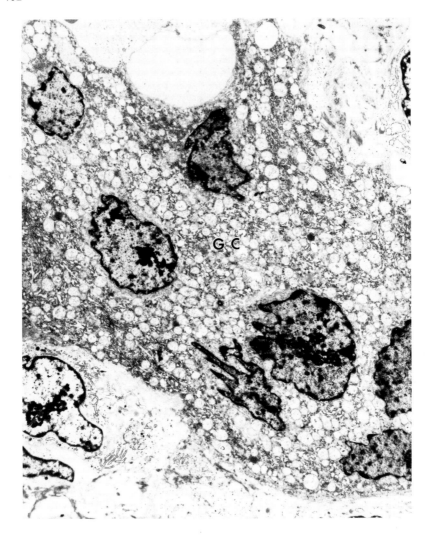

Fig. 3 Multinucleated cell (GC) without ruffled border, pseudopodia or visible relationship to bone in a giant cell tumor of bone. Note mitochondria are small, round and swollen due to anoxia or artefact of fixation. Magn. × 8,500

granulomatous lesions such as tuberculosis, or sarcoid (Abdelwahib and Norman, 1988).

Macrophage

Macrophages are cells specialized in the phagocytosis of foreign particles, including devitalized bone particles from which they release calcium and hydroxyproline (Teitelbaum, 1979). Both mononucleated and multinucleated macrophages lack a true ruffled border although they have specialized membrane infoldings that participate in phagocytosis. An abundance of cell processes is thought to be an indicator of heightened phagocytic activity (Ghadially, 1985). They do not excavate bone slices readily attacked by osteoclasts (Chambers and Horton, 1984). Others disagree and find that bone marrow contains monocytic cells that are osteoclast-like precursors that when cultured form multinucleated cells that resorb sperm whale dentine (Takahashi *et al.*, 1989). Macrophages contain specific antigenic markers absent from osteoclasts (Hume, 1984).

Histiocyte

The histiocyte is found in tissues and serves the function of a sedentary, local macrophage. The term originated from the tissue where the immobile macrophage was observed. The term "macrophage" is now preferred by most writers although genetic and neoplastic bone lesions are described using this term (McCarthy *et al.*, 1979).

Osteocyte

The osteocyte is the bone cell sometimes classified as a bone resorbing cell when it is found in an area of bone resorption and has an enlarged lacunae or is associated with roughened bone matrix channels encasing cellular extensions (observed in the electron microscope, Fig. 4). The term "osteocytic osteolysis" has been proposed by Belanger (1971) for this phenomenon. The cells responsible produce alkaline phosphatase and protease. Osteolysis is enhanced by a variety of stimuli, notably hyperparathyroidism (McClean, 1968).

Resorption in the Healthy Human

Environmental Factors

Environmental factors may cause skeletal damage in the healthy individual. Bone responds with a healing mechanism appropriate to the kind and severity of the damage. The healing process removes dead bone or other

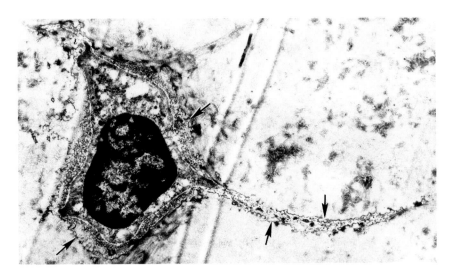

Fig. 4 Osteocytic osteolysis showing roughening of walls of matrix channels of cellular extensions (arrows) and accumulation of lead stained debris probably protein or lipid containing, in space surrounding osteocyte in bone of patient with medullary carcinoma. Magn. × 18,000

foreign debris by means of resorbing cells and remodels the new bone according to the mechanical lines of stress (Bogumill and Schwam, 1984).

Fractures

The process of replacement and repair is going on continuously in the normal skeleton and the mechanisms involved in fracture healing are no different (McKibben, 1978) other than for differences depending on whether the proces occurs in compact or cancellous bone. Osteoclasts must ream out a tunnel in dead compact bone down which a blood vessel follows. In trabecular bone the cells are never far from blood vessels and the process takes place on the surface of the trabeculae. Bone debris, dead tissue and foreign bodies are removed by a foreign body response while callus remodeling is accomplished primarily by chondroclasts or osteoclasts. However, dead bone may form a mechanical link to living tissue if the dead bone is in normal alignment in accordance with Wolff's law (McKibben, 1978). Simmons (1980) describes bone of the osseous callus becoming trabecularized even beyond the zone of osteoclastic activity and suggests that 1% of osteocytes are normally in a resorptive phase. Stress or fatigue fractures, although caused by less severe trauma, normally heal at the same rate and by the same mechanism as other fractures. Non-unions are the result of a failure to replace the injured tissue by the normal bony callus and usually are devoid of resorbing cells.

Osteomyelitis

Osteomyelitis may occur as sequelae of traumatic injury, especially following vehicular and industrial accidents. The association of neurovascular and soft tissue injury increases the risk of recurrent sepsis, Fitzgerald, 1986. Postoperative wound infection and septic arthritis may produce secondary sepsis. Infections around implants consist of a rich cellular matrix of polymorphonuclear leukocytes and lymphocytes located between the acrylic cement and the osseous tissue. Infections are sometimes walled off by new bone or contain dead bone (involucrum). Osteoclastic resorption of cancellous bone occurs adjacent to the acrylic cement and fibrous membrane (Fitzgerald, 1986).

Granuloma

Multinucleate giant cells (central giant cell granuloma) are formed by cell fusion of mononuclear cells (Schulz et al., 1976). The giant cells are localized at trabecular surfaces of newly formed woven bone and have a high dehydrogenase activity and lack alkaline phosphatase activity. The multinucleate giant cells associated with soft tissue granulomas such as granulomatous myositis, familial granulomatosis, lymphogranuloma, and granulomatous cholangitis are characterized by increased activities of nonspecific esterase and tartrate-sensitive acid phosphatase (Elleder, 1986). There are no peptidases, nor any tartrate-resistant acid phosphatase. In contrast, the subgroup of osteoclasts, giant cell tumors of bone, and giant cell tumors of soft parts have low activity of nonspecific esterase, high tartrate resistent acid phosphatase and peptidases. These giant cell containing granulomas are not believed to be identical with non-ossifying fibromas, Slootweg, 1988. However, the granuloma giant cells are thought to be identical with osteoclasts, Chambers, 1988.

Nutritional Inadequacy

Nutritional inadequacy or abnormality may have the effect of inducing abnormal bone resorption, often coupled with inadequate bone production or accumulation of uncalcified or abnormal matrix that cannot be remodeled normally. Dietary osteopenia can also occur due to inadequate mastication in the elderly, fad diets or malabsorption in chronic illness (Aegerter and Kirkpatrick, 1968).

Calcium

Measurements of metacarpal bone loss in adults of three countries differing markedly in calcium intake (Guatamala, El Salvador, and the United States) have failed to reveal any differences in aging osteopenia. It was concluded that aging bone loss is universal and independent of diet (Draper, 1986). Arctic Eskimo diet has changed since the abandonment of bone chewing in modern times and the higher serum phosphorus and lower serum calcium levels suggest that parathyroid stimulation and increased bone resorption account for the unusually rapid rate of bone loss recorded in adults (Mazess and Mathur, 1974).

Phosphorus

Experiments on human adults indicate that they may be more tolerant of phosphate loads than adult non-human animals. However, high phosphate diets in man stimulate parathyroid activity and bone resorption in man, resulting in increases in urinary hydroxyproline and cyclic AMP, Draper, 1986.

Vitamin A

Vitamin A deficiency causes decreased resorption of bone, concurrent with retarded growth (Sidransky, 1985). Moreover the coupled replacement of cancellous bone by compact bone ceases to operate. Osteopenia results because remodeling fails to replace the trabecular bone with cortical bone. Excess vitamin A stimulates those osteoclasts involved in modeling and produces rapid consumption of epiphyseal cartilage and acceleration of the remodelling processes in linear growth of bones, according to Wolbach (1947). However, in another study excess vitamin A produced no permanent deformities in 27 children and 9 adults with the exception of one infant given excessive vitamin A (Ruby and Mitel, 1974).

Vitamin D

Vitamin D acts synergistically with parathyroid hormone in its physiologic function and its metabolites are potent stimuli of bone resorption (Teitelbaum, 1985). Calcium is mobilized from bones, resulting in osteoporosis (Sidransky, 1985).

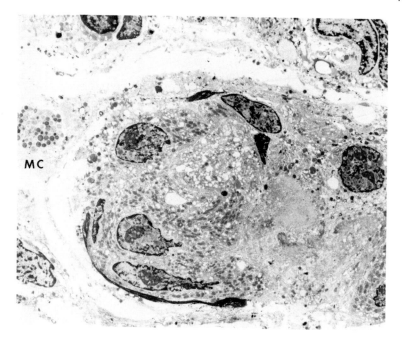

Fig. 5 Cluster of abnormal osteoclast-like cells from osteopenic bone of a patient with severe malabsorption syndrome. Disorganization of the remodeling process is apparent. Note pycnotic appearance of some nuclei and proximity of mast cell (MC). Magn. × 9,000

Inadequate ultraviolet light exposure or inadequate vitamin D intake or food fads can cause primary vitamin D deficiency manifested as rickets and osteomalacia. In children, the ricketic bone does not mineralize, is not resorbed, and results in a weak structure with widened physes and bowed legs.

Decreased circulating vitamin D metabolites resulting from liver disease or kidney disease contribute to secondary vitamin D deficiency. In addition, secondary hyperparathyroidism accompanies the osteomalacia induced by low serum calcium levels (Teitelbaum, 1985). Abnormal vitamin D absorption following gastrectomy can be so severe that pseudo-fractures develop (Eddy, 1971) (Fig. 5). Vitamin D dependent rickets is an inborn error in metabolism that results in defective conversion of 25-hydroxy-vitamin D to 1,25-dihydroxy-vitamin D with all the characteristics of the deficient state including osteomalacia and failure to resorb unmineralized bone (Fraser *et al.*, 1973; Figs 6A and 6B).

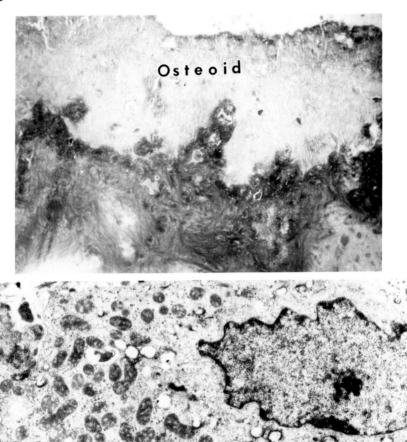

Fig. 6 A. Vitamin D resistent rickets produced this example of osteomalacia (thick layer of [osteoid] layered on surface of bone). Marrow space is seen in upper left. Magn. × 300 **B.** Part of an osteoclast resting on osteomalacic bone surface but not exhibiting a ruffled border or evidence of active resorption. Magn. × 18,000

Chronic Alcoholism

In patients aged 24 to 62 years chronic alcoholism produced radiographic evidence of extensive bone loss in 47 percent of those studied. Bone biopsy specimens confirmed the radiographic diagnosis of osteoporosis (Spencer *et al.*, 1986).

Smoking has also been implicated in bone loss (Daniell, 1976).

Industrial Toxic Chemicals

Lead

During lead intoxication severe damage can be done to osteoclasts, either by uptake of circulating lead or by removal of lead from matrix undergoing resorption. As a result of this accumulation most osteoclasts come to show characteristic nuclear and cytoplasmic inclusion bodies resembling those found in renal tubular cells (Bonucci, 1981). Intranuclear and intracytoplasmic inclusion bodies appear as roundish structures with a central, dense core from which thin filamentous projections radiate outwards (Choie *et al.*, 1975; Eisenstein and Kawanowe, 1975).

Radiation Injury

Necrosis of mature bone and cartilage is unusual and usually related to vascular injury caused by the radiation although there may also be destruction of cells (Vaughan, 1977). Bone-seeking radionuclides and external irradiation produce arrested maturation of growing bone or localized regions of bone resorption, foci of sclerosis, bone necrosis and pathologic fractures in mature bone. Radium produces the same effects. Long term induction of malignant tumors has been documented in radium dial painters (Anderson, 1985).

Radionuclides such as ^{85}Sr and ^{67}Ga are used in clinical diagnosis of necrotic lesions. It has been shown by scanning scintigraphy that ^{67}Ga localizes to Pagetic lesions and can be used to follow the effects of therapy (Waxman, *et al.*, 1980). Ultrastructural radioautography has localized the ^{67}Ga to the nuclei of osteoclasts (Mills *et al.*, 1988a; Figs 7A and 7B).

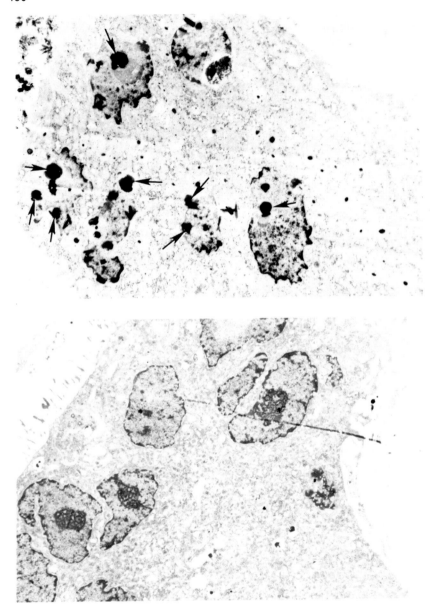

Fig. 7 A. Radioautograph of osteoclast from patient with Paget's disease of bone immediately following bone scan with ^{67}Ga illustrating gallium isotope induced silver grains (arrows) localized over nuclei. Magn. × 6,750 **B.** Same bone sample as above following demineralization and removal of radiogallium prior to autoradiography as negative control. Magn. × 6,750

Degenerative Conditions

Normal Aging

Remodeling continues throughout life but the rate slows as the individual ages. There is an age-related reduction in final bone resorption depth in both sexes but a relative hyper-resorptive state in females aged 31-60 which may be of importance in relation to the accelerated bone loss around the menopause according to Eriksen *et al.* (1985). In young adults it was found that although the osteoclast and osteoblast numbers were normal, the metabolic activity of the osteoblasts was impaired (Hills *et al.*, 1989). On the other hand Melsen and Mosekilde (1978), using tetracycline double-labeling of the iliac trabecular bone in 41 normal adults, found that resorptive surfaces were unrelated to age but higher in males than in females under age 55. Lips *et al.* (1978) agreed that the resorption surfaces are constant with advancing age and that the number of osteoclasts within resorption lacunae remain constant. In contrast Jowsey (1960) found that individuals over 70 years of age may have up to 25 per cent of bone surface occupied by resorption and the resorption cavities are typical of "fast resorption". There is considerable variation among individuals however (Marcus *et al.*, 1983).

Postmenopausal and Senile Osteoporosis

There was no correlation with the patient's age or severity of the bone lesions among postmenopausal women (Fallon *et al.*, 1983). Morphometric heterogeneity was found within a group of 17 osteoporotic women aged 64 ± 7 years compared to age matched normal women and between sequential biopsies (de Vernejoul *et al.*, 1988). The morphologic basis of rapid postmenopausal bone loss is an increase in both the number and the depth of resorption cavities (Parfitt, 1981b) although Eriksen *et al.* (1985) found that the resorption depth below osteoclasts did not vary with age in both men and women.

Over the time period of a year, bone histology showed an annual bone loss in women with postmenopausal osteoporosis that was significantly greater than premenopausal women and healthy postmenopausal women (Elias *et al.*, 1985). Trabecular bone was studied in women aged 53-81 years and by the criteria of acid phosphatase content only 39% of osteoclasts were multinucleate. Even though the osteoclasts were not numerous, the osteoclast activity (in square millimeters of bone resorbed per osteoclast cell unit per day) was significantly greater than the osteoblast activity (Gruber *et al.*, 1986).

Osteoporosis and Osteopenia

Osteoporosis and osteopenia are associated with a number of abnormalities as well as with "normal" aging. Kumar and Riggs (1980) define osteoporosis as a decrease in the amount of bone below the level required to maintain skeletal integrity. The pathogenesis of osteoporosis is determined by an imbalance between whole body rates of resorption and formation according to Parfitt (1982). It is believed to be a heterogeneous condition. In a study comparing biopsies of femoral neck fractures and iliac crest biopsies, it was found that there was a virtual absence of osteoblasts and osteoclasts in the femoral neck of half of the biopsies compared to the iliac crest biopsies. The osteopenia was of the "high turnover" type in the iliac crest and of the "low turnover" type in the femoral neck which suggests that there is different remodeling in different skeletal sites (Frisch and Evantov, 1986). Increased numbers of marrow mast cells have been reported in the osteoporosis of aging (Frame and Nixon, 1968).

Idiopathic Osteoporosis

Less than 45 patients have been reported with this rare condition which is characterized by the development in a previously normal subject of osteoporosis with bone pain shortly before puberty. Quantitative bone histology showed no evidence of excessive active resorption (Smith, 1980). The osteoporosis appeared to be related to an uncoupling of formation from resorption (Perry *et al.*, 1982; Barzel, 1982). There is no apparent increased bone resorption, but rather a decreased bone synthesis (Evans, 1983).

Rheumatoid Arthritis

Patients with long standing rheumatoid arthritis develop thin bones adjacent to the sites of the joint disease as well as in distant, unaffected areas (Duncan, 1972). Destruction of the subchondral bone by pannus is marked by osteoclastic bone resorption at the contact zone (Hough and Sokoloff, 1985). However, the course of rheumatoid arthritis is variable and in one study of newly diagnosed patients, 80% had no evidence of bone erosion after 5 years (Lipsky, 1985). Juvenile degenerative arthritis is often accompanied by juxtaarticular osteoporosis. These bone changes are generally regarded as being due to inflammatory hyperemia and disuse (Bunger, 1984).

Osteoarthritis

Osteoarthritis produces changes due to degeneration and results in painful joints, sometimes relieved by joint replacement. The bone adjacent to the joint may show little change from normal or may show resorption (Fig. 8).

Functional Failure

Metabolic Bone Disease

Metabolic bone disease is the term used to describe bone disease associated with failure of a system or organ that normally helps control bone metabolism. Marked increases occur in osteoblasts and osteoclasts together with the formation of a loose meshwork of undifferentiated mesenchymal cells, fibroblasts, macrophages and capillaries within the osseous spicules or trabeculae. In those diseases characterized by increased remodeling the osteoclastic activity is generally confined to the surface. However, in disturbances of mineral homeostasis the osteoclasts are seen to burrow or tunnel into mineralized bone matrix. In all pathologic resorptive states, the architecture of the bone will be distorted (Bullough *et al.*, 1987). Mesenchymal activation reaches a stage in which orderly osseous remodeling is completely abolished in such disorders as renal osteodystrophy (Fig. 9), primary hyperparathyroidism (Fig. 10), osteomyelitis, plasmacytoma, Paget's disease and metastatic carcinoma (Burkhardt *et al.*, 1984). Bordier and Tun Chot (1973) commented that there are very few histological characteristics specific to metabolic bone disease. Most changes consist of an increase or decrease of the amount of resorption and/or formation. They therefore proposed to use quantitative histology to analyze and record these changes.

Circulatory Disturbances

Increased blood flow is associated with bone loss in several conditions. Hyperemia: Osteolysis is associated with increasing the blood supply above the optimum (Aegerter and Kirkpatrick, 1968). Hemangioma: The so called disappearing bone is caused by an expanding hemangioma (Aegerter and Kirkpatrick, 1968).

Avascular Necrosis

In avascular necrosis subchondral fractures occur. Repair involves living tissue which includes osteoclastic resorption of the subchondral plate and overlying cartilage (McKibben, 1974). When there is avascular necrosis there

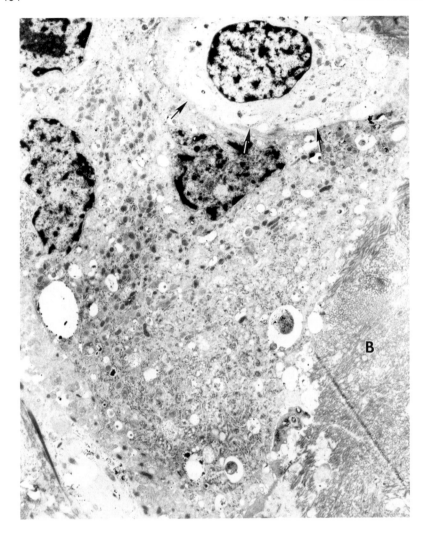

Fig. 8 Cells on bone (B) surface from the head of the femur of a patient with osteoarthritis undergoing a total hip replacement. Note cell being engulfed by osteoclast (arrows). Magn. × 11,000

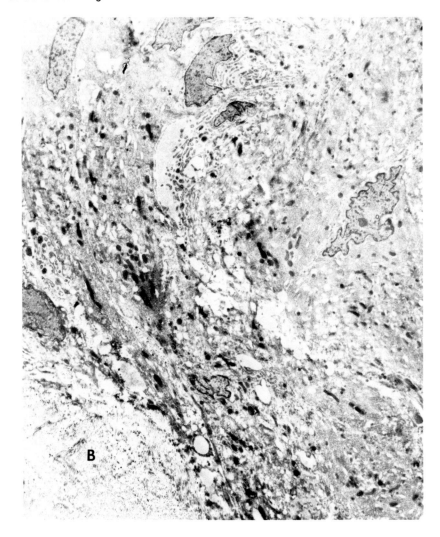

Fig. 9 Disorganization of orderly process of osseous remodeling of bone from a biopsy of the iliac crest of a patient with renal osteodystrophy (bone [B] lower left corner). Magn. × 6,200

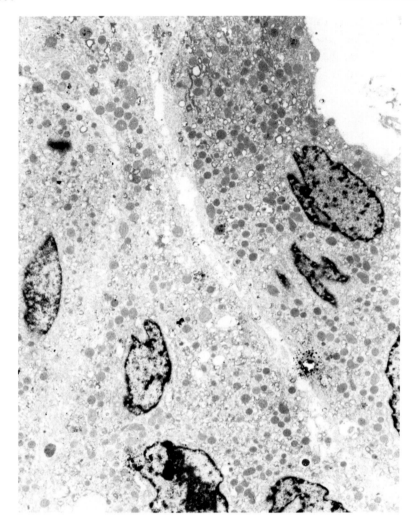

Fig. 10 Multiple osteoclasts and multinucleated cells several layers deep on surface of bone of patient with hypercalcemia due to a parathyoid adenoma prior to treatment. Magn. × 12,500

is very little resorption of dead trabeculae which had not been first, at least partially, encased in living woven bone. In cases where a portion of the femoral head remains viable, other regions of the subchondral plate are reached and resorbed. Repair processes include the appearance of blood vessels and mesenchymal cells (Glimcher and Kinzora, 1979).

Blood Dyscrasias

Abnormalities in the hematologic diseases are often associated with bone destruction because of impingement of marrow or bleeding into bone or joint spaces which in turn stimulates cartilage or bone remodelling to accommodate the mass.

Sickle Cell Disease

In the early stages of sickle cell osteopathy there is little evidence of ischemic necrosis in the bone marrow biopsy. Medullary extension, osteoporosis and necrosis are detected on X-ray. It is during this phase that there is extensive bone destruction (Cabannes and Mambo-Sambo, 1984).

Hemophilia

Bleeding into joints results in the architecture of the articular cartilage being severely disrupted. Hemarthrosis persisting for some days may have mechanical effects on articular cartilage that produce changes in the subchondral layer of bone similar to those of rheumatoid arthritis (Stein and Duthie, 1981).

Gastrointestinal Disorders

Malabsorption of Vitamins and Minerals

Intestinal bypass for the treatment of obesity has resulted in accelerated loss of bone due to persistent intestinal malabsorption of vitamin D and calcium, causing increased net endosteal resorption (Parfitt et al., 1978). According to Teitlebaum et al. (1977) the mechanism is not clear but reflected a defect in bone synthesis rather than over-stimulation of osteoclastic resorption. Bone biopsy failed to reveal changes in bone resorbing cells.

Chronic Liver Disease

Hepatic osteodystrophy (osteoporosis and osteomalacia) has been attributed to a deficiency in vitamin D in chronic liver disease, especially in primary biliary cirrhosis (Long et al., 1978). Cuthbert et al. (1984) described symptoms including fractures and bone pain. In this study, although there was no osteomalacia, histomorphometry detected increased bone resorption which was resolved after vitamin D therapy. Another study found no osteomalacia or osteoporotic bone but a high bone turnover rate which was attributed to the aging process (Shih and Anderson, 1987).

Hormonal Disorders

Diabetes Mellitus

Both insulin-dependent and adult-onset diabetic patients have diminished bone mass whether measured by densitometric or by roentgenographic techniques (Levin et al., 1976). Osteopenia may appear within 5 years after the onset of hyperglycemia (McNair, 1978). Significant loss of trabecular bone mass was found in 37% of male and 25% of female juvenile diabetics. No correlation was found between duration and loss of trabecular bone (Seidl, 1982).

Estrogen

The menopause is the event in women in which ovarian failure is associated with a loss of bone. It can be prevented to some extent by estrogen treatment (Lindsay et al., 1980). For a review see Nordin et al. (1983).

Testosterone

Male hypogonadism causes both cortical and trabecular osteoporosis and altered trabecular architecture. A major risk factor for the development of osteoporosis is a reduction in plasma $1,25(OH)_2D_3$ (Francis et al., 1986).

Adrenal Hormones

Cushing's syndrome is associated with osteoclastic bone resorption (Sissons, 1956). Upon initiating a heavy corticosteroid program a dramatic resorption of bone occurs that diminishes in intensity until a steady state is reached weeks or months later. According to Duncan (1972) there is no therapy such as androgen, estrogens, calcitonin or fluorides that can ameliorate the resorptive stimulus of steroids on bone.

Thyroid Excess and Deficiency

Thyroid hormone stimulates osteoblasts and osteoclasts (Mundy *et al.*, 1976). The mechanism of the calcium disturbance is not clear but parathyroid function is involved. There is a reduced level of 1,25(OH)$_2$ vitamin D but no evidence of a mineralization defect (Goldring and Krane, 1986).

Hyperthyroidism

As early as the 1930s there were reports of excessive bone destruction in hyperthyroidism, with eroded areas of bone filled with connective tissue and osteoclasts. Changes typical of osteitis fibrosa were described (Goldring and Krane, 1986). Histomorphometry has shown increased bone turnover with active bone resorption in cortical bone 16-26 times normal (Melsen and Moskilde, 1977; Mosekilde and Melsen, 1978a, b). Hyperthyroidism results in a shortening of the remodeling period in cortical and trabecular bone (Meunier *et al.*, 1972). The osteoclasts were uniform in size and contained 1 to 5 nuclei per section which is in sharp contrast to hyperparathyroidism or Paget's disease.

Hypothyroidism

Hypothyroidism lengthens the time of remodeling, as determined by tetracycline double labeling (Mosekilde and Melsen, 1978a; Mosekilde, 1979). It was concluded that hypothyroidism decreases the recruitment, maturation and activity of bone cells. Decreased bone resorption and bone formation per unit time results. The reduction in final resorption depth and the increase in the thickness of the bone laid down leads to a positive bone balance (Eriksen *et al.*, 1986a).

Calcitonin

The calcitonin responsive cells are the osteoclast-like cells. Osteoclasts retract their ruffled borders on the side of the cell in contact with bone in response to calcitonin. For this reason calcitonin is used to treat Paget's disease and osteoporosis when it is desired to depress osteoclastic activity.

Parathyroid Function

Normal osteoclastic function, as determined by quantitative histomorphometry, was found in osteoporosis of 57 patients including some with mild suppression of parathyroid function as well as mild secondary hyperparathyroidism (Kleerekoper *et al.*, 1986).

Primary Hyperparathyroidism

Using quantitative histomorphometry, Schenk *et al.* (1973) found that in hyperparathyroidism osteoclast numbers lie, without exception, beyond the normal range by two standard deviations (Fig. 10). Charhon *et al.* (1982) reported a significant increase in remodeling surfaces associated with osteoclasts. The osteoclasts are not markedly different, morphologically, from those found in controls except that there is often a more highly developed brush border, and a greater number of cytoplasmic vacuoles in the hyperparathyroid osteoclasts. Since these findings are considered to be ultrastructural evidence of increased resorption it is probable that osteoclast function is enhanced (Bonucci *et al.*, 1978). Scanning electron microscopy revealed enlarged resorbing surfaces over bone trabeculae (Lindenfelser *et al.*, 1973). Eriksen *et al.* (1986) using histomorphometry, reported that the active resorption period (the function period of osteoclasts and mononuclear cells) was reduced to 19 days, compared to 29 days in normal subjects. However, no difference from normal resorption rates could be detected. The only difference was the significantly shorter quiescent remodeling sequence in the hyperparathyroid patients compared to the matched controls. Thus, there is an indication that the reduction in bone mass observed in hyperparathyroidism may be caused by an irreversible bone loss rather than a more intense cellular resorptive activity during the observed more frequent remodeling cycles. Schulz and colleagues (1977) observed increased numbers of osteoclasts. They attributed the increased numbers of lysosomal vacuoles concentrated at the basal portion of the osteoclast adjacent to the ruffled border as evidence of stimulation of the lysosomal system. The vacuoles represented secondary lysosomes or phagosomes. In another study, daily urinary cyclic AMP levels were compared to PTH plasma levels and to bone resorption parameters by histomorphometry. There was a significant correlation between bone resorption surfaces and urinary cyclic AMP (Bernard *et al.*, 1976).

Hypoparathyroidism

Spontaneous hypoparathyroidism is an uncommon disorder. The bones may be denser than normal, owing to a low rate of osteoclastic resorption. Defective calcification of the dentin is seen in young adults (McClean, 1968). These patients are so sensitive to vitamin D that a sunbath can produce hypercalciuria (Granstrom and Hed, 1966).

Chronic Renal Failure, with Uremia

Renal Osteodystrophy

This term refers to the effect of failing renal function on bone. It includes a complex of osteomalacia, osteitis fibrosa, osteosclerosis and osteoporosis. Sometimes it is impossible to separate the effects in a single patient. The bone usually contains degenerating cells with pycnotic nuclei and loss of organelles and cytoplasm. Bone resorbing cells are often prominent and the osteoclasts may be enlarged, with increased numbers of nuclei and a prominent ruffled border overlying a brush border on the bone surface (Fig. 11). Mononuclear cells testing positive for tartrate resistant acid phosphatase and non-specific esterase negative believed to be precursors to osteoclasts are found on the trabecular surface (Kaye and Henderson, 1988). Renal osteomalacia is a bone disease consisting of an increased accumulation of organic matrix (osteoid) with a reduction in the extent of the calcification front, as a consequence of a defective activity of vitamin D on the osteoblasts and is the commonest complication of chronic renal failure. Osteomalacia was the main pathological feature in 60% of the patients (Maschio et al., 1974). Osteomalacia was associated with increased osteoclastic activity and some degree of bone resorption and bone marrow fibrosis in 13% of the patients. In 27% of the patients the bone tissue was normal.

Nephrotic Syndrome

In adult patients with the nephrotic syndrome, 7% of those with normal renal function had associated bone resorption. Patients with persistent proteinuria are at high risk of osteodystrophy even in the early phases of renal failure (Tessitore et al., 1984).

Treatment by Chronic Dialysis

In a recent study of 59 patients undergoing hemodialysis symptomatic patients demonstrated a three-fold increase in active resorption, a twofold increase in osteoclast numbers and a threefold increase in double label surfaces (Coburn et al., 1983). This increased bone resorption is due to both osteoclastic activity and osteocytic osteolysis according to (Bonucci et al., 1976). All patients in this series showed an increase in bone resorption to such an extent as to be predominant over the observed osteomalacia (Bonucci, 1977a). Osteoclasts were often smaller than normal and present within the trabeculae, which consequently were more or less completely dissected

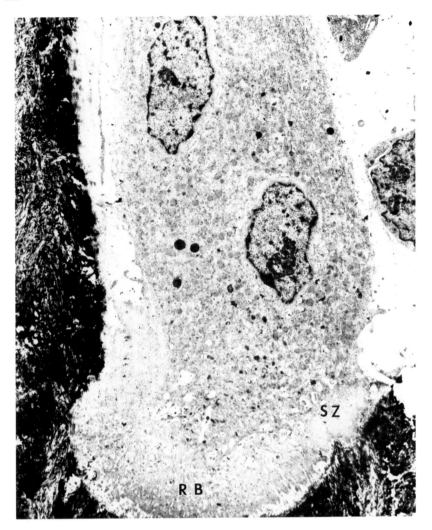

Fig. 11 Osteoclast from an iliac crest biopsy of a patient with chronic renal failure, and secondary hyperparathyroidism. There is a prominent ruffled border (RB) and sealing zones (SZ) are apparent in this undecalcified specimen. Magn. × 7,700

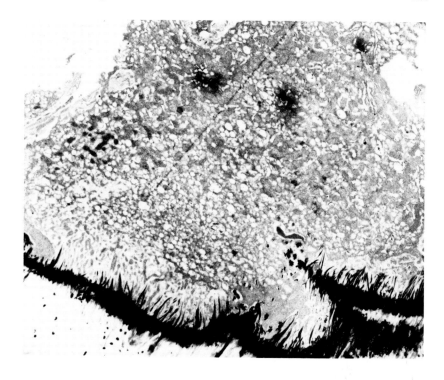

Fig. 12 Electron micrograph of an osteoclast and the brush border on bone following long term hemodialysis illustrating continuing renal osteodystrophy. Magn. × 4,500

(Bonucci, 1977b). Under the electron microscope, the osteoclasts displayed normal morphology. Usually there was a well developed ruffled border which was in contact with disrupted and disaggregated bone matrix (Fig. 12). From 3 to 6 or more nuclei were present in each osteoclast. Mitochondria were numerous and were usually collected in a cytoplasmic area opposite to that of the ruffled border. In some cases, giant cells were found near, but not in contact with the bone matrix. In these cases, the ruffled border was lacking and mitochondria were present throughout the cytoplasm. In cases where the osteoclasts were in contact with osteoid tissue the matrix was not usually resorbed but in some cases uncalcified collagen fibrils were contained within the channels of the ruffled borders as if they were reabsorbed by the osteoclasts. Bone fractures that develop only in patients on hemodialysis were attributed to the failure of hemodialysis to adequately remove the inhibitor(s)

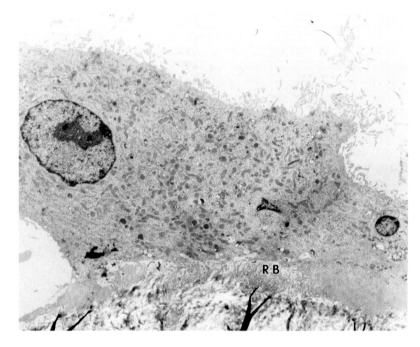

Fig. 13 Long term (more than 5 years) clinically successful renal transplants did not reduce the numbers or activity of osteoclasts in most patients as shown in this electron micrograph of an active osteoclast with ruffled border (RB) from an iliac crest follow-up biopsy. Magn. × 9,000

of calcification which appear to be removed by peritoneal dialysis (Oreopoulos *et al.*, 1971).

In the presence of osteoclasts, most of the osteocytes showed enlarged and irregular lacunae, and the lacunae often seemed to coalesce. The osteocyte canaliculi, too, were enlarged and coalescing. The osteocyte lacunae contained irregularly distributed filamentous and flocculent material and small fragments of collagen fibrils in the pericellular space. However, as emphasized by Sissons (1969), when hyperparathyroidism and osteomalacia are found together in the same subject, osteolytic-like changes of the lacunae could be produced by defective calcification, rather than by periosteocytic osteolysis.

Renal Transplants

Long term results following renal transplants indicated that despite marked chemical and clinical improvement the dystrophic bone did not return to normal even after several years (Fig. 13).

Hypophosphatemic Rickets and Osteomalacia

The circumlacunar, hypomineralized zones found in this disease were shown by scanning electron microscopy to consist of unfused mineral particle clusters. The osteocytes may retard the mineralization apparent in hypophosphatemic rickets rather than act as resorbing cells as in osteocytic osteolysis (Steendijk and Boyde, 1973). Osteoclasts had no characteristics specific to the disease and were adjacent to a brush border (Fig. 14).

Results of Therapeutic Intervention

Immobilization or Disuse

In most cases prolonged immobilization, including paralysis, leads to disuse osteoporosis. The age of space flight has increased interest in the loss of bone due to inactivity or the absence of gravity in healthy individuals (Parfitt, 1981a). The rapid bone loss (1%/week, Mazess and Whedon, 1983) appears to be due to unrestrained osteoclastic activity without controls and regulation (Young et al., 1986), although the resorbing cells are not abnormal. In non-weight bearing bones, there is apparently little loss of compact bone (Mazess and Whedon, 1983). Minaire and colleagues also observed an early increase in the trabecular osteoclastic resorption surfaces and later an increase in size of periosteocytic lacunae, after immobilization (Minaire et al., 1974). In healthy volunteers, osteoclast number was highly increased but after bisphosphonate in treated subjects, the osteoclasts number and osteoid was markedly reduced (Chappard et al., 1989).

Heparin Therapy

Osteoporosis and spinal fractures in patients receiving extended heparin anticoagulant therapy has been described by Griffith et al. (1965) and by Squires and Pinch (1979). Multiple fractures were observed by Jaffee and Willis (1965). However the mechanism of action of heparin in these instances is not entirely clear. Excessive resorption and bone loss has been attributed to a solubilizing effect of heparin on membranes resulting in local collagenase release (Asher and Nichols, 1965).

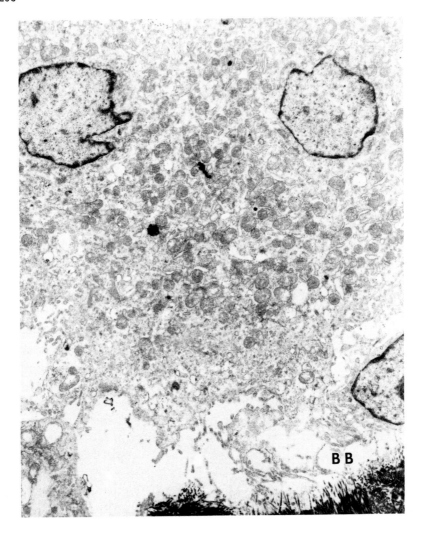

Fig. 14 Osteoclast from a patient with hypophosphatemia adjacent to the brush border (BB) of bone (lower right) with no unusual characteristics. Magn. × 10,000

Prostheses and Implants

Various materials have been used to replace lost bone or provide structural support following skeletal failure, such as produced by avascular necrosis. In allogeneic grafts only bone is formed and it is subsequently resorbed (Friedenstein and Petrakova, 1968). When demineralized bone powders are used "matrix-clasts", defined as foreign body-type multinucleated cells by Urist (1980a), appear and participate in the remodeling process. The rate of resorption of an alloimplant is proportional to the surface area. "Autodigestion" of dead cells leaves empty osteocyte lacunae and is not evidence of cellular activity such as osteocytic osteolysis.

The term "implant" refers to placing nonviable materials such as treated dead bone or metal prostheses in bony defects. Even when the implanted material is biocompatible it is recognized as "foreign" by the immune system and normal reparative mechanisms are activated to wall off or degrade the foreign material. If an infection occurs in the area of an implant it can cause loosening of the implant. Even in the absence of infection, it is usually possible to find some degree of increased bone resorption at the ultrastructural level (Ohlin and Kindblom, 1988). Active osteoclasts and histiocytes are present in the bone removed from the "normal" areas of bone-cement interface from a failed hip prosthesis (Fig. 15). Macrophages and giant cells which ingested material particles in loosening of total hip prostheses did not form pits or resorption lacunae on the bone substrates in tissue culture compared to osteoclasts as the control (Pazzaglia and Pringle, 1989).

Chronic Drug Intake

Fluorides

Chronic fluorosis causes exostoses in long and flat bones. Distorted bony trabeculae and poorly developed haversian systems are present (Hennigar and Gross, 1985). The benefit of sodium fluoride therapy of osteoporosis is still controversial. A three year study of 29 patients aged 51 to 76 years showed that continuous treatment with 80 mg NaF/day produced, after 3 years, a trabecular bone density in the treated patients which was 8% higher than that of untreated patients. The incidence of osteoarticular side effects and the increased number of new crush fractures of the spine raised the possibility of fluoride-induced microfractures (Dambacher et al., 1986). In another study, 33% of patients receiving sodium fluoride, calcium and vitamin D therapy for osteoporosis experienced pain and swelling of the large joints (Schnitzler and

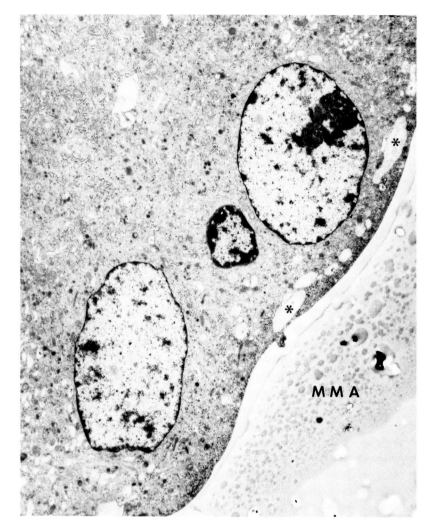

Fig. 15 Multinucleated giant cell between bone and methyl methacrylate cement from the femoral component of a hip prosthesis removed because of failure of the acetabular component. Note particles of methyl methacrylate (MMA) within the cytoplasm of the giant cell (asterisks) but lack of a ruffled border. Magn. × 15,000

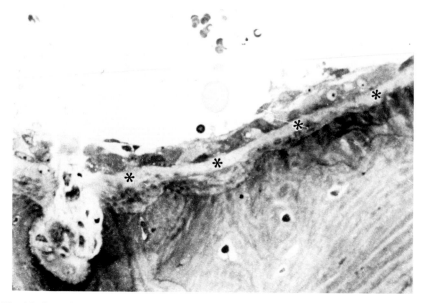

Fig. 16 Light micrograph of bone from patient whose osteoporosis was treated with fluoride. Note unmineralized layer of osteoid (asterisks) underlying plump osteoblasts and partially filling the resorption cavities. Howship's lacuna lower left. Magn. × 520

Salomon, 1986). Bone biopsy showed a trabecular fissure fracture and large intratrabecular resorption cavities surrounded by microcallus in a calcaneous fracture. There are often many osteoclasts and the number of haversian remodeling sites is increased (Rosenquist, 1975; Fig. 16).

Anticonvulsants

Anticonvulsant drugs such as diphenyl hydantoin and phenobarbital disturb bone metabolism by the induction of increased hepatic catabolism of hormones (estrogens) and of vitamin D and its biologically active products, as well as by direct effects on membrane cation transport systems (Hahn, 1976). Children may have deformities, hypocalcemia, hypophosphatemia and adults severe osteopenia, with pseudofractures. Osteoclastic activity may also be part of the histologic pattern of anticonvulsant-induced osteomalacia (Campbell *et al.*, 1977).

Diphosphonates

Intravenous etidronate is an effective inhibitor of bone resorption. Studies of etidronate in hypercalcemia suggest that the response is sustained for several weeks (Kanis *et al.*, 1987). Recent evidence suggests that the diphosphonates directly affect the activity of osteoclasts as well as the interaction between mononuclear cells and their recruitment to the osteoclast pool(Bijvoet *et al.*, 1980). One apparent difference between etidronate and other diphosphonates is that it also delays the mineralization of bone at high doses (Mundy *et al.*, 1983). However, at 5 mg/kg/day for six months, etidronate did not significantly inhibit bone mineralization in pagetic patients, although it induced a focal mineralization in a few (Meunier *et al.*, 1987).

Corticoids

Osteoporosis as a result of corticosteroid excess, both endogenous and exogenous is a well recognized syndrome. Low dose prednisone for as long as seven months produces a dramatic loss of trabecular bone (Lo Cascio *et al.*, 1984). These authors emphasize that the dramatic loss of bone occurs in the early treatment period. Aseptic necrosis of the head of the femur is also correlated with the use of corticosteroid drugs. Such osteolysis involves the trabeculae of the epiphysis (Hennigar and Gross, 1985). In another histomorphometric study of trabecular bone volume, cortocosteroid treated patients also had a significantly reduced trabecular bone volume. Since formation is tightly coupled in space and time to resorption the bone loss is accounted for by an uncoupling of the process. The result is that osteoclasts differentiate and remove bone in the face of a normal osteoblastic appositional rate (Dempster *et al.*, 1983).

Idiopathic

Cytotoxic Drugs

Aseptic necrosis, leading to cell death, has also been reported in patients receiving cytotoxic agents (cyclophosphamide and methotrexate) for malignant disease or psoriasis (Fechner, 1982). There is a good correlation between methotrexate toxicity and enzymatic tetrahydrofolate dehydrogenase expression in osteoclasts (Miszta *et al.*, 1988).

Idiopathic

Genetic

The sclerosing bone dysplasias are characterized by increased bone density and abnormalities of skeletal modeling. For a review see Beighton (1982).

Osteogenesis Imperfecta Congenita and Tarda

Recent studies identify four general types of osteogenesis imperfecta based on groups of characteristics (Sillence and Danks, 1979; Kirsch *et al.*, 1987). Only one of these groups (Type III) have fractures. A history of high fracture rates which can occur *in utero* is designated "congenita". In the milder form "tarda" in addition to high fracture rates, there are blue sclerae, and deafness (Doty and Matthews, 1971). A decreased amount of bone and an abnormal bone matrix is also associated with both (Baron *et al.*, 1983). The pathogenesis is not well understood but has been attributed either to decreased bone formation with or without decreased resorption, or to increased bone resorption, with or without decreased formation. The ultrastructure and enzymatic activity of osteoclasts and osteocytes was found to be normal by Doty and Baron although the osteoblasts were abnormal and there was a high bone turnover.

Osteopetrosis

This heterogeneous, heritable syndrome of unknown etiology is chiefly characterized by abnormal bone density and brittleness with pathologic fractures. There is imperfect orientation of collagen fibers and obliteration of the medullary spaces by calcified osteocartilagenous trabeculae (Shapiro *et al.*, 1980). Failure to resorb calcified cartilage during ossification leads to abnormally contoured bone in the metaphyseal region. Osteoclast numbers are often increased but when the disease is active they may lack ruffled borders and clear zones (Bonucci *et al.*, 1975). In malignant osteopetrosis there is a variable spectrum of osteoclast abnormalities (Shapiro *et al.*, 1988). Ultrastructurally normal osteoclasts with ruffled borders (Teitelbaum *et al.*, 1981) and containing acid phosphatase (van Tran *et al.*, 1985) have been reported as well as huge abnormal osteoclasts closely applied to bone but without resorption bays (Teitelbaum *et al.*, 1981). Mills (unpublished) has observed that the thick amorphous layer on the surface of the bone underlying inactive multinucleated cells contains antigens to osteonectin. Of interest is the recent finding of nuclear inclusions (Figs 17A and 17B) identical in

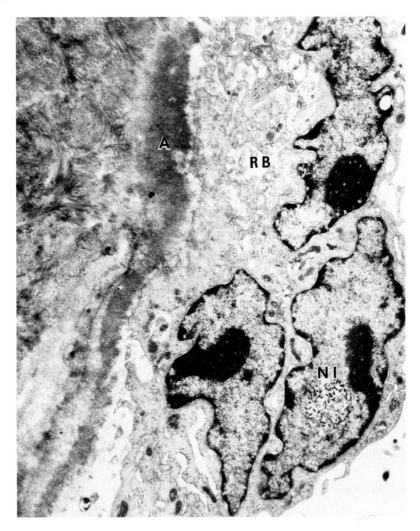

Fig. 17 A. Osteopetrosis showing osteoclast applied to bone but not resorbing thick layer of amorphous substance (A) covering surface of bone. Cytoplasmic extensions (RB) present at top of electron micrograph do not have collagen fibrils within their folds. Note nuclear inclusion (NI) in nucleus at lower right. Magn. × 15,000

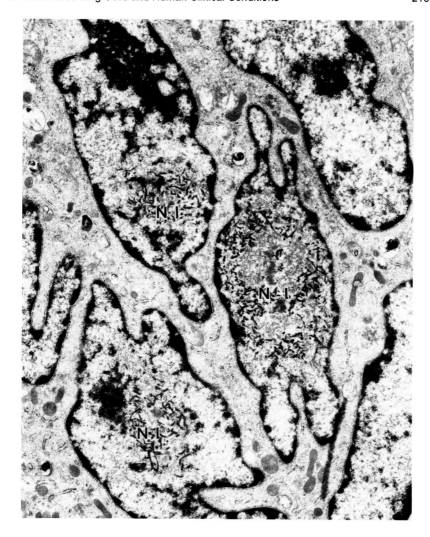

Fig. 17 B. Higher power electron micrograph of another osteoclast to illustrate the Paget-like nuclear inclusions (NI) (both smooth and rough) to be found in the osteoclasts of some osteopetrosis patients. Magn. × 15,000

morphology and size to those in Paget's disease of bone that are labeled with antibodies to paramyxoviruses (Mills, 1988a).

Pycnodysostosis

This rare osteopetrosis-like bone disease of unknown etiology is characterized by short stature, failure of closure of the cranial sutures, open fontanelles, obtuse mandibular angles, partial or total aplasia of the terminal phalanges, and generalized osteopenia with a predisposition to bone fractures (Elmore, 1967; Everts *et al.*, 1985). The osteoclasts have several peculiarities, including vacuoles filled with bone collagen fibrils (Elmore, 1967) and nuclei containing Paget-like inclusions (Beneton *et al.*, 1987).

Lower Motor Neuron Degeneration with Skeletal Manifestations

This is a familial disorder characterized by combined lower motor neuron degeneration and X-ray evidence of skeletal disorganization accompanied by elevation of alkaline phosphatase. Bone scans showed areas of increased uptake where previous X-rays had shown coarseness of trabeculation (Tucker *et al.*, 1982). Osteoclasts in the lesion contained nuclear inclusions typical of those in Paget's disease of bone (Yabe *et al.*, 1986; Fig. 18).

Skeletal Dysgenesis

One rare form, geroderma osteodysplastica hereditaria is characterized by severe osteoporosis with spontaneous fractures of multiple bones. Other conditions with similar findings include osteogenesis imperfecta, osteodysplasia, progeria, cutis laxa syndrome, acrogeria, Bonnevie-Alrich and Ehlers-Danlos syndrome (Suter *et al.*, 1982). Dysplastic changes can also occur in the dentin but usually the two conditions are not related and there is no abnormality of remodeling in the healing process (Wannfors *et al.*, 1985).

Klinefelter's Syndrome

Osteoporosis and hypogonadism are characteristic of Klinefelter's syndrome. Histomorphometric data confirmed the osteoporosis primarily as a depressed osteoblastic activity and resultant rarefied spongy bone (Delmas and Meunier, 1981). The osteopenia is believed to be related to low androgen levels rather than to the chromosomal abnormality. Osteoclastic resorption occurs however (Fig. 19).

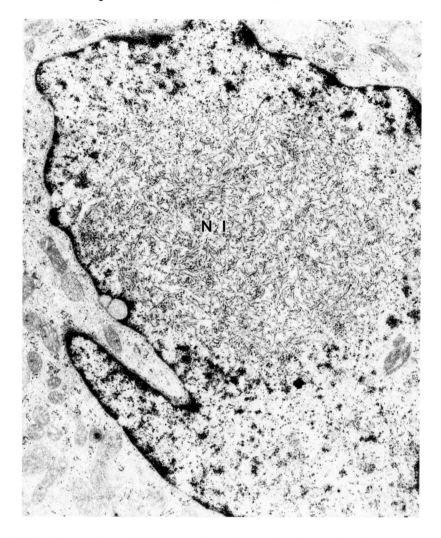

Fig. 18 Electron micrograph of nucleus of osteoclast from bone biopsy of patient with lower motor neuron disease with skeletal manifestations. Microtubular filaments (NI) are the same dimensions and identical in morphology with those of Paget's disease of bone. Magn. × 30,000

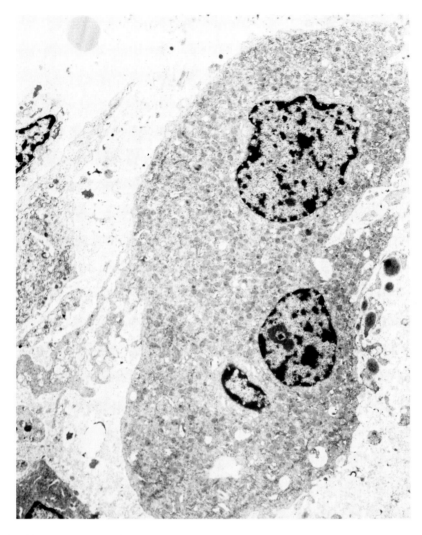

Fig. 19 Multinucleated giant cell located near bone surface of bone biopsy of patient with Kleinfelter's disease. Osteopenia is characteristic of this disorder. Magn. × 26,500

Storage Diseases

There are a number of congenital, hereditary storage diseases in which mucopolysaccharides, lipids and other substances occupy the cytoplasm of cells. The bones do not form normally and the result is osteoporosis, often due to disuse of the abnormally formed bones that will not support body weight. Accumulations of mucopolysaccharides in cells may be accompanied by the presence of macrophages or giant cells. Osteoclasts may be difficult to find.

Hypophosphatemia

This congenital, lethal, autosomal-recessive disorder maintains a low alkaline phosphatase in serum and tissues. The skeletal manifestations include disturbed bone formation, large areas of irregular unmineralized osteoid and lacunae with osteoblastoid cells. An unusual feature is areas of active osteoclastic resorption of unmineralized osteoid close to the growth plate (Burck et al., 1982). Increased activity of osteoclasts, identified by increased numbers of mitochondria, intracytoplasmic vacuoles, extensive ruffled borders and underlying bone surfaces with collagen fibrils exposed are seen in the electron microscope.

Hyperphosphatasia

This bone dysplasia is characterized by excessive bone resorption early in life with resulting severe skeletal deformity. It can be ameliorated by treatment with human calcitonin (Nunez et al., 1979). These authors found that osteoclasts contained dense intramitochondrial microcrystal deposits that disappeared after calcitonin treatment. The ultrastructure of osteocytes was profoundly affected by calcitonin. Following therapy, the osteocyte lacunae which previously contained a flocculent material but few collagen fibrils were filled with mature collagen, and the intramitochondrial microcrystal deposits were gone. Although this disorder is sometimes referred to as "juvenile Paget's disease", it is characterized by a lack of normal cortical remodeling and there is none of the classical mosaic pattern of Paget's disease (Krane, 1977; Fig. 20).

Systemic Mastocytosis

In mastocytosis mast cells are found, which might suggest a common ancestry with tissue macrophages and reticulum cells. In 21 cases the bone lesions were of two types. The first was a cystic osteoporosis of the ribs and skull with thickening of bone trabeculae and generalized sclerosis of the

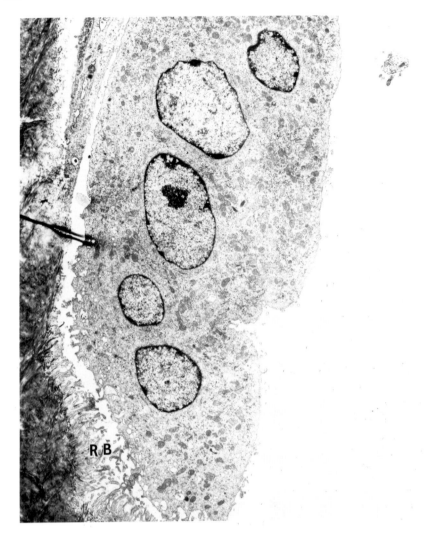

Fig. 20 Hyperphosphatasia, illustrating osteoclast with well developed ruffled border (RB) from a biopsy of a child. Separation of ruffled border from body of osteoclast is artefactual. Magn. × 8,200

pelvis and vertebrae. The second form was localized, with radiolucent areas in humerus, radius, femur, skull and shoulder (Bendel and Race, 1963). Gallium-67 scans localized the bone lesions and bone marrow biopsy confirmed mastocytosis (Ensslen *et al.*, 1983; Rebel and Malkani, 1974; Malkani and Rebel, 1974).

Hyperoxaluria

This genetic disorder, transmitted as an autosomal recessive trait, is characterized by deposition of calcium oxalate throughout the body. The result is bone oxalosis and renal osteodystrophy (Gherardi *et al.*, 1980). In the electron microscope large Howship's lacunae were found along the borders of the bone trabeculae. They often contained large osteoclasts that had two or more nuclei and a cytoplasm with many mitochondria and vacuoles that contained inorganic material. There was a well developed ruffled border in the resorption zone, and there were free crystals and a few isolated collagen fibrils between the bone matrix and the ruffled border. The finding of concomitant osteomalacia is consistent with the coexistence of two disorders.

Osteitis Deformans

The incidence of Paget's disease of bone is about 4.5% in Latin America, as in the United States (Schajowicz *et al.*, 1988). During its acute stage there is an increase in osteoblastic activity and osteoclastic bone resorption accompanied by defects in the calcification of the newly formed bone matrix which is not remodeled adequately according to lines of stress (Bonucci, 1981; Johnson, 1964). An interesting peculiarity is the presence in osteoclast nuclei of characteristic inclusion bodies consisting of microtubular filaments which are often arranged in parallel and sometimes form paracrystalline structures (Rebel *et al.*, 1976; Malkani *et al.*, 1976; Mills and Singer, 1976; Schultz *et al.*, 1977; Schajowicz *et al.*, 1985). They are also present in osteoclast cytoplasm (Gherardi *et al.*, 1980a; Figs 21 A-E). The fine structure of these inclusions suggested that they might be viral nucleo-capsids (Howatson and Fournasier, 1982) an hypothesis that has received strong support from the observation that paramyxovirus antigens can be demonstrated in pagetic osteoclasts by immunofluorescence and immunoperoxidase (Rebel *et al.*, 1979; Mills *et al.*, 1980a, 1984). The hypothesis that Paget's disease of bone is a viral disease is supported by the fact that *in situ* hybridization studies of osteoblasts, osteocytes, and other skeletal cells detects the measles genome (Basle *et al.*, 1986), and that, by dot blot, the mRNA for the nucleocapsid

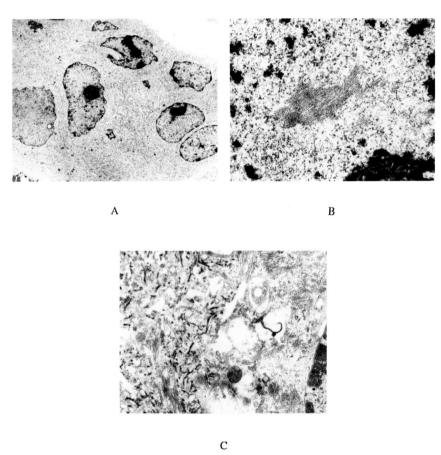

A   B

C

Fig. 21 Paget's disease of bone. **A.** Osteoclast from a Paget's disease patient illustrating multiple nuclei and nuclear inclusions characteristic of the lesion. Magn. × 3,500 **B.** Nucleus of osteoclast illustrating paracrystalline array of microtubular filaments in longitudinal section. Magn. × 36,000 **C.** Cytoplasmic inclusions illustrating both smooth and rough varieties of filaments. Magn. × 27,000

D

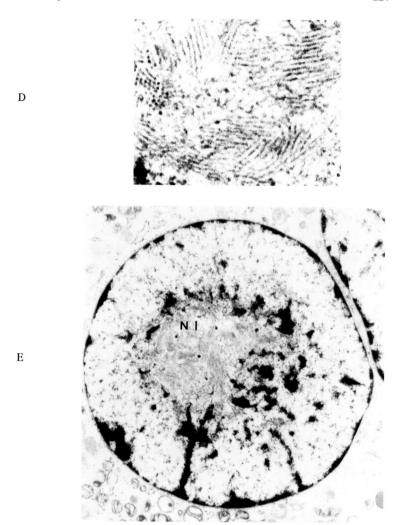

E

Fig. 21 D. Microtubular filaments of nuclear inclusions illustrating both cross-sections and longitudinal sections of the tubular structures. Magn. × 150,000 **E.** Nucleus of an osteoclast illustrating microtubular filaments (NI) in center of chromatin clumps in osteoclast. Magn. × 27,000

protein of respiratory syncytial virus can also be detected (Mills *et al.*, 1988; Lai *et al.*, 1989).

Inclusions morphologically and dimensionally identical with those described in Paget's disease of bone have also been found in malignant giant cell tumors (Welsh and Meyer, 1970; Mills, 1981), benign giant cell tumors (Abelanet *et al.*, 1986; Fournasier *et al.*, 1985; Mirra *et al.*, 1981), in pyc-nodysostosis (Beneton *et al.*, 1987), in osteopetrosis (Mills *et al.*, 1988), in lower motor neuron degeneration with skeletal manifestations (Mills *et al.*, 1988a) and in inclusion body myositis (Chou, 1968; Yunis and Smaha, 1971; Schochet and McCormick, 1973; Mills (unpublished)).

There are no changes in blood vessels. Shrunken osteoclasts which detach from the bone matrix and have pycnotic nuclei are often found (Bonucci, 1981). This is interesting in that it might illustrate what happens in normal bone just before osteoclast death. The fact that inclusion bodies are found in some but not all of the nuclei of the affected osteoclasts could explain why these osteoclasts maintain their resorbing activity and survive. The presence of normal and diseased nuclei seems to be confirmation that the nuclei represent fusion of cells incorporated at various stages. Isolated osteoclasts showed many of the enzymatic characteristics of osteoclasts in Paget's bone *in situ* (Basle *et al.*, 1988).

Fibrogenesis Imperfecta Ossium

This rare, acquired, disorder of bone mineralization is characterized by an abnormality of bone collagen with bone pain and tenderness leading to incapacity and severe morbidity. There is increased bone turnover with increased numbers of both osteoblasts and osteoclasts. Few of the Howship's lacunae are empty and the osteoclasts occasioned no comment in the report of Lang *et al.* (1986).

Ectopic Bone Resorption

Urist (1980b) distinguishes heterotopic or ectopic bone formation from pathologic calcification by describing heterotopic bone as an organized matrix containing living cells. Heterotopic bone formation is a benign, self-limiting growth with no obvious function. Morphologically, heterotopic bone is indistinguishable from other bone and is resorbed by apparently normal osteoclasts (Fig. 22).

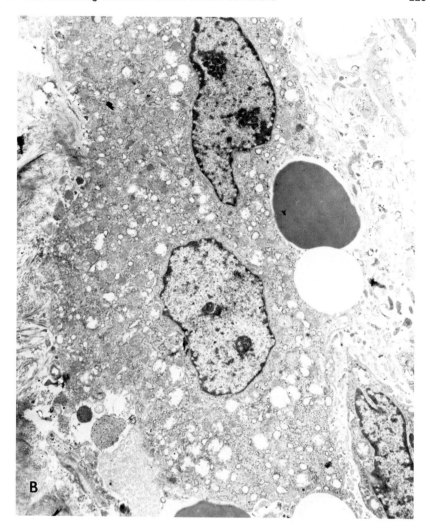

Fig. 22 Heterotopic bone (B) surface illustrating osteoclast with resorptive activity. Note the similarity to osteoclasts in bone at other sites. Magn. × 9,400

Bone Cysts

Simple

The etiology of the simple bone cyst is still unknown. Based on a study of fluid contents it was proposed that a focus of fibrous tissue is formed in an area of rapid resorption which could represent the initial lesion (Cohen, 1960). Correlation of ultrastructure with simple cysts in the jaw suggested that the alkaline and acid phosphatase contents of the fluid (more than 10 times that of serum, Neer *et al.*, 1973) correlated well with the cellular activity of osteoclasts and osteoblasts (Mills *et al.*, 1979). The ratio of alkaline to acid phosphatase in another series of simple cysts of long bone correlated well with the progress of the lesion. A low ratio had a poor prognosis for healing and a high ratio was found in the lesions that healed (Mills *et al.*, 1980a; Fig. 23).

Aneurysmal Bone Cysts

The aneurysmal bone cyst (Jaffe and Lichtenstein, 1942) is a benign non-neoplastic lesion of unknown etiology most often occurring in patients less than 15 years of age. The cyst wall and septa consist of a superficial layer of cellular fibroblastic and histiocytic tissue in which multinuclear giant cells are present, covering a deeper layer of less cellular fibrous tissue. This architecture was found in 88.6% of 105 cases (Rutter *et al.*, 1977; Aho *et al.*, 1982). In the active lesion that continues to expand, the osteoclasts are large, display an extensive ruffled border and are associated with a fluid high in acid phosphatase, up to 10 times normal (Mills *et al.*, 1979, 1980b). The osteoclasts are inhibited by calcitonin, resorb bone and contain acid phosphatase but have no Fc receptors, DrW(Ia) or common leucocyte antigenic markers (Horton *et al.*, 1984).

Florid Osseous Dysplasia

Osseous dysplasia is a fibroosseous disease limited to jaw bone and ranging from localized periapical involvement to multiquadrant involvement (Fig. 24). Occurrence of simple bone cysts with florid osseous dysplasia is uncommon (Melrose *et al.*, 1976). Active bone resorption associated with numerous osteoclasts is seen but there was no elevation of parathyroid hormone levels in the normocalcemic patients.

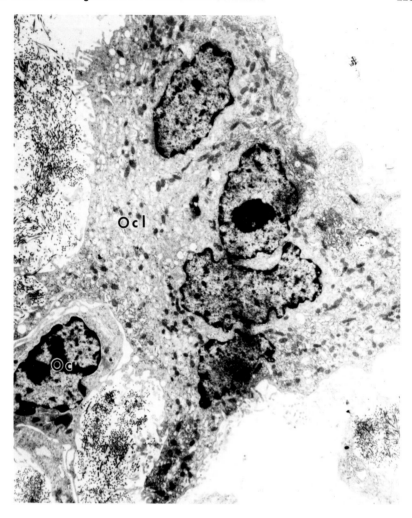

Fig. 23 Lining of cyst in distal radius of 6 year old boy. Osteoclast (Ocl) is interdigitated with bone and surrounding half buried osteocyte (Oc). There is no evidence of cell fusion in this instance. Magn. × 9,400

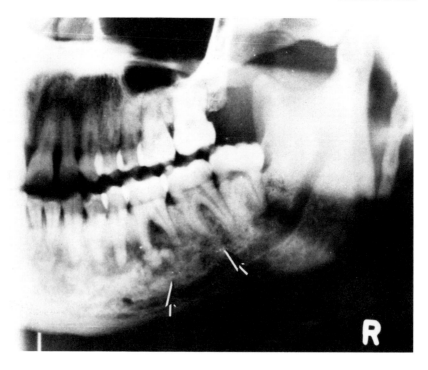

Fig. 24   Florid osseous dysplasia. Roentgenogram illustrating multiple small cystic lesions (arrows) in mandible.

Neoplasms

Neoplasms may contain any or all of the kinds of bone resorbing cells described in non-neoplastic conditions. In addition bizarre forms of multinucleated cells or abnormal organelles may be present in bone resorbing cells. Increased numbers of osteoclasts that conform to all the criteria of a strict definition can occur on the surface of bone in the vicinity of a giant cell tumor or neoplasm that is as much as 500 microns distant (Kulenkampff *et al.*, 1986). Other metastatic neoplasms may secrete substances that stimulate bone resorption by multinucleated cells (Burkhart *et al.*, 1984). Tumors of bone or cartilage containing multinucleated giant cells include: Chondroblastoma, chondromyxoid fibroma, chondroma, chondrosarcoma, enchondromtosis, giant cell granuloma of the mandible, giant cell tumor of bone, non-ossifying fibroma, osteoblastoma, osteoclastoma, osteoid osteoma, osteosarcoma and extraosseous chondrosarcoma and osteosarcoma (Evans, 1968). Areas of osteoclastic bone absorption are frequently seen at the periphery of any bone lesion (Thomson and Turner-Warwick, 1955).

Benign

It is difficult to generalize about the characteristics of the bone resorbing cells associated with tumors due to the many forms to be found. Tumors containing multinucleated cells were studied to correlate size with enzyme activities (tartrate-resistant acid phosphatase, NADH-tetrazolium-oxidoreductase and non-specific esterase). In 6 tumors containing giant cells it was found that large cells had a reduced enzyme activity and showed signs of degeneration while medium sized cells showed an increase in activity in the tumors (Metze et al., 1987).

Histiocytosis X (eosinophilic granuloma, Hand-Schuller-Christian disease, and Letterer-Siwe disease). These diseases have in common an accumulation of histiocytes. Eosinophilic granulomas are bone destroying lesions occurring in children. Multinucleated cells are frequent. All three diseases have a distinctive ultrastructural rod-shaped inclusion (Birbeck granule) in the cytoplasm of the histiocytes (Rywlin, 1985).

Fibrous Dysplasia

This condition develops when the remodelling process results in an excess of fibrous tissue in which are embedded spicules of bone, usually in a growing young person. Giant cells may be present and typical osteoclasts can be found resorbing bone spicules (Aegerter and Kirkpatrick, 1968). The osteoclasts appear normal, with deep ruffled borders and sealing zone. The underlying bone matrix has a brush border, with collagen fibrils apparent within the membranous channels of the ruffled border of the osteoclast (Fig. 1). Fibrous dysplasia can undergo malignant transformation (Yabut et al., 1988).

Osteochondroma

The osteochondroma has the gross appearance of regular cortical and underlying medullary bone with a fatty or hematopoietic component underlying a lobulated cartilaginous cap (Dahlin, 1967). The trabecular component is well organized and the cells are normal in appearance. Bone remodeling is carried out by normal-appearing osteoclasts (Fig. 25). Exostoses are very

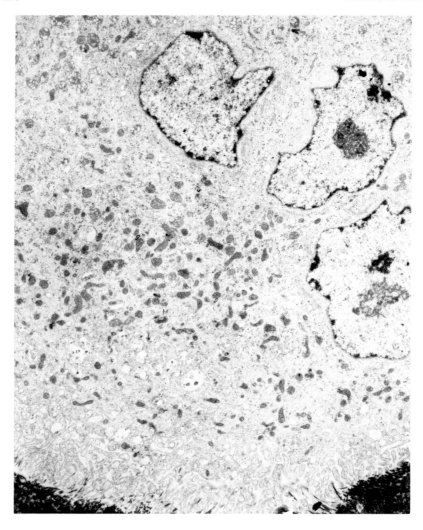

Fig. 25 Osteochondroma. Typical osteoclast on bone surface in proximity of lesion. Osteoclast shows no abnormal characteristics. Magn. × 11,000

similar lesions, frequently occurring in the distal phalanges and often associated with trauma.

Benign Osteoblastoma

These tumors produce bone and osteoid. They are usually vascular. There may be numerous giant cells and macrophages which can cause confusion with a giant cell tumor. However giant cell tumors do not produce bone (Lichtenstein and Sawyer, 1964).

Giant Cell Tumor

This tumor contains multinucleated cells with some of the morphologic and histochemical characteristics found in osteoclasts (Hanaoka et al., 1970; Aparisi et al., 1977a; Gothlin and Ericsson, 1976). However, the two types of multinucleated cells differ in many respects but in particular, the giant cells of the tumor have no ruffled border and do not appear to participate in active bone resorption (Bonucci, 1981; Aparisi et al., 1977b; Steiner et al., 1972; Figs 26 A-D). However, some resorption is indicated when scanning electron microscopy reveals a resorption pit on the bone surface adjacent to a giant cell, although these cells are poorly phagocytic, Wood et al., 1978. These multinucleated cells respond to calcitonin. The only monocyte antigens detected on these cells by Horton and colleagues (1984) were My-7, MCS.2 and DuHL60. However, others using a battery of monoclonal antibodies against a variety of lymphoid and non-lymphoid antigens compared osteoclasts from fetal long bones with giant cells from a giant cell tumor of bone. Finding only one cross-reacting antibody to macrophages, they concluded that osteoclasts and tumor-derived giant cells are derived from a similar mononuclear precursor (Athanasou et al., 1985). Cells cultured from human giant cell tumors respond to PTH by increased synthesis of cyclic adenosine monophosphate but this is not a unique skeletal property Goldring et al., 1978.

Virus-like, filamentous intranuclear inclusions have been described in giant cell tumors of bone not associated with Paget's disease (Welsh and Meyer, 1970; Abelanet et al., 1986; Schajowicz et al., 1985; Fournasier et al., 1985; Mills (unpublished); Figs 27 A-D). However the incidence in the unpublished study was only 8% of 13 patients, 2% of 201 giant cells examined and 0.3% of 1,316 nuclei surveyed at a magnification of 8,000 or greater. This is in contrast to the incidence of 49% reported by Abelanet et al. (1986) but confirms earlier work by that group.

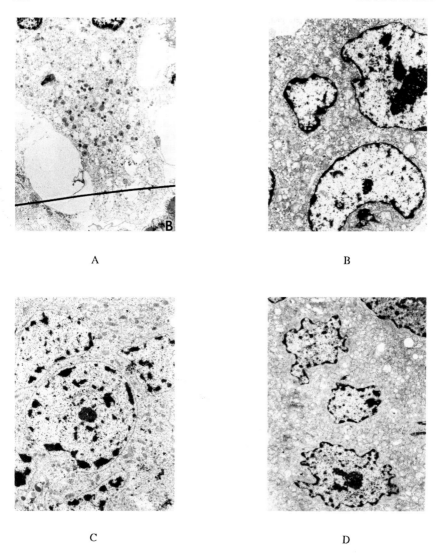

Fig. 26 Benign giant cell tumor. **A.** Osteoclast-like cell on bone surface. Magn. × 4,000 Examples of differing morphology: **B.** Giant cell showing 4 nuclei with clumped chromatin and relatively smooth surfaces. Cell surface without filopodia. Magn. × 7,200 **C.** Giant cell with pale nuclei and smooth surfaces, note clumped but not marginated chromatin. Cytoplasm fewer mitochondria with more varied shapes than tumor B. Magn. × 12,000 **D.** Nuclei of giant cell are invaginated, chromatin is clumped and nucleoli are prominent. Cytoplasm contains large numbers of small round mitochondria and vacuoles. Magn. × 6,600

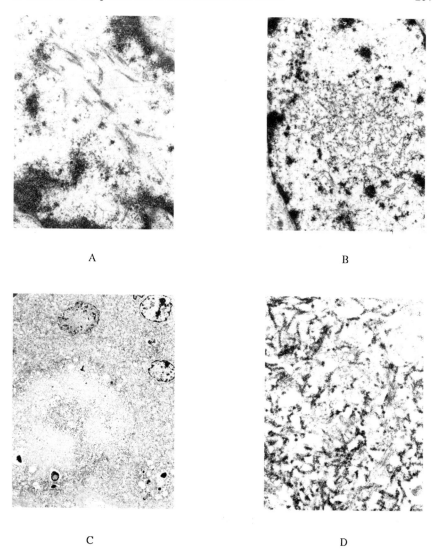

A   B

C   D

Fig. 27 Inclusions found in benign giant cell tumors. **A.** Harani bodies found in nucleus, dissimilar to inclusions found in Paget's osteoclasts. Magn. × 36,400 **B.** Nuclear inclusions identical in morphology and dimensions to those found in Paget's disease of bone. Magn. × 27,000 **C.** Giant cell tumor developing in Paget's bone lesion. Multinucleated cell on bone surface. Note heterogeneity of nuclei, large area of disorganized cytoplasm, "ghost" of nucleus (arrow) and cell engulfed but not assimilated into giant cell. Magn. × 3,200 **D.** Cytoplasm of giant cell illustrating smooth and "rough" filaments. Magn. × 31,000

Giant cell tumor of tissues other than bone such as breast, thyroid, parotid gland, colon, dermis, myometrium, heart, and other soft tissues occur very rarely and their histogenesis is controversial. The osteoclast-like giant cells of a breast carcinoma did not possess a ruffled border or clear zone and failed to respond to calcitonin, however when transplanted to cortical bone resorbed bone in a manner similar to osteoclasts (Athanasou *et al.*, 1989). These tumors are named "osteoclast-type giant cell tumors" on the basis of their histologic resemblance to skeletal giant cell tumors ("osteoclastomas") (Berendt *et al.*, 1987). Since these tumors are non-skeletal and may be of epithelial derivation they will not be discussed further.

Malignant

Tumors are termed malignant because of their unremitting course, invasiveness and tendency to metastasize. Bone resorbing cells are stimulated to resorb bone by osteolytic neoplasms. Primary malignant skeletal tumours include osteosarcoma, chondrosarcoma, fibrosarcoma, spindle cell sarcoma and giant cell tumours (Thomson and Turner-Warwick, 1955). The American Cancer Society has listed and described malignant bone tumors (Copeland and Geschickter, 1971).

Medullary Thyroid Cancer

This cancer secretes calcitonin which can be stimulated by calcium and pentagastrin. In spite of the excessive amounts of the hormone in the blood and the renal effects there is no detectable effect on the skeleton (Singer and Krane, 1973). At the ultrastructural level there is some evidence of cellular degeneration with possible "death" of osteoclasts (Fig. 28).

Fibrosarcoma

This malignant tumor invades and destroys bone (McLeod *et al.*, 1957). Benign multinucleated cells are sometimes found, although these are more commonly a characteristic of osteogenic sarcomas (Dahlin, 1967b).

Osteosarcoma

Structural variation from case to case and even within a single specimen causes difficulty in describing the typical morphology of osteosarcomas (Ferguson, and Yunis, 1978). There are at least two morphologically distinct types of multinucleated giant cells. One type resembles osteoclasts and has nuclei with marginated chromatin and prominent nucleoli. The cytoplasm contains small mitochondria and interspersed dense bodies. The rough endoplasmic

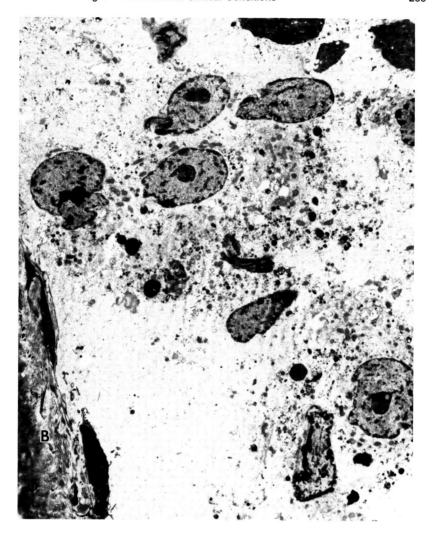

Fig. 28 Medullary carcinoma. Bone surface without active appearing cells and clusters of nuclei lacking a cell membrane with the appearance of degeneration of a giant cell. Magn. × 6,600

reticulum is in the form of narrow bands, often located at the periphery of the cell. A second type of multinucleated giant cell has a very anaplastic malignant appearance. These cells contain multiple nuclei, with no margination of chromatin, and the cytoplasm contains very few mitochondria, occasional dense bodies and tightly packed smooth endoplasmic reticulum. They also have lipid and glycogen deposits. Many of these cells show degenerative changes, including cytoplasmic vacuolation, chromatin condensation and disrupted mitochondria. At the ultrastructural level all osteosarcomas contain numerous primitive cells (Fig. 29).

An osteosarcoma arising in Paget's disease of bone has an incidence of 6.28% in Latin America (Schajawicz et al., 1988).

Malignant Giant Cell Tumor

In 1922, Stewart described the histogenesis of "myeloid sarcoma" stating that there is almost "complete unanimity of opinion as to the clinical behaviour and appropriate treatment of the lesion". He described the giant cells of the malignant giant cell tumor as corresponding very closely in their microscopic characters to the osteoclasts of normal bone and commented that "there seems no reason to doubt that they are just as essential and specific a constituent of the tumour as the osteoclasts are of bone". He differentiates the two multinuclear cells sharply; the giant cell never forms bone, and is an integral part of the tumor. The osteoclast is found only in bone and arises from the reticulum of the marrow as an end product. These definitions are relevant to present controversies.

One malignant giant cell tumor of bone was reported to have nuclear clusters of fibrils 80 to 120Å in diameter in nuclei which appeared otherwise normal (Welsh and Meyer, 1970). It was suggested that these fibrils resembled those found in polymyositis described as "myxovirus-like". Morphologically these are identical with the nuclear inclusions of Paget's disease of bone (Mills, 1981; Figs 30A and 30B).

Multinucleated Giant Cells in the Stroma of Malignant Tumors

The phagocytic function of multinucleated giant cells of the foreign body type was described in ten cases of oral squamous cell carcinomata treated by bleomycin. Their genesis was from macrophages and they represent a unique form of phagocytosis ("giganto-phagocytosis") (Burkhardt and Gebbers, 1977). The mononuclear macrophage and the giant cell interlock by closely

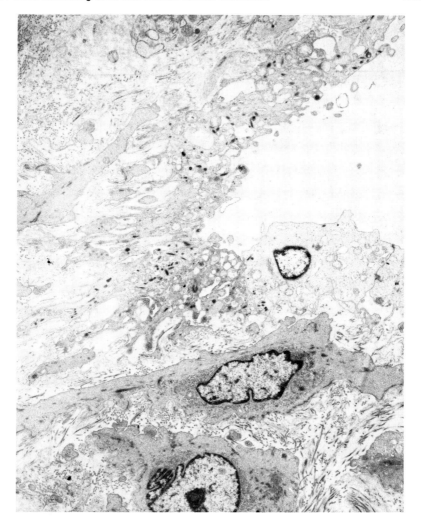

Fig. 29 Osteosarcoma. Grossly abnormal cells and disorganization of tumor bone. Normal osteoclastic function is not observed. Magn. × 8,750

A

B

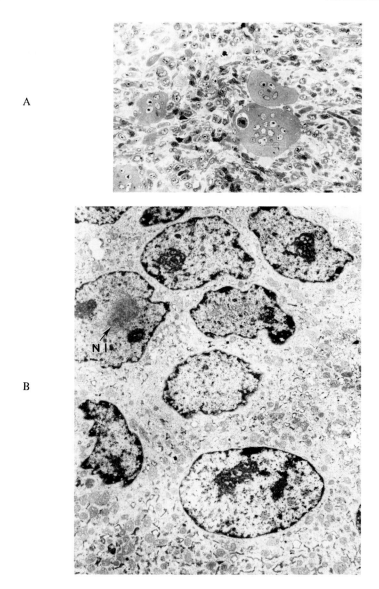

Fig. 30 Malignant giant cell tumor. **A.** Section of tumor stained with toluidine blue illustrating variety of cells, numerous mitoses, giant cells containing engulfed cells and disorganization. Magn. × 525 **B.** Electron micrograph of giant cell with nuclear inclusion resembling nuclear inclusion (NI) of Paget's disease of bone in patient with no known symptoms or signs of Paget's disease. Magn. × 10,000

apposed interdigitations of the cellular membranes thereby enclosing the keratinized cells of the carcinoma through fusion with the giant cell.

Malignant Giant Cell Tumors of Soft Tissues

The tumor consists a mixture of osteoclast-like and pleomorphic malignant type multinucleated giant cells, histiocytes, and fibroblasts (Angervall et al., 1981). Differentiating the malignant giant cell tumor of soft tissues from osteogenic sarcoma of soft tissues may present a problem if the osteogenic sarcoma has many multinucleated osteoclast-like giant cells and little osteogenic activity (Alguacil-Garcia et al., 1977). Since soft tissue tumors are not located within bone and have no apparent local bone resorbing activity they will not be discussed further.

Ewing's Sarcoma

This name persists because of the controversy concerning the histiogenesis and nature of this neoplasm. It occurs in adolescents and is highly malignant. Although producing osteolytic lesions, no giant cells are present (Evans, 1968; Friedman and Gold, 1968).

Hematologic Malignancy

These neoplasms may be associated with bone destruction.

Multiple Myeloma

Secretion of a soluble factor by myeloma cells stimulates osteoclastic activity in adjacent bone (Mundy, 1974; Josse, 1981) and correlated well with the number of osteoclasts and lytic bone defects (Thiele et al., 1988).

Lymphoma

Lympho-proliferative disorders such as Hodgkin's disease, lymphocytic lymphoma, Burkitt's lymphoma and acute lymphoblastic leukemia occasionally develop bone lesions. Increased osteoclast activity occurs adjacent to the malignant cells (Mundy et al., 1981).

Leukemia

A study of 18 autopsy cases of adult T-cell leukemia revealed proliferation of osteoclasts, bone resorption and fibrous replacement of bone in 8 patients of 13 with hypercalcemia. No osteoclast proliferation was found in 9 normocalcemic patients. The hypercalcemia could not be accounted for by parathyroid hormone levels or prostaglandin E levels, which were in the normal range, or vitamin D metabolites which were low (Kiyokawa *et al.*, 1987).

Metastatic Bone Disease

Most bone metastases arise from carcinomas, usually arising in breast, prostate, thyroid, kidney and bronchus (Mundy and Spiro, 1981). In a study of 267 cases of metastatic bone disease three developmental stages were identified. No bone resorption takes place in the first phase of early appearance. Stimulation of osteoclastic resorption in the bone surrounding tumor tissue is typical of the second phase. The third phase consists of atrophy, aseptic necrosis and "osteolysis" by the tumor cells themselves. Direct contact of tumor cells with trabecular surfaces can be seen only in the last phase of metastatic development. Tumor cells could cause bone resorption by a direct effect on bone. The mechanism is postulated to be a release of lysosomal enzymes and collagenase (Eilon and Mundy, 1979).

Activated osteoclasts in metastatic disease are larger and have more nuclei. The numbers of osteoclasts and nuclei per osteoclast are significantly higher in renal than in breast carcinoma. Osteoclasts can be activated at distances of more than 500 μm from tumor tissue (Kulenkampff *et al.*, 1986). In metastatic bone disease either more osteoclasts are created under the influence of tumor cells or the life span of multinucleated cells is exceeded by continuous activation from the malignancy (Galasko, 1981; Bonucci, 1981). Baron (1977) suggested that coupling messages get lost if the reversal phase is too long and remodeling resumes with a new resorption phase. Others found no uncoupling of bone formation and resorption (Scher, 1987). Metastases have a predilection for certain sites within the skeleton, particularly the axial skeleton and the proximal ends of long bones (Mundy and Spiro, 1981).

Metastases of Carcinoma in Pagetic Bone

Despite the high incidence of Paget's disease and metastatic carcinoma in bone in elderly people, it is infrequent for both to occur in the same patient (Schajowicz *et al.*, 1988). However, biopsy confirmed only Paget's disease in these patients.

Hypercalcemia of Malignancy

The pathophysiology of this complication of malignancy is incomplete but there is evidence that tumor cells, having taken up residence in bone, stimulate (by cytokines) osteoclasts in their vicinity to resorb bone (Canfield, 1987) suggesting that osteoclast inhibitors can benefit these patients (Fig. 31).

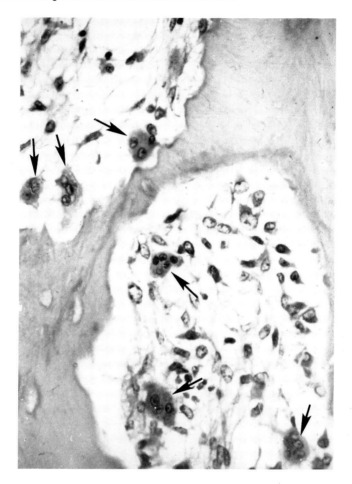

Fig. 31 Hypercalcemia of malignancy. Patient with carcinoma of the lung and hypercalcemia. Note numerous osteoclasts (arrows). Magn. × 300

Summary and Conclusion

In clinical medicine one of the most distressing aspects of "too thin bones" is the hazard to the patient of even minor trauma or the edentulous dental arch. Falls in the very elderly can lead to a fatal downhill course which is very difficult to treat or reverse. Loss of teeth produces a slower decline. As with other chronic diseases, prevention is the most rational approach to this problem.

As becomes obvious from a clinical survey such as has been presented in this chapter, there are innumerable causes of osteopenia many of which involve bone resorbing cells of the kinds described. However, resorption is rarely present without accompanying malfunction of the precursor generating or maturation systems. Likewise, bone forming cells usually are also involved either as contributing cause or are affected by the resorption process. It can be concluded that study of the involved bone by any of the present diagnostic techniques or those now being perfected can help the clinician both with prognosis and treatment planning. The future should bring better methods for preventing bone loss when the proper diagnosis has been made.

Acknowledgements

The author wishes to express her gratitude to James Alexander, whose expertise made the illustrations possible. Special thanks to many collaborators, especially Frederick M. Singer who shared his clinical acumen and resources as well as providing patients with a wide spectrum of metabolic bone disease for study. Thanks also to David B. N. Lee, M. D., nephrologist, Donald Cooksey, D. M. D., oral surgeon, Roger Terry, M. D., C. P. Schwinn, M. D., M. A. Abrams, D. D. S., and R. Melrose, D. D. S., pathologists; J. V. Luck, M. D., both senior and junior, A. Sarmiento, M. D., S. Noel, M. D., orthopaedic surgeons and fellows M. McKenna, M. D. and H. Yabe, M. D. The interest of, and contributions of bone specimens form, colleagues in the medical community world-wide has made this study possible.

References

Abdelwahab, I.F. and Norman, A. (1988) Osteosclerotic sarcoidosis. *AJR* **150**: 161-162

Abelanet, R., Daudet-Monsac, M., Laoussadi, S., (1986) *et al.*, Frequency and diagnostic value of the virus-like filamentous intranuclear inclusions in giant cell tumor of bone not associated with Paget's disease. *Virchows Arch.* **410**: 65-68

Addison, W. C. (1978) The distribution of nuclei in human odontoclasts in whole cell preparations. *Arch. Oral Biol.* **23**: 1167-1171

Aegerter, E. and Kirkpatrick, J. A. Jr., (1968) The skeletal dysplasias. Chapter 6. pp 95-221. **In:** *Orthopedic Diseases, Physiology, Pathology, Radiology. 3rd Ed.* W.B. Saunders Co. Philadelphia, London, Toronto.

Aegerter, E. and Kirkpatrick, J. A. Jr. (1968) Metabolic disease of bone. Chapter 11 pp 369-424. **In:** *Orthopedic diseases, Physiology, Pathology, Radiology. 3rd Ed.* W.B. Saunders Co. Philadelphia, London, Toronto

Aho, H. J., Aho, A. J. and Einola, S. (1982) Aneurysmal bone cyst. A study of ultrastructure and malignant transformation. *Virchows Arch.* **A 395**: 169-179

Alguacil-Garcia, A., Unni, K. K. and Goellner, J. R. (1985) Malignant giant cell tumor of soft parts. *Cancer* **40**: 244-253

Anderson, R. E. (1985) Radiation injury. Chapter 6. pp 239-277. In: *Anderson's Pathology. 8th Ed.* (John M. Kissane, Ed.) C. V. Mosby, St. Louis.

Angervall, L., Hagman, B. and Kudblom, L-G. (1981) *et al.*, Malignant giant cell tumor of soft tissue. *Cancer* **47**: 736-747

Aparisi, T., Arborgh, B. and Ericsson, J. L. E. (1977a) Giant cell tumor of bone. *Virchows Arch. A* **376**: 299-308

Aparisi, T., Arborgh, B. and Ericsson, J. L. E. (1977) Giant cell tumor of bone. Detailed fine structural analysis of different cell components. *Virchows Arch. A* **376**: 273-298

Ascenzi, A. (1979) A Problem in Palaeopathology. The origin of thalassemia in Italy. *Virchows Arch A* **384**: 121-130

Asher, J. D. and Nichols, G. Jr. (1965) Heparin stimulation of bone collagenase activity. *Fed. Proc.* Abstr. *459 p 211*

Athanasou, N. A., Bliss, E., Gatter, K. C. (1985) *et al.*, An immuno-histological study of giant-cell tumor of bone: Evidence for an osteoclast origin of the giant cells. *J. Pathol.* **147**: 153-158

Athanasou, N. A., Wells, C. A. and Quinn, J., (1989) *et al.*, The origin and nature of stromal osteoclast-like multinucleated giant cells in breast carcinoma: implications for tumor osteolysis and macrophage biology. *Br. J. Cancer* **59**: 491-498

Barlow, T., (1883) *Med. Chir. Trans.* **66**: 159

Baron, R. (1977) Importance of intermediate phase between resorption and formation in the measurement and understanding of the bone remodeling sequence. pp 179-183. In: *Bone histomorphometry, Second International Workshop.* (P. J. Meunier, Ed.). Societe' de la Nouvelle Imprimerie Fournce. Toulouse France.

Baron, R., Gertner, J. M., Lang, R. (1983) *et al.*, Increased bone turnover with decreased bone formation by osteoblasts in children with osteogenesis imperfecta tarda. *Pediatr. Res.* **17**: 204-207

Barzel, U. S. (1982) Osteoporosis in young men. Editorial. *Arch. Intern. Med.* **142**: 2079-2080

Basle, M. F., Fournier, J. G., Rozenblatt, S. (1986) *et al.*, Measles virus RNA detected in Paget's disease bone tissue by *in situ* hybridization. *J. Gen. Virol.* **67**: 907-913

Basle, M. F., Mazud, P., Malkani K., (1988) *et al.*, Isolation of osteoclasts from Pagetic bone tissue: morphometry and cytochemistry on isolated cells. *Bone* **9**: 1-6

Beighton, P., (1982) Sclerosing bone dysplasias. pp 173-194. In: *International Clinical Genetics Seminar.* Alan R. Liss Inc. New York

Belanger, L. F. (1971) Osteocytic resorption. In: *The biochemistry and physiology of bone.* (G. H. Bourne, Ed.) p 239. Vol 3 Academic Press, New York and London

Bendel, W. L. and Race, G. J. (1963) Urticaria pigmentosa with bone involvement. *J. Bone Jt. Surg.* **45A**: 1043-1056

Beneton, M. N. C., Harris, S. C. and Kanis, J. A. (1987) Paramyxovirus-like inclusions in two cases of pycnodysostosis. *Bone* **8**: 211-217

Berendt, R. C., Shnitka, T. K., Wiens, E., (1987) *et al.*, The osteoclast-type giant cell tumor of the pancreas. *Arch. Pathol. Lab. Med.* **111**: 43-48

Berglund, G. and Lindquist, B. (1960) Osteopenia in adolescence. *Clin. Orthop.* **17**: 259-264

Bernard, J., Chapuy, M-C., David, L. (1976) *et al.*, L'AMP cyclique urinaire et la parathomone plasmatique confrontes aux parameters histomorphometriques osseux de resorption. *Path. Biol.* **24**: 343-347

Bijvoet, O. L. M., Frijlink, W. E., Jie, K. (1980) *et al.*, APD in Paget's disease of bone: role of the mononuclear system. *Arthritis Rheum.* **23**: 1193-1204

Bogumill, G. P. and Schwamm, H. A. (1984) Trauma. **In**: *Orthopaedic Pathology. A synopsis with clinical and radiographic correlation.* Chapter 3, pps 70-110. W. B. Saunders Co. Philadelphia

Bonucci, E. (1977a) Ultrastructural aspects of bone mineralization in renal osteodystrophy. *Adv. Exptl. Med.* **81**: 477-491

Bonucci, E. (1977b) Ultrastructural aspects of bone mineralization in renal osteodystrophy. **In**: *Phosphate Metabolism.* (Massry, S. G. and Ritz, E., Eds.), pp 477-491, Plenum Press, New York

Bonucci, E. (1981) New knowledge on the origin, function and fate of osteoclasts. *Clin. Orthop.* **158**: 252-269

Bonucci, E. and Gherardi, G. (1977c) Osteocyte ultrastructure in renal osteodystrophy. *Virchows Arch.* **A. 373**: 213-231

Bonucci, E., Gherardi, G. and Faraggiana, T. (1976) Bone changes in hemodialyzed uremic subjects. Comparative light and electron microscopic investigations. *Virchows Arch.* **A. 371**: 183-198

Bonucci, E., LoCascio, V. and Adami S. (1978) *et al.*, The ultrastructure of bone cells and bone matrix in human primary hyperparathyroidism. *Virchows Arch.* **A. 379**: 11-23

Bonucci, E., Sartori, E. and Spina, M. (1975) Osteopetrosis Fetalis. *Virchows Arch.* **A. 368**: 109-121

Bordier, P. and Tun Chot, S. (1973) Histologic aspects of bone remodeling with special reference to the effects of parathyroid hormone and vitamin D. **In**: *Clinical Aspects of Metabolic Bone Disease.* (Frame, B., Parfitt, A. M. and Duncan, H. Eds.). pp 95-102. Excerpta Medica Amsterdam

Boyce, B.F., Fogelman, I. and Ralston, S. (1984) *et al.*, Focal osteomalacia due to a lower dose diphosphonate therapy in Paget's disease of bone. *Lancet* **1**: 821-824

Broadus, A. E., Magee, J. S., Mallette, L. E. (1983) *et al.*, A detailed evaluation of oral phosphate therapy in selected patients with primary hyperparathyroidism. *J. Clin. Endocrinol. Metab.* **56**: 953-961

Bullough, P. G., Bansal, M. and DiCarlo, E. F. (1987) Morphology of the Metabolic Diseases of Bone. **In**: *A CPC Series: Cases in Metabolic Bone Disease.* (Zackson, D. A., Ed.). Part I pp 1-11. Publications Triclinica Communications. New York

Bunger, C. (1984) Regional blood flow and intraosseous pressure changes of the juvenile knee in experimental arthritis. **In**: *Bone Circulation.* (Arlet, J., Ficat, R. P. and Hungerford, D. S. Eds.). Chapter 36, pp 216-221. Williams and Wilkins, Baltimore.

Burck, U., Kaitila, I. I., Goebel, H. H. (1982) *et al.*, Clinical, radiological and biochemical data on fetal congenital hypophosphatasia. **In**: *International Clinical Genetics Seminar.* pp 149-154. Alan R. Liss, New York

Burkhardt, R., Bartl, R. and Frisch, B. (1984) *et al.*, The structural relationship of bone forming and endothelial cells of the bone marrow. **In**: *Bone Circulation.* (Arlet, J., Ficat, R. P. and Hungerford, D. S. Eds.). Chapter 1, pp 2-13. Williams and Wilkins, Baltimore.

Burkhardt, A. and Gebbers, J-O. (1977) Giant cell stromal reaction in squamous cell carcinomata. *Virchows Arch.* **A. 375**: 263-280

Cabannes, R. and Mambo-Sambo, F. (1984) Anatomical and pathological aspects of bone changes in Sickle Cell disease. **In**: *Bone Circulation.* (Arlet, J., Ficat, R. P. and Hungerford, D. S. Eds.). Chapter 45, pp 265-273. Williams and Wilkins, Baltimore.

Campbell, J. E., Tam, C. S. and Sheppard, R. H. (1977) "Brown tumor" of hyperparathyroidism induced with anticonvulsant medication. *J. Can. Assoc. Radiol.* **28**: 73

Canfield, R. E. (1987) Introduction: Rationale for diphosphonate therapy in hypercalcemia of malignancy. *Am. J. Med.* **82**: (Suppl 2A) 1-5

Chambers, T. J. (1985) Review Article: The pathobiology of the osteoclast. *J. Clin. Pathol.* **38**: 241-252

Chambers, T. J. (1988) The regulation of osteoclastic development and function. In: *Cell and molecular biology of vertebrate hard tissues.* pp 92-107. Ciba Foundation Symposia 136. Wiley, Chichester.

Chambers, T. J. and Horton, M. A. (1984) Failure of cells of the mononuclear phagocyte series to resorb bone. *Calcif. Tiss. Int.* **36**: 556-558

Chambers, T. J. and Magners, C. J. (1982) Calcitonin alters behavior of isolated osteoclasts. *J. Pathol.* **136** 27-40

Chappard, D., Alexandre, C., Palle, S. (1989) *et al.*, Effects of a biphosphonate (1-hydroxy ethylidene-1,1 biphosphonic acid) on osteoclast number during prolonged bed rest in healthy humans. *Metabolism* **38**: 822-825

Charhon, S. A., Chavassieux, P. M., Chapuy, M. C. (1986) *et al.*, Case Report: High bone turnover associated with an aluminum-induced impairment of bone mineralization. *Bone* **7**: 319-324

Charhon, S. A., Edouard, C. M., Arlot, M. E. (1982) *et al.*, Effects of parathyroid hormone on remodeling of iliac trabecular bone packets in patients with primary hyperpara-thyroidism. *Clin. Orthop.* **162**: 255-263

Chavassieux, P. M., Arlot, M. E. and Meunier, P. J. ((1985) Inter-sample variation in bone histomorphometry: Comparison between parameter values measured on two contiguous transiliac bone biopsies. *Calcif. Tissue Int.* **37**: 345-350

Choie, D. D., Richter, G. W. and Young, L. B. (1975) Biogenesis of intranuclear lead-protein inclusions in mouse kidney. *Beitr. Path. Bd.* **155**: 197-203

Chou, S. M. (1968) Myxovirus-like structures and accompanying nuclear changes in chronic polymyositis. *Arch. Pathol.* **86**: 649-658

Coburn, J., Kanis, J., Popovtzer, M. (1983) *et al.*, Pathophysiology and treatment of uremic bone disease. *Calcif. Tissue Int.* **35**: 712-714

Cohen, J. (1960) Simple bone cysts. Studies of cyst fluid in six cases with a theory of pathogenesis. *J. Bone Joint. Surg.* **42A**: 609-616

Copeland, M. M. and Geschickter, C. F. (1971) Malignant bone tumors, Primary and Metastatic. In: *CA - A Cancer Journal for Clinicians* **13**: No 4-6, American Cancer Soc. Inc. 2nd Ed.

Cuthbert, J. A., Pak, C. Y. C., Zerioekh, J. E. (1984) *et al.*, Bone disease in primary biliary cirrhosis: Increased bone resorption and turnover in the absence of osteoporosis or osteomalacia. *Hepatology* **4**: 1-8

Dahlin, D. C. (1967a) Osteochondroma. In: *Bone Tumors 2nd Ed.* Chapter 2, pp 18-27, Charles C. Thomas, Springfield Il.

Dahlin, D. C. (1967b) Fibrosarcoma and desmoplastic fibroma. In: *Bone Tumors 2nd Ed.* Chapter 22 pp 212-221. Charles C. Thomas, Springfield Il.

Dambacker, M. A., Ittner, J. and Ruegsegger (1986) Long-term fluoride therapy of postmenopausal osteoporosis. *Bone* **7**: 199-205

Daniell, H. W. (1976) Osteoporosis of the slender smoker. *Ann. Int. Med.* **136**: 298-304

Delmas, P. and Meunier, P. J. (1981) L'osteoporose au cours du syndrome de Klinefelter. *La Nouvelle Presse Medicle* **10**: 687-690

Dempster, D. W., Arlot, M. A. and Meunier, P. J. (1983) Mean wall thickness and formation periods of trabecular bone packets in corticosteroid-induced osteoporosis. *Calcif. Tissue Int.* **35**: 410-417

de Vernejoul, M. C., Belenguer-Prieto, R., Kuntz, D. (1988) *et al.*, Bone histological heterogeneity in postmenopausal osteoporosis: A sequential histomorphometric study. *Bone* **8**: 339-342

Doty, S. B. and Mathews, L. 91971) Electron microscopic and histochemical investigation of osteogenesis imperfecta tarda. *Clin. Orthop.* **80**: 191-201

Draper, H. (1986) Nutritional aspects of aging. In: *Nutritional Aspects of Aging Vol. II.* (Linda H. Chen, Ed.). Chapter 6 pp 152-157. CRC Press Inc. Boca Raton, Florida

Duncan, H. (1972) Osteoporosis in rheumatoid arthritis and corticosteroid induced osteoporosis. *Orthop. Clinics of N. Am.* **3**: 571-583

Eddy, E. R. L. (1971) Metabolic bone disease after gastrectomy. *Am. J. Med.* **50**: 442-449

Eilon, G. and Mundy, G. R. (1979) Increases in cyclic AMP in human breast cancer cells causes release of hydrolytic enzymes and bone resorbing activity. *First Ann. Meeting ASBMR Anaheim CA.*

Eisenstein, R. and Kawanowe, S. (1975) The lead line in bone -A lesion apparently due to chondroblastic indigestion. *Am. J. Path.* **80**: 309-316

Elias, C., Heaney, R. P. and Recker, R. R. (1985) Placebo therapy for postmenopausal osteoporosis. *Calcif. Tissue Int.* **37**: 6-13

Elleder, M. (1986) Enzyme patterns in human endocytotic multinucleate giant cells - a histochemical study. *Acta Histochem (Jena)* **79**: 1-10

Elmore, S. M. (1967) Pycnodysostosis: A review. *J. Bone Joint Surg.* **49**A: 153-162

Ensslen, R. D., Jackson, F. I. and Reid, A. M. (1983) Bone and gallium scans in mastocytosis: Correlation with count rates, radiography and microscopy. *J. Nucl. Med.* **24**: 586-588

Erickson, E. F., Mosekilde, L. and Melsen, F. (1985) Trabecular bone resorption depth decreases with age: Differences between normal males and females. *Bone* **6**: 141-146

Ericksen, E. F., Mosekilde, L. and Melsen, F. (1986a) Kinetics of trabecular bone resorption and formation in hypothyroidism: Evidence for a positive balance per remodeling cycle. *Bone* **7**: 101-108

Ericksen, E. F., Mosekilde, L. and Melsen, F. (1986b) Trabecular remodeling and balance in primary hyperparathyroidism. *Bone* **7**: 213-221

Evans, R. A., Dunstan, C. R. and Hills, C. (1983) Bone metabolism in idiopathic juvenile osteoporosis: A case report. *Calcif. Tissue Int.* **35**: 5-8

Evans, R. W. (1968) Tumors of cartilage and bone. In: *Histological Appearances of Tumors 2nd Ed.* Chapter IX pp 164-215. Williams and Wilkins Co. Baltimore

Everts, V., Aronson, D. C. and Beertsen, W. (1985) Phagocytosis of bone collagen by osteoclasts in two cases of pycnodysostosis. *Calc. Tissue Int.* **37**: 25-31

Fallon, M. D., Whyte, M. P., Craig, R. B. Jr (1983) *et al.*, Mast-cell proliferation in postmenopausal osteoporosis. *Calcif. Tissue Int.* **35**: 29-31

Fechner, R. E. (1982) Bones and joints. In: *Pathology of Drug-induced and Toxic Diseases.* (Riddell, R. H., Ed.). pp 71-85. Churchill Livingstone, New York

Ferguson, R. J. and Yunis, E. J. (1978) The ultrastructure of human osteosarcoma. *Clin. Orthop.* **131**: 234-246

Fitzgerald, R. H. (1986) Pathogenesis of musculoskeletal sepsis. In: *Musculoskeletal Infections.* (Hughes, S. P. and Fitzgerald, R. H., Eds.). Chapter 1 p. 20. Year Book Medical Publishers Inc. Chicago.

Flanagan, A. M., Nui, B., Tinkler, S. M. (1988) *et al.*, The multinucleate cells in giant cell granulomas of the jaw are osteoclasts. *Cancer* **15**: 1139-1145

Fournasier, V. L., Flores, L., Hastings, D. (1985) *et al.*, Virus-like filamentous intranuclear inclusions in a giant cell tumor not associated with Paget's disease. A case report. *J. Bone Jt. Surg.* **67**A: 333-336

Frame, B. and Nixon, R. K. (1968) Bone marrow mast cells in osteoporosis of aging. *N. Engl. J. Med.* **279**: 626-630

Francis, R. M., Peacock, M., Aaron, J. E. (1986) *et al.*, Osteoporosis in hypogonadel men: Role of decreased plasma 1,25-dihydroxyvitamin D, calcium malabsorption and low bone formation. *Bone* **7**: 261-268

Fraser, D. (1973) *et al.*, Pathogeneisi of hereditary vitamin-D-dependent rickets: an inborn error of vitamin D metabolism involving conversion of 25-hydroxyvitamin D to 1, 25 dihydroxy vitamin D. *New Engl. J. Med.* **289**: 817-822

Friedman, B. and Gold, H. (1968) Ultrastructure of Ewing's sarcoma of bone. *Cancer* **22**: 307-322

Friedenstein, A. J., Petrakova, K. V., Kurossova, I. (1968) *et al.*, Heterotopic transplants of bone marrow. *Transplantation* **6**: 230-247

Frisch, B. and Eventov, I. (1986) Hematopoiesis in osteoporosis - preliminary report comparing biopsies of the femoral neck and iliac crest. *Isr. J. Med. Sci.* **22**: 380-384

Galasko, C. S. B. (1981) The development of skeletal metastases. In: *Bone metastases.* (Weiss, L. W. and Gilbert, H. A., Eds.). pp 49-63. G. K. Hall , Medical Publ. Boston

Ghadially, F. N. (1985) *Diagnostic electron microscopy of tumors. 2nd Ed.* p 219. Buttersworths, Boston.

Gherardi, G., LoCascio, V. and Bonucci, E. (1980a) Fine structure of nuclei and cytoplasm of osteoclasts in Paget's disease of bone. *Histopathology* **4**: 63-74

Gherardi, G., Pogge, A., Sisca, S. (1980b) *et al.*, Bone oxalosis and renal osteodystrophy. *Arch. Pathol. Lab. Med.* **104**: 105-111

Glimcher, M. J. and Kinzora, J. E. (1979) The biology of osteonecrosis of the human femoral head and its clinical implications. III. The pathological changes in the femoral head as an organ and in the hip joint. *Clin. Orthop.* **139**: 283-312

Goldring, S. R., Dayer, J-M., Russell, R. G. G. (1978) *et al.*, Response to hormones of cells cultured from giant cell tumors of bone. *J. Clin. Endocrinol. Metab.* **46**: 425-433

Goldring, S. R. and Krane, S. M. (1986) The skeletal system. In: *Werner's The Thyroid A Fundamental and Clinical Test. 5th Ed.* (Ingbar, S. H. and Braverman, L. E., Ed). pp 930-948. J. B. Lippincott Co. New York

Gothlin, G. and Ericcsson, J. L. E. (1976) The osteoclast. Review of ultrastructure, origin and structure-function relationship. *Clin. Orthop.* **120**: 201-230

Granstrom, K. O. and Hed, R. (1966) Idiopathic hypoparathyroidism with cataract and spontaneous hypocalcemic hypercalciuria. *Acta Med. Scand.* **178**: 417-421

Griffith, G. C., Nichols, G., Asher, J. D. (1965) *et al.*, Heparin osteoporosis. *JAMA* **193**: 85-88

Gruber, H. E., Ivey, J. L., Thompson, E. R. (1986) *et al.*, Osteoblast and osteoclast cell number and cell activity in postmenopausal osteoporosis. *Miner. Electrolyte Metab.* **12**: 246-254

Hahn, T. J. (1976) Bone complications of anticonvulsants. *Review. Drugs* **12**: 201-211

Ham, A. W. and Cormack, D. H. (1979) *Histology. 8th Ed.* Chapters 14, 15, 16. pp 367-485. J. B. Lippincott Co. Philadelphia

Hall, B. K. (1975) The origin and fate of osteoclasts. *Anat. Rec.* **183**: 1-11

Hanaoka, H., Friedman, B. and Mack, R. P. (1970) Ultrastructure and histogenesis of giant-cell tumor of bone. *Cancer* **25**: 1408-1423

Hills, E., Dunstan, C. R., Wang, S. Y. (1989) *et al.*, Bone histology in young adult osteoporosis. *J. Clin. Pathol.* **42**: 391-397

Hennigar, G. R. and Gross, P. (1985) Drug and chemical injury-environmental pathology. In: *Anderson's Pathology. 8th Ed.* (Kissane, J. M., Ed.). Chapter 5 pp 147-235. C. V. Mosby Co. St. Louis.

Hogg, N., Shapiro, I. M., Jones, S. J. (1977) *et al.*, Lack of Fc receptors on osteoclasts. *Cell Tissue Res.* **212**: 509-510

Holtrop, M. E. and King, G. J. (1977) The ultrastructure of the osteoclast and its functional implications. *Clin. Orthop.* **123**: 177-196

Horton, M. A., Rimmer, E. F., Lewis, D. (1984) *et al.*, Cell surface characterization of the human osteoclast: Phenotypic relationship to other bone marrow-derived cell types. *J. Pathol.* **144**: 281-194

Hough, A. J. and Sokoloff, L. (1986) Pathology. In: *Rheumatoid Arthritis*. (Utsinger, P. D., Zvaifler, N. J. and Ehrlich, G. F., Eds.). Chapter 4, pp 49-69. J. B. Lippincott Co. New York

Howatson, A. F. and Fournasier, V. L. (1982) Microfilaments associated with Paget's disease of bone: Comparison with nucleocapsids of measles virus and respiratory syncytial virus. *Intervirology* **18**: 150-159

Hume, D. A., Loutit, J. F. and Gordon, S. (1984) The mononuclear phagocyte system of the mouse defined by immunohistochemical localization of antigen F4/80. *J. Cell Sci.* **66**: 189-194

Jaffe, H. L. and Lichtenstein, L. (1942) Solitary unicameral bone cyst with emphasis on the roentgen picture, the pathologic appearance and pathogenesis. *Arch. Surg.* **44**: 1004-1025

Jaffee, M. D. and Willis, P. W. (1964) Multiple fractures associated with long-term sodium heparin therapy. *JAMA* **193**: 152-154

Johnson, L. C. (1964) Morphologic analysis in pathology. In: *Bone Biodynamics*. (Frost, H. M., Ed.). Chapter 29, pp 543-654. Little Brown and Co., Boston

Josse, R. G., Murray, T. M., Mundy, G. R. (1981) *et al.*, Observations on the mechanism of bone resorption induced by multiple myeloma marrow culture fluids and partially purified osteoclast-activating factor. *J. Clin. Invest.* **67**: 1472-1481

Jowsey, J. (1960) Age changes in human bone. *Clin. Orthop.* **17**: 210-217

Kanis, J. A., Irwin, G. H., Gray, R. E. S. (1987) *et al.*, Effects of intravenous etidronate disodium on skeletal and calcium metabolism. *Am. J. Med.* **87**: Suppl 2A 55-88

Kaye, M. and Henderson, J. (1988) The nature of mononuclear cells positive for acid phosphatase activity in bone marrow of patients with renal osteodystrophy. *J. Clin. Pathol.* **41**: 277-279

Kirsch, E., Krieg, T., Nerlich, A. (1987) *et al.*, Compositional analysis of collagen from patients with diverse forms of Osteogenesis Imperfecta. *Calcif. Tissue Int.* **41**: 11-17

Kiyokawa, T., Yamaguchi, K., Takeya, M. (1987) *et al.*, Hypercalcemia and osteoclast proliferation in adult T-cell leukemia. *Cancer* **59**: 1187-1191

Kleerekoper, M., Bernstein, R. S., Crouch, M. (1986) *et al.*, Parathyroid function in osteoporosis: Lack of correlation with skeletal histology. *J. Pathol.* **150**: 239 Abstract *78*

Kolliker, A. (1956) Die normale Resorption des Knocnengewebes und ihre Bedentung fur die Entstehung der typischen Knochenformen. Leipzig, Vogel 1873, Cited: N. Hancox, The Osteoclast p 249. In: *The Biochemistry and Physiology of Bone*. (Bourne, G. F., Ed.). Academic Press Inc. New York

Krane, S. M. (1977) Paget's disease of bone. *Clin. Orthop.* **127**: 24-36

Kulenkampff, H-A., Dreyer, T., Kersjes, W. (1986) *et al.*, Histomorphometric analysis of osteoclastic bone resorption in metastatic bone disease from various primary malignomas. *Virchows Arch.* **A 409**: 817-828

Kumar, R. and Riggs, B. L. (1980) Pathologic bone physiology. In: *Fundamental and clinical bone physiology*. Chapter 13, pp 394. J. B. Lippincott Co. Philadelphia

Lai, M. M. C., Wang, Y-J. and Mills, B. (1989) Molecular cloning and characterization of paramyxovirus RNA sewuences in Paget's disease of bone. *J. Bone Miner. Res.* **4**: S198

Lang, R., Vignery, A. M. C. and Jensen, P. S. (1986) Case Report: Fibrogenesis imperfecta ossium with early onset: Observation after 20 years of illness. *Bone* **7**: 237-246

Levin, M. E., Boisseau, V. C. and Avioli, L. V. (1976) Effects of diabetes mellitus on bone mass in juvenile and adult-onset diabetes. *N. Engl. J. Med.* **294**: 241-245

Lindenfelser, R., Schmitt, H. P. and Haubert, P. (1973) Vergleichende raslerelektronenmikroskopische Knochenuntersuchungen bei promarem und sekundarem hyperparathyreoidismus. *Virchows Arch* **A. 360**: 114-154

Lindsay, R., Hart, D. M. and Forrest, C. (1980) *et al.*, Prevention of spinal osteoporosis in oophrectomised women. *Lancet* **2**: 1151-1153

Lips, P., Courpron, P. and Meunier, P. J. (1978) Mean wall thickness of trabecular bone packets in the human iliac crest: Changes with age. *Calcif. Tissue Res.* **26**: 13-17

Lipsky, P. E. (1985) Disease-modifying Drugs. In: *Rheumatoid Arthritis*. (Utsinger, P. D., Zvaifler, N. J. and Ehrlich, J. E., Eds.). pp 601-634. J. B. Lippincott Co., Philadelphia

LoCascio, V., Bonucci, E., Imbimbo, B. (1984) *et al.*, Bone loss after glucocorticoid therapy. *Calc. Tiss. Int.* **36**: 435-438

Long, R. G., Memhard, E., Skinner, R. K. (1964) *et al.*, Clinical biochemical and histological studies of osteomalacia, osteoporosis and parathyroid function in chronic liver disease. *Gut* **19**: 85-90

Lichtenstein, L. and Sawyer, W. R. (1964) Benign osteoblastoma. *J. Bone Jt. Surg.* **46A**: 755-765

Malkani, K., Basle, M. and Rebel, A. (1976) Goniometric observation of nuclear inclusions in osteoclasts in Paget's bone disease. *J. Submicro. Cytol.* **8**: 229-236

Malkani, K. and Rebel, A. (1974) Etude au microscope electronique des rapports entre mastocytes et tissu osseux au cours des remaniements osteomalaciques de l'osteodystrophe renale. *Path. Biol.* **22**: 393-400

Marcus, R., Kosek, J., Pfefferbaum, A. (1983) *et al.*, Age-related loss of trabecular bone in premenopausal women: A biopsy study. *Calcif. Tiss. Int.* **35**: 406-409

Mariano, M. and Spector, W. G. (1974) The formation and properties of macrophage polykaryons (inflammatory giant cells). *J. Path.* **113**: 1-19

Maschio, G., Bonucci, E., Mioni, G. (1974) *et al.*, Biochemical and morphological aspects of bone tissue in chronic renal failure. *Nephron* **12**: 437-448

Mazess, R. B. and Mathur, W. (1974) Bone mineral content of Northern Alaskan Eskimos. *Am. J. Clin. Nutr.* **27**: 916-925

Mazess, R. B. and Whedon, G. D. (1983) Editorial: Immobilization and bone. *Calcif. Tiss. Int.* **35**: 265-267

McCarthy, E. F., Matsuno, T. and Dorfman, H. D. (1979) Malignant fibrous histocystoma of bone: a study of 35 cases. *Hum. Pathol.* **10**: 57-70

McClean, F. C. (1968) Resorption of bone. In: *Bone: fundamentals of skeletal tissue*. p 108.

McLeod, J. J., Dahlin, D. C. and Ivins, J. C. (1957) Fibrosarcoma of Bone. *Am. J. Surg.* **94**: 431-437

McKibben, B. (1978) The biology of fracture healing in long bones. *J. Bone Jt. Surg.* **60B**: 150-162

McKibben, B. and Ralis, Z. (1974) Pathological changes in a case of Perthe's disease. *J. Bone Jt. Surg.* **56B**: 438-447

McNair, P. (1978) *et al.*, Osteopenia in insulin-treated diabetes mellitus: its relation to age at onset, sex and duration of disease. *Diabetologia* **15**: 87-90

Meema, H. E. and Meema, S. (1988) Longitudinal microradioscopic comparisons on endosteal and juxtaendosteal bone loss in premenopausal and postmenopausal women, and those with end-stage renal disease. *Bone* **8**: 343-350

Melrose, R. J., Abrams, A. M. and Mills, B. G. (1976) Florid osseous dysplasia. *Oral Surg.* **41**: 62-82

Melsen, F. and Mosekilde, L. (1977) Morphometric and dynamic studies of bone changes in hyperthyroidism. *Acta Pathol. Microbiol. Scand. S(A)* **85**: 141-150

Melsen, F. and Mosekilde, L. (1978) Tetracycline double-labeling of iliac trabecular bone in 41 normal adults. *Calcif. Tiss. Res.* **26**: 99-102

Metze, K., Ciplea, A. G., Hettwer, H. (1987) *et al.*, Size dependent enzyme activities of multinucleated (osteoclasts) giant cells in bone tumors. *Pathol. Res. Pract.* **182**: 214-221

Meunier, P. J., Bianchi, G. G. S., Edouard, C. M. (1972) *et al.*, Bony manifestations in thyrotoxicosis. *Orthop. Clin. North Am.* **3**: 745-774

Meunier, P. J., Chapuy, M-C., Delmas, P. (1987) *et al.*, Intravenous disodium etidronate therapy in Paget's disease of bone and hypercalcemia of malignancy. Effects on biochemical parameters and histomor-phometry. *Am. J. Med.* **82**: (Suppl. 2A), 71-78

Meunier, P. J. and Chavassieux, P. (1985) Histomorphometry. Method for evaluating the bone mass. *Rev. Rhum. Mal. Osteoartic.* **52**: 669-673

Mills, B. G. (1981) Comparison of the ultrastructure of a malignant tumor of the mandible containing giant cells with Paget's disease of bone. *J. Oral Pathol.* **10**: 203-215

Mills, B. G., Hendricks, D. and Singer, F. R. (1988) Evidence for nucleocapsid gene of respiratory syncytial virus in Paget bone derived cells. *J. Bone Min. Res.* **3**: S93 Abstract 97

Mills, B., Holst, P. and Graham, C. (1979) Correlation of ultrastructure with phosphatase activity in cyst fluid of jaw lesions. *J. Dental Res.* **58**: 355

Mills, B. G. and Lee, D. B. N. (1984) Ultrastructure of bone following renal transplatation compared to osteodystrophy. **In**: *Endocrine control of bone and calcium metabolism.* (Cohn, D. V., Potts, J. R. Jr. and Fujita, T., Eds.). pp 158-160. Elsevier Science Publ. Co. Amsterdam.

Mills, B. G., Masuoka, L. S., Graham, C. C. (1988a) *et al.*, Gallium-67 citrate localization in osteoclast nuclei of Paget's disease of bone. *J. Nucl. Med.* **29**: 1083-1087

Mills, B. G., Moore, T. M. and Holst, P. A. (1980b) Phosphatase levels in fluid from unicameral bone cysts. *Am. Soc. Bone Min. Res.* Abstract *70, p IX*

Mills, B. G. and Singer, F. R. (1976) Nuclear inclusions in Paget's disease of bone. *Science* **194**: 257-261

Mills, B. G., Singer, F. R., Weiner, L. P. (1980a) *et al.*, Cell cultures from bone affected by Paget's disease. *Arthritis and Rheumatism* **23**: 1115-1120

Mills, B. G., Singer, F. R., Weiner, L. P. (1984) *et al.*, Evidence for both respiratory syncytial virus and measles virus antigens in the osteoclasts of patients with Paget's disease of bone. *Clin. Orthop.* **183**: 303-311

Mills, B. G., Yabe, H. and Singer, F. R. (1988b) Osteoclasts in human osteopetrosis contain viral-nucleocapsid-like nuclear inclusions. *J. Bone and Min. Res.* **3**: 101-106

Minaire, P., Meunier, P., Edouard, C. (1974) *et al.*, Quantitative histologie data on disuse osteoporosis. Comparison with biologie data. *Calcif. Tiss. Res.* **17**: 57-73

Minkin, C. and Shapiro, I. M. (1986) Editorial: Osteoclasts, mononuclear phagocytes and physiologic bone resorption. *Calcif. Tissue Int.* **39**: 357-359

Mirra, J. M., Bauer, F. C. H. and Grant, T. T. (1981) Giant-cell tumor with viral-like inclusions associated with Paget's disease. *Clin. Orthop.* **158**: 243-251

Miszta, H., Dabrowski, Z. and Lanotte, M. (1988) *in vitro* patterns of enzymic tetrahydrofoliate dehydrogenase (EC 1.5.1.3) expression in bone marrow stromal cells. *Leukemia* **2**: 754-759

Moskilde, L. and Melsen, F. (1978a) Morphometric and dynamic studies on bone changes in hypothyroidism. *Acta. Pathol. Microbiol. Scand. S(a)* **86**: 56-62

Moskilde, L. and Melsen, F. (1978b) A tetracycline-based histomorphometric evaluation of bone resorption and bone turnover in hyperthyroidism and hyperparathyroidism. *Acta Med. Scand.* **204**: 97-102

Moskilde, L. (1979) *Effects of thyroid hormones on bone remodeling and bone mass and calcium phosphorous homeostasis in man.* Thesis, University of Aarhus, Denmark

Mundy, G. R., Raisz, L. G., Cooper, RT. A. (1974) *et al.*, Evidence for the secretion of an osteoclast stimulating factor in myeloma. *N. Engl. J. Med.* **291**: 1041-1046

Mundy, G. R., Shapiro, J. L., Bandelin, J. G. (1976) *et al.*, Direct stimulation of bone resorption by thyroid hormones. *J. Clin. Invest.* **58**: 529-534

Mundy, G. R. and Spiro, T. P. (1981) The mechanisms of bone metastasis and bone destruction by tumor cells. **In**: *Bone Metastases.* (Weiss, L. and Gilbert, H. A., Eds.). G. K. Hall Publ. Boston

Mundy, G. R., Wilkinson, R. and Heath, D. A. (1983) Comparative study of available medical therapy for hypercalcemia of malignancy. *Am. J. Med.* **74**: 421-437

Murrills, R. J., Shane, E., Lindsey, R. (1989) *et al.*, Bone resorption by isolated human osteoclasts *in vitro*: effects of calcitonin, *J. Bone Miner. Res.* **4**: 259-268

Neer, C. S. II, Francis, K. C., Johnston, A. D. (1973) *et al.*, Current concepts on the treatment of solitary unicameral bone cyst. *Clin. Orthop.* **97**: 40-51

Nordin, B. E. C. (1960) Osteomalacia, osteoporosis and calcium deficiency. *Clin. Orthop.* **17**: 235-257

Nordin, B. E. C., Aaron, J. E., Makins, N. B. (1983) *et al.*, Bone formation and resorption in postmenopausal osteoporosis. **In:** *Osteoporosis. A Multidisciplinary Problem.* (Dixon, A. St. J., Russell, R. G. G. and Stamp, T. C. B., Eds.). pp 1612-1710. Royal Society of Medicine International Congress and Symposium Series No. 55. Royal Society of Medicine/Academic Press, London

Nunez, E. A., Horwith, M., Krook, L. (1979) *et al.*, An electron microscopic investigation of human familial bone dysplasia. Inhibition of osteocytic osteolysis and induction of osteocytic formation of elastic fibers following calcitonin treatment. *Am. J. Pathol.* **94**: 1-18

Ohlin, A. and Kindblom, L. G. (1988) The ultrastructure of the tissue surrounding the Christiansen total hip. *Acta Orthop. Scand.* **59**: 629-634

Oreopoulos, D. G., Rabinovich, S., Meema, H. E. (1973) *et al.*, Contrasting bone changes in patients on chronic hemodialysis and chronic peritoneal dialysis. **In:** *Clinical Aspects of Metabolic Bone Disease.* (Frame, B., Parfitt, A. M. and Duncan, H., Eds.). Excerpta Medica, Amsterdam (1973).

Parfitt, A. M. (1981a) Bone effects of space flight: analysis by quantum concept of bone remodelling. *Acta Astronautica* **8**: 1083-1090

Parfitt, A. M. (1981b) Bone remodeling in the pathogenesis of osteoporosis. *Resident and Staff Physician.* pp 60-72.

Parfitt, A. M. (1982) The coupling of bone formation to bone resorption: A critical analysis of the concept and of its relevance to the pathogenesis of osteoporosis. *Metab. Bone Dis. and Rel. Res.* **4**: 1-6

Parfitt, A. M., Miller, M. J. and Frame, B. (1978) *et al.*, Metabolic bone disease after intestinal bypass for the treatment of obesity. *Ann. Int. Med.* **89**: 193-199

Pazzaglia, U. E. and Pringle, J. A. (1989) Bone resorption *In vitro*: macrophages and giant cells from failed total hip replacement versus osteoclasts. *Biomaterials* **10**: 286-288

Perry, H. M. III, Fallon, M. D., Bergfeld, M. (1982) *et al.*, Osteoporosis in young men. *Arch. Intern. Med.* **142**: 1295-1298

Podenphant, J., Gotfredsen, A., Nilas, L. (1986) *et al.*, Iliac crest biopsy: Representative for the amount of mineralized bone. *Bone* **7**: 427-430

Rebel, A., Basle, M. and Pouplard, R. (1979) Paget's disease of bone: First immunological evidence of viral antigen in osteoclasts. *14th European Symposium on Calcified Tissues,* Rhodes, Greece,

Rebel, A. and Malkani, K. (1974) Ultrastructure des mastocytes dans des biopsies de la crete iliaque au cours de l'osteodystrophie renale. *Path. Biol.* **22**: 221-228

Rebel, A., Malkani, K., Basle, M. (1976) *et al.*, Osteoclast ultrastructure in Paget's disease. *Calcif. Tiss. Res.* **20**: 187-199

Remagen, W., Hohling, H. J., Hall, T. T. (1969) *et al.*, Electron microscopical and microprobe observations on the cell sheath of stimulated osteocytes. *Calcif. Tiss. Res.* **4**: 60-68

Rigby, P. J. and Papadimitriou, J. M. (1984) Cytoskeletal control of nuclear arrangement in Langhans multinucleate giant cells. *J. Path.* **143**: 17-29

Rosenquist, J. B. (1975) Effects of supply and withdrawal of fluoride. *Acta Pathol. Microbiol. Scand.* **83**: 628-632

Ruby, L. K. and Mital, M. A. (1974) Skeletal deformities following chronic hypervitaminosis A. *J. Bone Jt. Surg.* **56A**: 1283-1287

Rutter, D. J., Rijssel, T. G. and van der Velde, E. A. (1977) Aneurysmal bone cysts. A clinicopathological study of 105 cases. *Cancer* **39**: 2231-2239

Rywlin, A. M. (1985) Hemopoietic System: Reticuloendothelial system, spleen, lymph nodes, bone marrow and blood. In: *Anderson's Pathology 8th Ed.* (Kissane, J. M., Ed.) Chapter 30 pp 1257-1351. C. V. Mosby Co. St. Louis.

Schajowicz, F., Ubios, A. M., Ararujo, E. S. (1985) *et al.*, Virus-like intranuclear inclusions in giant cell tumor of bone. *Clin. Orthop.* **201**: 247-250

Schajowicz, F., Velen, O., Aranjo, E. S. (1988) *et al.*, Metastases of carcinoma in the Pagetic bone. A report of two cases. *Clin. Orthop.* **228**: 290-296

Schenk, R. K., Olah, A. J. and Merz, W. A. (1973) Bone cell counts. In: *Clinical aspects of metabolic bone disease.* (Frame, B, Parfitt, A. M. and Duncan, H. Ed.). pp 103-114. Excerpta Medica, Amsterdam

Scher, H. I. (1987) Bone metastases: Pathogenesis, treatment and rationale for use of resorption inhibitors. *Am. J. Med.* **82**: 6-11

Schnitzler, C. M. and Salomon, L. (1986) Histomorphometric analysis of a calcaneal stress fracture: A possible complication of fluoride therapy for osteoporosis. *Bone* **7**: 193-198

Schochet, S. S. Jr. and McCormick, W. F. (1973) Polymyositis with intranuclear inclusions. *Arch Neurol.* **28**: 280-283

Schulz, A., Bressel, M. and Delling, G. (1977a) Activity of osteoclastic bone resorption in primary hyperparathyroidism-comparative electronmicroscopic and histomorphometric study. *Calcif. Tiss. Res.* **22**: (Suppl) 307-310

Schulz, A., Delling, G. and Ringe, J-D. (1977b) *et al.*, Morbus Paget des Knochens. *Virchows Arch. A.* **376**: 309-328

Schulz, A., Maerker, R. and Delling, G. (1976) Das zentrale Reisen-zellgranulom. *Virchows Arch A.* **371**: 161-170

Sedlin, E. D., Frost, H. M. and Villanueva, A. R. (1963) Variations in cross section area of rib cortex with age. *J. Gerontol.* **18**: 9-13

Seidl, K., Harmut, M., Kostial, K. (1982) *et al.*, Changes of bone mass in diabetes mellitus. *Periodicum Biologorum* **84**: 13-21

Shapiro, F., Glimcher, M. J., Holtrop, M. E. (1980) *et al.*, Human osteopetrosis. A histological, ultrastructural and biochemical study. *J. Bone and Jt. Surg.* **62A**: 384-399

Shapiro, F., Key, L. L. and Anast, C. (1988) Variable osteoclast appearance in human infantile osteopetrosis. *Calcif. Tissue Int.* **43**: 67-76

Shih, M-S. and Anderson, C. (1987) Does "hepatic osteodystrophy" differ from peri- and postmenopausal osteoporosis? A histomorphometric study. *Calcif. Tiss. Int.* **41**: 187-191

Sidransky, H. (1985) Malnutrition and deficiency diseases. In: *Anderson's Pathology 8th Ed.* (Kissane, J. M., Ed.). Chapter 14 pp. 495-513.

Sillence, D. O., Danks, S. A. (1980) Genetic heterogeniety in osteogenesis imperfecta. *J. Med. Genetics* **16**: 101-116

Simmons, D. J. (1980) Fracture healing. In: *Fundamental and Clinical Bone Physiology.* (Urist, M. R., Ed.). Chapter 10 pp 283-332. J. B. Lippincott Co. Philadelphia

Singer, F. R. and Krane, S. M. (1973) Skeletal resistance to salmon calcitonin in patients with medullary carcinoma of the thyroid. *55th Annual Meeting of the Endocrine Society* pp A-184

Sissons, H. A. (1969) Les changements peri-osteocytaires dans l'osteomalacie. *Rev. Chir. Orthop. Appl Moteur (Paris)* **55**: 284

Sissons, H. A. (1956) The osteoporosis of Cushing's syndrome. *J. Bone and Jt. Surg.* **38B**: 417-433

Slootweg, P. J. (1989) Comparison of giant cell granuloma of the jaw and non-ossifying fibroma. *J. Oral Pathol. Med.* **18**: 128-132

Smith, R. (1980) Idiopathic osteoporosis in the young. *J. Bone Jt. Surg.* **62B**: 417-427

Spencer, H., Rubio, N., Rubio, E. (1986) et al., Chronic alcoholism. Frequently overlooked cause of osteoporosis in men. Am. J. Med. 80: 393-397

Squires, J. W. and Pinch, L. L. (1979) Heparin-induced spinal fractures. JAMA 241: 2417-2418

Stark, A., Aparisi, T. and Ericsson, J. L. E. (1985) Human osteogenic sarcoma: Fine structure of hard tissue areas. Ultrastr. Pathol. 8: 83-102

Steendijk, R. and Boyde, A. (1973) Scanning electron microscopic observations on bone from patients with hypophosphataemic (Vitamin D resistent) rickets. Calc. Tiss. Res. 11: 242-250

Stein, H. and Duthie, R. B. (1981) The pathogenesis of chronic haemophilic arthropathy. J. Bone Jt. Surg. 63B: 601-609

Steiner, G. C., Ghosh, L. and Dorfman, H. D. (1972) Ultrastructure of giant cell tumors of bone. Human Pathol. 3: 569-586

Stewart, M. J. (1922) The histogenesis of myeloid sarcoma. Lancet 1106-1108, Nov. 25

Suter, H., Tonz, O. and Scharli, A. (1982) Geroderma osteodysplastica hereditaria (GOH) in a girl. In: Skeletal Dysplasias. (Papadatos, C. J. and Bartsocas, C. S., Ed.). Progress in Clinical Biological Research. Vol 104 Alan R. Liss Inc. New York

Takahashi, N., Kukita, T., MacDonald, B. R. (1989) et al., Osteoclast-like cells form in long-term human bone marrow but not in peripheral blood culture, J. Clin. Invest. 83: 543-550

Teitelbaum, S. L. (1985) Metabolic and other nontumerous disorders of bone. In: Anderson's Pathology. 8th Ed. Vol. 2. (Kissane, J. M., Ed.). Chapter 40 pp 1705-1777. C. V. Mosby Co. St. Louis

Teitelbaum, S. L., Coccia, P. F., Brown, D. M. (1981) et al., Malignant osteopetrosis: A disease of abnormal osteoclast proliferation. Metab. Bone Dis. and Rel. Res. 3: 99-105

Teitelbaum, S. L., Halvason, J. D. and Bates, M. (1977) et al., Abnormalities of circulating 25-OH vitamin D after jejunal-ileal bypass for obesity. Ann. Int. Med. 86: 289-293

Teitelbaum, S. L., Stewart, C. C. and Kahn, A. J. (1979) Rodent peritoneal macrophages vs bone resorbing cells. Calcif. Tiss. Int. 27: 255-261

Tessitore, N., Bonucci, E., D'Angelo, A. (1984) et al., Bone histology and calcium metabolism in patients with nephrotic syndrome and normal or reduced renal function. Nephron 37: 153-159

Thiele, T., Arenz, B, Klein, H. (1988) et al., Differentiation of plasma cell infiltrates in the bone marrow. A clinicopathological study on 80 patients including immunohistochemistry and morphometry Virchows Arch. [A] 412: 553-562

Thomson, A. D. and Turner-Warwick, R. T. (1955) Skeletal sarcomata and giant cell tumour. Bone Jt. Surg. 37B: 266-303

Tucker, W. S, Hubbard, W. H., Stryker, T. D. (1982) et al., A new familial disorder of combined lower motor neuron degeneration and skeletal disorganization. Tran. Assoc. Am. Physic. 1005: 126-134

Urist, M. R. (1980a) Bone transplants and implants. In: Fundamental and clinical bone physiology. (Urist. J. B., Ed.). Chapter 11 pp 331-368. Lippincott Co. Philadelphia

Urist, M. R. (1980b) Heterotopic bone formation. In: Fundamental and Clinical Bone Physiology. (Urist, M. R., Ed.). Chapter 12 pp 369-393. J. B. Lippincott Co. Philadelphia

van Tran, P., Dryll, A., Lausaman, J. (1985) et al., Osteoclast abnormalities in ideopathic osteopetrosis. Virchows Arch. A 408: 269-280

Vaughan, J. M. (1977) External irradiation. In: The effects of irradiation on the skeleton. Chapter 5 pp 51-93. Clarendon Press, Oxford

Wannfors, S., Lindskog, S., Olander, K. J. (1985) et al., Fibrous dysplasia of bone and concomitant dysplastic changes in the dentin. Oral Surg. Oral Med. Oral Pathol. 59: 394-398

Waxman, A. D., McKee, D., Seimsen, J. K. (1980) et al., Gallium scanning in Paget's disease of bone: Effect of calcitonin. AJR 134: 303-306

Wellesley, D. (1964) The significance of paleopathology. In: *Bones, Bodies and Disease.* (Wells, C., Ed.). Frederick A. Praeger Co., New York

Welsh, R. A. and Meyer, A. T. (1970) Nuclear fragmentations and associated fibrils in giant cell tumor of bone. *Lab. Invest.* **22**: 63-72

Wolbach, S. B. (1947) Vitamin A deficiency and excess in relation to skeletal growth. *J. Bone Jt. Surg.* **29**: 171-192

Wood, G. W., Nett, J. R., Gollahon, K. A. (1978) *et al.,* Macrophages in giant cell tumors of bone. *J. Pathol.* **125**: 53-58

Yabe, H., Singer, F. R., Tucker, W. S. (1986) *et al.,* Paget-like inclusions in osteopetrosis and hereditary neuromuscular and skeletal disease. *J. Bone Min. Res.* **1**: Suppl. p 221

Yabut, S. M., Kinan, S., Sissons, H. A. (1988) *et al.,* Malignant transformation of fibrous dysplasia. *Clin. Orthop.* **228**: 281-289

Young, D. R., Niklowitz, W. J., Brown, R. J. (1986) *et al.,* Immobilization-associated osteoporosis in primates. *Bone* **7**: 109-117

Young, R. Y. (1962) Cell proliferation and specialization during endochondral osteogenesis in young rats. *J. Cell Biol.* **14**: 357-370

Yunis, E. J. and Smaha, F. J. (1971) Inclusion body myositis. *Lab. Invest.* **25**: 240-248

8

Mutations Affecting Osteoclasts

SANDY C. MARKS, JR.
Department of Cell Biology
University of Massachusetts Medical School
Worcester, Massachusetts

Introduction
Example - Mammalian Osteopetrosis
Overview and General Features
Mechanisms of Pathogenesis
Direct
Indirect
Summary
References

Introduction

As with other cells and tissues, studies of mutations have illuminated our understanding of bone biology including the osteoclast. The possible effects of mutations on osteoclast function are to increase, decrease or to produce no change in osteoclast function. As one would expect, the likelihood of discovering a mutation without change in osteoclast function is less than either of the other possibilities. With respect to increased skeletal resorption, the *Brachyury* allele in the mouse is presumed to result from a localized tail shortening due to increased resorption of developing tail structures (Wittman *et al.*, 1972). However, this involves non-mineralized tissues and there is no evidence for direct activation of osteoclasts. It is unfortunate that mutations characterized by increased osteoclast function are not available because they could potentially be excellent models for exploring pathogenetic mechanisms in osteoporosis. Mutations involving osteoclast hypofunction are numerous and result in a generalized accumulation of skeletal mass. These mutations in mammals represent interceptions of osteoclast development or function as depicted in Fig. 1 and discussed in previous chapters of this volume.

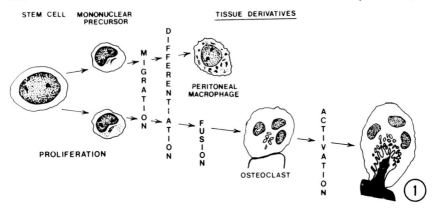

Fig. 1 Diagram indicating related but separate lineages for osteoclasts and macrophages and the processes involved in their ontogeny. (Reproduced from Marks, *Am. J. Medical Genetics*, (1989), with permission of the publisher A.R. Liss).

For our purposes osteoclast biology can be divided into osteoclast development (consisting of proliferation of stem cells, migration of their progeny from sites outside the endosteum to skeletal sites where they differentiate and fuse to form osteoclasts) and osteoclast activation to resorb bone. The structural hallmarks of active osteoclasts (see Chapter 1) include a well developed ruffled border and cytoplasmic vacuolization next to bone surfaces. These features have been exaggerated in Fig. 1. The ruffled border is an area of intense plasma membrane infolding and lies over bone surfaces undergoing degradation. Peripheral areas of cytoplasmic contact with bone surfaces, called clear zones, are devoid of organelles and inclusions. Serial-section reconstructions of ruffled borders and clear zones (Lucht, 1972; Malkani *et al.*, 1973) have shown that the ruffled border of an osteoclast is surrounded in 3-dimensions by the clear zone, effectively sealing off the confines of the ruffled border-bone surface region from the surrounding extracellular space. Thus, the osteoclast functions as a local recycling center (Marks and Popoff, 1988,1990).

The broad outlines of osteoclast function are summarized in Fig. 2. Enzymes (acid hydrolases) made on the rough endoplasmic reticulum are packaged in the perinuclear Golgi complex (A in Fig. 2a) and delivered to the ruffled border where these lysosomes fuse with the plasma membrane and are emptied onto the bone surface. There the pH is lowered by the combined activities of carbonic anhydrase II and a Na^+/K^+ ATPase (Fig. 2b) located on

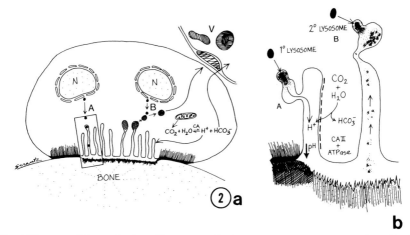

Fig. 2 Diagrams of the mechanism of bone resorption by osteoclasts. a. Enzymes packaged in the perinuclear Golgi region (A) move to the ruffled border region where they are released into the confined space next to mineralized tissue. Products of resorption are taken back up into the cell (B), further digested in secondary lysosomes, and released in adjacent venous sinuses (V). Products of cell respiration are catalized by carbonic anhydrase (CA-located in ruffled border) to produce hydrogen ions which acidify the confined extracellular compartment below the ruffled border, thus providing an optimal environment for the action of acid hydrolases. b. Higher magnification of rectangular area A in Fig. 2a, depicting the exocytic and endocytic pathways of bone resorption. (Reproduced from Marks and Popoff, *Am. J. Anat.*, (1988), with permission of the publisher A. R. Liss).

the ruffled border membrane (Anderson *et al.*, 1982; Baron *et al.*, 1985, 1986; Akisaka and Gay, 1986). Products of bone matrix and mineral degradation are taken back up into the osteoclast as digestive vacuoles and further digested through the action of secondary lysosomes. Thus, bone resorption involves both exocytosis and endocytosis at the ruffled border, processes that account for vacuolization of the vicinal cytoplasm.

The regulation of osteoclast function is poorly understood but presumed to involve local mediators (cytokines, growth factors and prostaglandins among others) produced in the skeletal microenvironment (Marks and Popoff, 1988). Osteoclasts, derived from the fusion of circulating mononuclear precursors (Marks, 1983), are among several distinct bone cell types. Because receptors for the classical hormones known to cause bone resorption (parathyroid hormone and 1,25(OH)2D) are found on osteoblasts not osteoclasts, a theory about osteoblast-directed osteoclast function has been developed (Rodan and Martin, 1981). Briefly, this states that osteoclasts are

Table 1. Congenital osteopetrosis in laboratory animals				
Species/Mutation	Genetic		Distinctive phenotype[*]	
	Symbol	Background (Chromosome)		
Mouse				
Grey-lethal	gl	GL/Le (10)	Grey coat	Lethal
Microphthalmia	mi	C57BL/6 (6)	Albino, blind	
Osteosclerosis	oc	B6C3 (19)		Lethal
Osteopetrosis	op	B6C3 (3)		
Rat				
Incisors-absent	ia	Long-Evans		
Osteopetrosis	op	Fatty/ORL		Lethal
toothless	tl	Osborne-Mendel		
Rabbit				
Osteopetrosis	os	Dutch/NZW		Lethal
[*] other than failure of postnatal eruption of some or all teeth				

activated indirectly by neighboring cells *via* the release of paracrine factors and osteoclasts are inactivated by direct contact with calcitonin and some prostaglandins for which they have receptors. There is increasing evidence for the indirect activation and direct inhibition of osteoclasts, including a role for both local cells (osteoblasts, osteocytes, hemopoietic cells, lymphocytes) and bone matrix components (osteonectin, osteocalcin, osteopontin, transforming growth factor-B, and various growth factors) in the recruitment and fusion of osteoclast precursors and their activation for bone resorption (Marks and Popoff, 1988). Thus, the ontogeny and function of osteoclasts involve a myriad of processes, events and mechanisms which must proceed smoothly for bone resorption to occur. Specific parts of this developmental cascade have been both intercepted and illuminated by mammalian osteopetrotic mutations, the best examples of mutations affecting osteoclast function.

Example - Mammalian Osteopetrosis

Overview and General Features

The mammalian osteopetroses are inherited disorders of bone metabolism resulting in osteoclast hypofunction and a net, generalized accumulation of skeletal mass (Marks and Walker, 1976). Mutations are found in both human beings and animals, the first having been described in an adult male in 1904

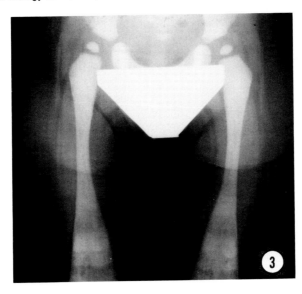

Fig. 3 Radiograph of a 1-year-old male with congenital osteopetrosis of recessive inheritance. Note the general skeletal sclerosis and the failure of development of marrow spaces in the femora. Taken from the Radiology Teaching Files, Univ. Massachusetts Medical School, Worcester, courtesy of P. Kleinman.

by the German radiologist Albers-Schönberg. The most severe forms of the disease in man and animals are of autosomal recessive inheritance. There are at least 8 distinct mutations in the common laboratory mammals and these are listed, along with their distinguishing features, in Table 1. Note that half these mutations are lethal. The earliest reports of the osteopetroses were essentially descriptive and it remained for Walker (1966) to provide the experimental bases for understanding the disease. His pioneering work set the stage for both the successful management of osteopetrotic children and modern osteoclast biology.

Osteopetrotic mutations have a number of biological and biochemical similarities. They invariably have a dense skeleton (Fig. 3). Characteristic radiographic features include generalized skeletal sclerosis and failure of development of marrow cavities. Surface contours of all bones are abnormal. Foramina are reduced in size and changes in bone shape (flares and curves) dependent upon bone resorption do not take place (Fig. 4). Instead, osteopetrotic mutants have club-shaped (4b) rather than flared (4a) ends of long

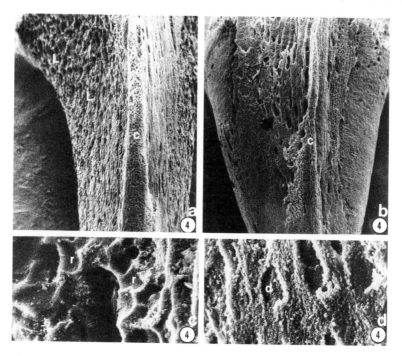

Fig. 4 Scanning electron micrographs of mineralized surfaces of anterior proximal tibiae from a 14-day-old normal mouse (4a,4c) and its osteopetrotic (op/op) littermate (4b,4d). Note that the concave, lateral flare (L) produced by surface resorption in the normal mouse (4a) is replaced by a convex surface in the mutant (4b). Vascular channels (arrows in 4b) penetrate both surfaces. At higher magnification, resorption pits (r) present in this area in normal mice are replaced in mutants (4d) by depressions (d) surrounded by knobby projections, characteristics of bone forming surfaces. c = tibial crest. a,b = 40X; b,d = 900X. (Reproduced from Marks, *Am. J. Anat.* **163**: 157, 1982 with permission of the publisher, A. R. Liss).

bones and bone surface features of resorption (4c) are replaced by bone formation (4d). Osteopetrotic individuals are resistant to the hypercalcemic effects of parathyroid hormone (Walker, 1966 a,b; Marks, 1977a) and 1,25 dihydroxyvitamin D ($1,25(OH)_2D$) (Key *et al.*, 1984; Popoff *et al.*, 1989). Reduced bone resorption is evident in both the failure of the features for which it is required in development (marrow cavity formation, long bone shape and tooth eruption; Marks, 1984) and in direct measurements of this parameter in several mutations (Marks, 1973, 1977a; Raisz *et al.*, 1977, 1981). A final common feature is significant elevations of blood levels of $1,25(OH)_2D$ (Fig.

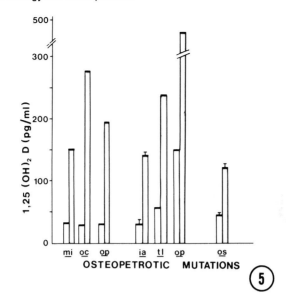

Fig. 5 Serum concentrations of 1,25 dihydroxyvitamin D in 7 mutations from 3 species. Data taken from Zerwekh *et al.*, *Bone and Mineral* **2**: 193, 1987 and figure reproduced from Marks, *Am. J. Medical Genetics*, (1989), with permission of the publisher A.R. Liss).

5) in all animal mutations (Zerwekh *et al.*, 1987) and children (Key *et al.*, 1984; Glorieux *et al.*, 1981) examined to date.

Significant differences among mutations include variations in severity of the disease (Table 1), blood calcium and phosphorus levels (Marks, 1990), rates of bone matrix formation (Marks and Walker, 1969, 1976), presence and degree of development of the ruffled border in osteoclasts (Fig. 6) and numbers of osteoclasts in several sites (Marks *et al.*, 1984). Some, but not all, hypocalcemic mutations have rickets (Ozdirim *et al.*, 1981; Reeves *et al.*, 1981; Zamboni *et al.*, 1977; Banco *et al.*, 1985; Milhaud *et al.*, 1981; Fig. 7).

The most significant discovery among the experimental manipulations of the osteopetroses was that parabiotic union of a mutant and a normal litter-mate (Fig. 8) dramatically reversed the skeletal sclerosis in the mutant without effect on the normal parabiont (Walker, 1972). Indeed, only temporary parabiosis was needed to cure osteopetrosis (Walker, 1973), a procedure which when transformed to bone marrow or spleen cell transplantation produced a cure in several animal (Walker, 1975 a,b,c; Marks, 1976; Milhaud

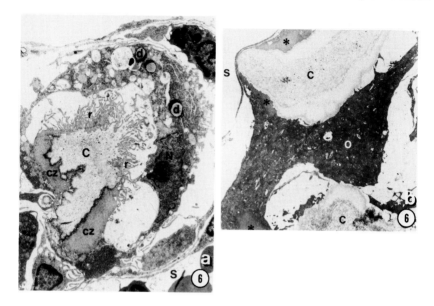

Fig. 6 Transmission electron micrographs of osteoclasts from op mice (6a) and *ia* rats (6b) illustrating the variable development of the ruffled border among osteopetrotic mutations. In *ia* rats (6b) osteoclasts (o) cannot develop ruffled borders next to bone or calcified cartilage (C) surfaces of metaphyseal trabeculae but instead exhibit extensive expanses of clear zones (asterisks). In op mice, on the other hand (6a), osteoclasts develop extensive ruffled borders (r) surrounded in 3-dimensions by clear zones (cz). Osteoclasts in both mutants are situated close to vascular sinuses (S) and op osteoclasts contain dense cytoplasmic vacuoles (d) of unknown composition. 6a = ×3000; 6b = ×2100. (Fig. 6a taken from Marks, *Am. J. Anat.* **163**: 157, 1982, with permission of the publisher A.R. Liss and Fig. 6b taken from Marks, *Clin. Orthop.* **189**: 239, 1984, with permission of the publisher J.B. Lippincott.)

et al., 1975) and human (Coccia *et al.*, 1980; Ballet *et al.*, 1977; Kaplan *et al.*, 1988) mutations. This cure did not prove to be universal as several mutations including those of children are not cured by these procedures (Marks, 1977b; Sorell *et al.*, 1981; Marks *et al.*, 1984; Seifert and Marks, 1987). This breakthrough, nevertheless, has been instructive in underscoring the heterogeneity of the osteopetroses and the complicated pathway of osteoclast ontogeny and function (see above).

This cursory overview of the mammalian osteopetroses illustrates their phenotypic heterogeneity. As demonstrated later a remarkable pathogenetic heterogeneity underlies this diversity of phenotype. Lest one conclude that the diversity is largely one of animal and not human mutations, consider that on

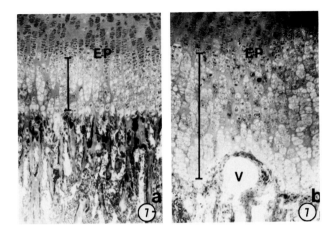

Fig. 7 Photomicrographs of the proximal tibial epiphyseal plate (EP) and metaphysis from a normal 10-day-old mouse and its osteosclerotic (*oc*) littermate. The zone of hypertrophic chondrocytes (vertical bar) is greatly increased and dilated subepiphyseal venous channels (V) are prominent in the *oc* mutant (7b) compared to its normal littermate (7a). These are cardinal histologic signs of rickets. ×75. (Reproduced from Seifert and Marks, *Am. J. Anat.* **172**: 141, 1985, with permission of the publisher A. R. Liss).

phenotype alone one can delineate at least ten different human osteopetroses as follows. Reports of juvenile forms have included lethal (Nussey, 1938) and non-lethal types (Loria-Cortes *et al.*, 1977), carbonic anhydrase isozyme II deficiency (Sly *et al.*, 1983) and parathyroid hormone resistance (Glorieux *et al.*, 1981), all inherited in an autosomal recessive manner. Adult expressions of the disease include severe (Lovisetto *et al.*, 1978), intermediate (Beighton *et al.*, 1979) and mild (Horton *et al.*, 1980) clinical forms of autosomal recessive inheritance, two different types of autosomal dominant inheritance (Johnston *et al.*, 1968; Bollerslev and Andersen, 1988) and a third one with viral inclusions in osteoclast nuclei (Mills *et al.*, 1988). Thus, a diversity of human osteopetroses can be identified using clinical, genetic and biochemical criteria. Unfortunately, little is known of the mechanism(s) of the human counterparts which are assumed, largely on extrapolations from animal studies, to be due to varieties of osteoclast incompetence. Most of these are indistinguishable radiographically (Graham *et al.*, 1973).

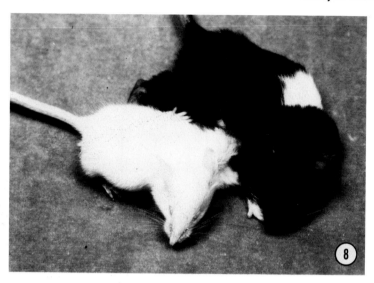

Fig. 8 Parabiotic union of a 6-week-old microphthalmic mouse (left) and its normal littermate (right). This treatment establishes a cross circulation between parabionts at the surgical site of union (arrows) and permits resorption of bone (cure of the disease) in the mutant without effect on the normal littermate. Reproduced from Marks and Walker, Ch. 6 of *The Biochemistry and Physiology of Bone*, vol. IV, 1976, with permission of the publisher Academic Press).

Mechanisms of Pathogenesis

The heterogeneous expression of the mammalian osteopetroses, illustrated above, becomes understandable within the context of osteoclast biology. Our present understanding suggests that osteoclast function in osteopetrosis is intercepted *via* two broad mechanisms; directly, by defects intrinsic to the osteoclast, and indirectly by defects extrinsic to osteoclasts, presumably involving cells and/or signals involved in osteoclast ontogeny or function. These categories correspond to those mutations cured by stem cell (bone marrow) transplantation from normal littermates (direct) and those not cured (indirect).

Direct

This category includes those mutations in which the defect resides in the osteoclast or its precursor (Fig. 1). As a result one would expect that these mutations are curable by a stem cell (bone marrow or spleen cell) transplant.

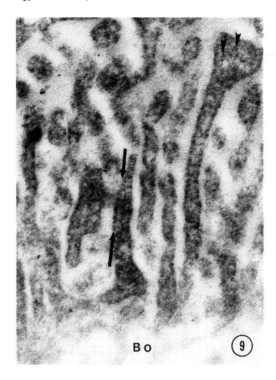

Fig. 9 Immunocytochemical localization of carbonic anhydrase on the cytoplasmic side of the ruffled border (arrow) membrane of an osteoclast. (Taken from Anderson *et al.*, *Anat. Rec.* **204**: 9-20, 1982 with permission of the authors and publisher, A. R. Liss. Kindly provided by C. Gay).

These situations are illustrated by the pioneering work of Walker (1973, 1975abc) which has been extended into clinical applications (Coccia *et al.*, 1980). Temporary parabiosis (Walker, 1972) of mutants and normal litter-mates or transplantation of normal spleen cells or bone marrow (Walker, 1975abc) has cured osteopetrosis in some animals (Marks, 1976; Milhaud *et al.*, 1975) and children (Coccia *et al.*, 1980; Sieff *et al.*, 1983; Kaplan *et al.*, 1988). Indeed the appearance in the recipient of both bone resorption and osteoclasts of donor origin (Coccia *et al.*, 1980; Sorrell *et al.*, 1981; Ash *et al.*, 1980; Marks and Walker, 1981) was sufficient evidence to establish that osteoclast progenitors were present in the spleen and bone marrow cells used for these transplants. The cure by temporary parabiotic union (Walker, 1972) was interpreted to mean that the cross-circulation provided by parabiosis for 2 weeks allowed competent osteoclast precursors to move from the normal to the mutant parabiont. The development of marrow spaces in the mutant two weeks after separation from parabiosis represented the time needed for the development of functional osteoclasts from circulating precursors which seeded to and differentiated in skeletal sites. The subsequent demonstration that normal spleen or bone marrow cells could cure osteopetrosis in a similar manner established these sites as sources of osteoclast precursors, at least under these conditions. Whether osteoclast precursors are continually derived from bone marrow and spleen throughout life, traveling to skeletal sites *via* vascular pathways, is at present only a presumption. Recent work using fluorescence-sorted cells has shown that those responsible for both the cure and the competent osteoclasts in treated mutants are hemopoietic stem cells (Schneider, 1985; Schneider *et al.*, 1986) of granulocyte-macrophage lineage (Schneider and Relfson, 1988a). These observations suggest that osteoclasts and macrophages may share a common progenitor early in development. Furthermore, future therapeutic options for certain osteopetroses may involve only transplantation of specific stem cell populations, reducing the risk of adverse consequences for the host. Considered together with data from mutations not cured by stem cell transplants (see below), we can look forward to treatment of osteopetrosis in the future by either specific stem cell transplant, infusion of a deficient matrix component into local sites or specific gene therapy, depending upon the nature of the lesion.

The significance of carbonic anhydrase in osteoclast function (see above) was solidified by its localization on the cytoplasmic surface of the ruffled border membrane (Anderson *et al.*, 1982; Fig. 9) and the demonstration that children without carbonic anhydrase exhibited osteopetrosis (Whyte *et al.*, 1980). The discovery of this recessive syndrome in children, consisting of renal tubular acidosis, calcification of the basal ganglia and osteopetrosis (Whyte *et al.*, 1980) secondary to a congenital absence of the second isozyme (CA II) of carbonic anhydrase (Sly *et al.*, 1983), underscored the importance of this enzyme. Osteoclasts in these patients fail to develop a ruffled border and the absence of CA II in these cells intercepts bone resorption. The identification of this syndrome showed not only the importance of CA II in resorption but spurred the subsequent identification of CA II as the isozyme in osteoclasts (Vaananen and Parvinen, 1983). While not specifically identified beforehand, it appears likely that one or more of the earliest osteopetrotic children treated successfully by bone marrow transplantation (Ballet *et al.*, 1977) could have had this syndrome of CA II deficiency.

Indirect

In these mutations, illustrated by resistance to cure by bone marrow transplantation, the defect is presumed to be extrinsic to the osteoclast. Potential candidates include matrix proteins and local factors (cytokines, growth factors) involved in the recruitment and activation of osteoclasts. Cellular candidates include osteoblasts, immune and mesenchymal cells known to produce numerous factors capable of affecting osteoclast function *in vitro* (Marks and Popoff, 1988). These mutations are excellent candidates for exploring the role of other cells/factors in osteoclast biology.

Numerous reports detail the matrix aberrations and mineralization abnormalities, including rickets (Fig. 7), in osteopetrotic mutations (Banco *et al.*, 1985, Ozdirim *et al.*, 1981; Bonucci *et al.*, 1975; Milhaud *et al.*, 1981; Van Slyke and Marks, 1987; Zamboni *et al.*, 1977) which cannot be explained on the basis of calcium and phosphorus levels alone. Furthermore, recent studies of bone and bone matrix have shown that macrophage colony stimulating factor (M-CSF) is markedly deficient in *op* mouse bone (Felix *et al.*, 1988), osteocalcin is reduced but osteopontin increased in bone from *tl* and *op* rat mutants (Lian *et al.*, 1987; 1988) and live *tl* rat metatarsals cannot support the development of normal osteoclasts *in vitro* (Osier *et al.*, 1987). All these mutations are resistant to cure by bone marrow transplantation. The significance of these findings remains to be established, but the emerging appreciation of the role of matrix products in cell differentiation and tissue development (Trelstad, 1985) underscore the significance that studies of osteopetrosis can play in determining the role of bone matrix as mentor in osteoclast biology.

The susceptibility to infection of osteopetrotic mutants (Reeves *et al.*, 1979; Marks, 1987) make them ideal candidates in which to explore immune influences on bone resorption. Immune dysfunction is suggested by reports of impaired intracellular bacterial killing (Reeves *et al.*, 1979; Coccia *et al.*, 1980; Key *et al.*, 1987) in children with osteopetrosis and reduced natural killer (NK) cell activity in osteopetrotic children (Sorell *et al.*, 1981; Key *et al.*, 1987) and animals (Schneider and Relfson, 1987; Stechschulte *et al.*, 1987; Popoff *et al.*, 1988). Interleukin-2 (IL-2) production by lymphocytes from one osteopetrotic child has been reported to be reduced (Key *et al.*, 1987), and infusions of recombinant IL-2 or normal bone marrow transplan-

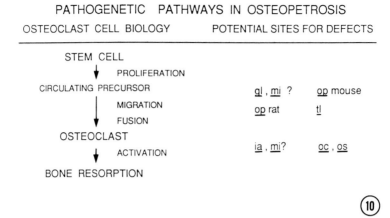

Fig. 10 Pathogenetic pathways for development of congenital osteopetrosis in 8 animal mutations based on interceptions of osteoclast development or function. Mutations are listed in two columns based on their ability to be cured (left) or not (right) by bone marrow (stem cell) transplantation from a normal littermate. Those cured by bone marrow transplants are presumed to have defects intrinsic to the osteoclast or its precursors. Those not cured by transplants are presumed to have defects extrinsic to these cells, presumably in the skeletal microenvironment. Mutations intercepting osteoclast development tend to have fewer osteoclasts whereas those involving osteoclast activation may have more osteoclasts per unit area of the skeleton than normal littermates. (Reproduced from Marks, *Am. J. Medical Genetics*, (1989), with permission of the publisher A. R. Liss).

tation can restore NK cell activity in *ia* rat mutants (Schneider *et al.*, 1988; Schneider and Relfson, 1988b). However, 1,25(OH)$_2$D is known to reduce IL-2 levels (Amento, 1987) and these effects could be secondary to the elevated blood levels of this hormone. Whether immune dysfunction in osteopetrosis is coincidental or causal remains to be established and will illuminate our understanding of the interactions of immune products and osteoclasts.

Reports of high blood levels of 1,25(OH)$_2$D in children (Glorieux *et al.*, 1981; Key *et al.*, 1984) and all animal mutations with osteopetrosis (Zerwekh *et al.*, 1987) coupled with their known resistance to the hypercalcemic effects of parathyroid hormone and 1,25(OH)$_2$D (see above) present unusual opportunities to explore the roles of these hormones in osteoclast ontogeny and biology. Studies of two other target tissues for these hormones, gut and kidney, have not shown resistance. Elevations of the renal 1-hydroxylase for 25 hydroxy-vitamin D in *oc* mice are proportional to the circulating levels of

1,25(OH)$_2$D, suggesting that increased synthesis is a major contributor to increased circulating levels. However, the renal enzyme is only partially suppressed by a high calcium diet suggesting aberrant regulation (Nesbitt *et al.*, 1988). In the intestine calcium binding protein levels in young *oc* mice and *tl* rats are significantly elevated commensurate with the elevations of 1,25(OH)$_2$D (Seifert *et al.*, 1986; 1988). Skeletal resistance to 1,25(OH)$_2$D has been reported in osteopetrotic rabbits (Popoff *et al.*, 1988) and some children (Key *et al.*, 1984; Key, 1987) where osteoclast numbers and bone resorption are variably elevated by chronic infusions of this metabolite. Osteoclast differentiation *in vitro* is known to depend upon 1,25(OH)$_2$D (Fuller and Chambers, 1987). Thus, the selective skeletal resistance of some mutants to 1,25(OH)$_2$D offers additional opportunities to explore the role of this hormone in osteoclast biology.

Summary

The potential sites/processes for interception of osteoclast development and function in congenital mammalian osteopetrosis are illustrated in Fig. 10. Reductions in osteoclast numbers can result from faulty migration, differentiation and/or fusion of precursors whereas small osteoclasts may represent a fusion disability (Fig. 1). With few exceptions, osteoclasts in osteopetrotic mutants have few cytoplasmic vacuoles and represent unactivated cells (Marks and Seifert, 1985). Fig. 10 also illustrates the probable sites of interception of osteoclast development and/or function represented by 8 osteopetrotic mutations in laboratory animals. The *gl* and *mi* mouse mutations have reduced numbers of osteoclasts which are smaller than those in normal littermates (Thesingh and Scherft, 1985; Green *et al.*, 1986) probably representing a defect in fusion. These mutants along with the *op* rat can be cured by bone marrow transplantation which suggests that the defect is intrinsic to the mutant osteoclasts. Osteoclasts in *op* mice and *tl* rats are small in both number and size. The reduction in G-CSF in *op* mouse bone, the inability of *tl* bone to support the development of normal osteoclasts *in vitro* (see above) and the failure of bone marrow transplants to cure either mutant suggest that matrix or microenvironmental factors (extrinsic to the mutant osteoclast) are responsible for reduced bone resorption. Osteoclasts in *ia* rats and *mi* mice cannot elaborate a ruffled border but resorption is restored and osteoclasts with ruffled borders appear after bone marrow transplantation (Marks and Walker, 1981; Marks and Schneider, 1982) showing that osteoclast stem cell incompetence underlies these two mutations. On the other hand osteoclasts in *oc* mice and *os* rabbits cannot be activated by PTH, 1,25(OH)$_2$D or bone marrow transplantation. These observations coupled with abnormalities of matrix in *oc* mice and osteoblasts in *os* rabbits (Marks *et al.*, 1987) strongly suggest matrix or microenvironmental defects.

Experimental investigations of osteopetrotic mutations have provided significant contributions to our understanding of osteoclast biology. Furthermore, the enduring enigmas of osteopetrosis bear witness to additional insights into osteoclast biology that studies of these mutations might provide.

References

Akisaka, T. and Gay, C. V. (1986) Ultracytochemical evidence for a proton-pump adenosine triphosphatase in chick osteoclasts. *Cell Tiss. Res.* **245**: 507-512

Amento, E. P. (1987) Vitamin D and the immune system. *Steroids* **49** :55-72

Anderson, R. E., Schraer, H. and Gay, C. V. (1982) Ultrastructural immunocytochemical localization of carbonic anhydrase in normal and calcitonin-treated chick osteoclasts. *Anat. Rec.* **204**: 9-20

Ash, P., Loutit, J. F. and Townsend, K. M. S. (1980) Osteoclasts derived from haematopoietic stem cells. *Nature* **283**: 669-670

Ballet, J., Griscelli, C., Courtris, C., Milhaud, G. and Maroteaux, P., (1977) Bone marrow transplantation in osteopetrosis. *Lancet* **ii**: 1137

Banco, R., Seifert, M. F., Marks, S. C. Jr. and McGuire, J. L. (1985) Rickets and Osteopetrosis: the osteosclerotic (*oc/oc*) mouse. *Clin. Ortho. Rel. Res.* **201**: 238-246

Baron, R., Neff, L., Louvard, D. and Courtoy, P. J. (1985) Cell-mediated extracellular acidification and bone resorption: Evidence for a low pH in resorbing lacunae and localization of a 100-kD lysosomal membrane protein at the osteoclast ruffled border. *J. Cell Biol.* **101**: 2210-2222

Beighton, P., Hamersma, H. and Cremin, B. 91979) Osteopetrosis in South Africa. The benign, lethal and intermediate forms. *S. Afr. Med. J.* **55**: 659-665

Bollerslev, J. and Andersen, P. E. Jr. (1988) Radiological, biochemical and hereditary evidence of two types of autosomal dominant osteopetrosis. *Bone* **9**: 7-13

Bonucci, E., Sartori, E. and Spina, M. (1975) Osteopetrosis fetalis. Report on a case, with special reference to ultrastructure. *Virchows Arch* **368**: 109-121

Coccia, P. F., Krivit, W., Cervenka, J., Clawson, C., Kersey, J. H., Kim, T. H., Nesbit, M. E., Ramsay, N. K. C., Warkentin, P. I., Teitelbaum, S. L., Kahn, A. J. and Brown, D. M. (1980) Successful bone-marrow transplantation for infantile malignant osteopetrosis. *New Engl. J. Med.* **302**: 701-7088

Felix, R., Hofstetter, W., Stutzer, A. and Fleisch, H., (1988) Impairment of macrophage colony-stimulating factor (M-CSF) production in the osteopetrotic *op/op* mouse. *J. Bone Min. Res.* **3**: Suppl 1, Abstr 264

Fuller, K. and Chambers, T. J. (1987) Generation of osteoclasts in cultures of rabbit bone marrow and spleen cells. *J. Cell. Physiol.* **132**: 441-452

Glorieux, F., Pettifor, J., Marie, P., Delvin, E., Travers, R. and Shepard, N. (1981) Induction of bone resorption by parathyroid hormone in congenital malignant osteopetrosis. *Metab. Bone Dis. Rel. Res.* **3**: 143-150

Green, P. M., Marshall, M. J. and Nisbet, N. W. 91986) A study of osteoclasts on calvaria of normal and osteopetrotic (*mi/mi*) mice by vital staining with acridine orange. *Br. J. Exp. Pathol.* **67**: 85-93

Horton, W., Schimke, R. and Iyama, T. (1980) Osteopetrosis: further heterogeneity. *J. Pediat.* **97**: 580-585

Johnson, C. C. Jr., Reeves, J. D., Wilson, D. W. and Wesenberg, R. L. (1968) Osteopetrosis: a clinical, genetic, metabolic, and morphologic study of the dominantly inherited, benign form. *Medicine (Baltimore)* **47**:149-167

Kaplan, F. S., August, C. S., Fallon, M. D., Dalinka, M., Axel, L. and Haddad, J. G. (1988) Successful treatment of infantile malignant osteopetrosis by bone-marrow transplantation. *J. Bone Joint Surg.* **70-A**: 617-623

Key, L. (1987) Osteopetrosis: A genetic window into osteoclast function. from: *CPC Series: Cases in Metabolic Bone Disease* **2**: 1-12

Key, L., Carnes, D., Cole, S., Holtrop, M., Bar-Shavit, Z., Shapiro, F., Arceci, R., Steinberg, J., Gundberg, C., Kahn, A., Teitelbaum, S. L. and Anast, C. (1984) Treatment of congenital osteopetrosis with high-dose calcitriol. *New Engl. J. Med.* **310**: 409-415

Key, L. L., Ries, W. L. and Schiff, R. (1987) Osteopetrosis associated with interleukin-2 deficiency. *J. Bone Min. Res.* **2**: Suppl 1, Abstr 85

Lian, J. B., Mackowiak, S., Teixeira, J. and Marks, S. C. (1988) Increased synthesis and accumulation of bone phosphoprotein in osteopetrotic mutants: Is this a consequence of elevated $1,25(OH)_2D_3$? *J. Bone Min. Res.* **3**: Suppl 1, Abstr 261

Loria-Cortes, R., Quesada-Calvo, E. and Cordero-Chaverri, C. (1977) Osteopetrosis in children: a report of 26 cases. *J. Pediatr.* **91**: 43-47

Lovisetto, P., Barese, V. and Marchi, L. (1978) Assay on the present clinical and nosographical aspects of osteopetrosis (Albers-Schünberg's disease). *Panminerva Med.* **20**: 213-222

Lucht, U. 91972) Osteoclasts and their relationship to bone as studied by electron microscopy. *Z. Zellforsch. Mikrosk. Anat.* **135**: 211

Malkani, K. , Luxembourger, M. M. and Rebel, A. (1973) Cytoplasmic modifications at the contact zone of osteoclasts and calcified tissue in the diaphyseal growing plate of foetal guinea-pig tibia. *Calcif. Tissue Res.* **11**: 258-264

Marks, C. R., Seifert, M. F. and Marks, S. C. III. (1984) Osteoclast populations in congenital osteopetrosis: additional evidence of heterogeneity. *Metab. Bone Dis. & Rel. Res.* **5**: 259-264

Marks, S. C. Jr. (1973) Pathogenesis of osteopetrosis in the *ia* rat: reduced bone resorption due to reduced osteoclast function. *Am. J. Anat.* **138**: 165-190

Marks, S. C. Jr. 91976) Osteopetrosis in the *ia* rat cured by spleen cells from a normal littermate. *Am. J. Anat.* **146**: 331-338

Marks, S. C. Jr. (1977a) Pathogenesis of osteopetrosis in the microphthalmic mouse: reduced bone resorption. *Am. J. Anat.* **149**: 269-276

Marks, S. C. Jr. (1977b) Osteopetrosis in the toothless (*tl*) rat: presence of osteoclasts but failure to respond to parathyroid extract or to be cured by infusion of spleen or bone marrow cells from normal littermates. *Am. J. Anat.* **149**: 289-297

Marks, S. C. Jr. (1983) The origin of osteoclasts: the evidence, clinical implications and investigative challenges of an extraskeletal sosurce. *J. Oral Pathol.* **12**: 226-256

Marks, S. C. Jr. (1984) Congenital osteopetrotic mutations as probes of the origin, structure and function of osteoclasts. *Clin. Ortho. Rel. Res.* **189**: 239-263

Marks, S. C. Jr. (1987) Osteopetrosis - multiple pathways for the interception of osteoclast function. *Appl. Pathol.* **5**: 172-183

Marks, S. C. Jr. (1989) Osteoclast biology: lessons from mammalian mutations. *Am. J. Med. Genetics* **34**: 43-54

Marks, S. C. Jr. (1990) Congenital Osteopetrosis, Mouse and Congenital Osteopetrosis, Rat. In: *Monographs on Pathology of Laboratory Animals. Vol 9, Skeletal System.* (Jones, T. C., Ed.) Springer-Verlag, New York, in press

Marks, S. C. Jr., MacKay, C. A. and Seifert, S. F. (1987) The osteopetrotic rabbit - skeletal cytology and ultrastructure. *Am. J. Anat.* **178**: 300-307

Marks, S. C. Jr. and Popoff, S. N. (1988) Bone Cell Biology: the regulation of development, structure and function in the skeleton. *Am. J. Anat.* **183**: 1-44

Marks, S. C. Jr. and Popoff, S. N. (1990) Ultrastructural biology and pathology of the osteoclast. In: *Ultrastructure of skeletal tissues. Bone and cartilage in health and disease.* (Bonucci, E. and Motta, P. M., Eds.). Boston: Kluwer Academic Publishers. pp. 239-252.

Marks, S. C. Jr. and Schneider, G. B. (1982) Transformations of osteoclast phenotype in *ia* rats cured of congenital osteopetrosis. *J. Morphol.* **174**: 141-147

Marks, S. C. Jr., Seifert, M. F. and McGuire, J. L. (1984) Congenitally osteopetrotic (*op/op*) mice are not cured by transplants of spleen or bone marrow cells from normal littermates. *Metab. Bone Dis. Rel. Res.* **5**: 183-186

Marks, S. C. Jr. and Seifert, M. F. (1985) The development and structure of osteoclasts in osteopetrosis. In: *The Chemistry and Biology of Mineralized Tissues.* (Butler, W. T., Ed.) Birmingham: EBSCo Media:408-410

Marks, S. C. Jr. and Walker, D. G. (1969) The role of the parafollicular cell of the thyroid gland in the pathogenesis of congenital osteopetrosis in mice. *Am. J. Anat.* **126**: 299-314

Marks, S. C. Jr. and Walker, D. G. (1976) Mammalian osteopetrosis: a model for studying cellular and humoral factors in bone resorption. In: *The Biochemistry and Physiology of Bone.* (Bourne, G. Ed.). Chap 6, Vol 4, 227-301. New York: Academic Press:

Marks, S. C. Jr. and Walker, D. G. (1981) The hematogenous origin of osteoclasts: experimental evidence from osteopetrotic (microphthalmic) mice treated with spleen cells from beige mouse donors. *Am. J. Anat.* **161**: 1-10

Milhaud, G., Labat, M., Graf, B., Juster, M., Balmain, N., Moutier, R. and Royama, K. 91975) Demonstration cinetique, radiographique et histologique de la guerison de l'osteopetrose congenitale du rat. *C. R. Hebd. Scanc. Acad. Sci. Paris* **280**: 2485-2488

Milhaud, G., Labat, M., Litwin, I., Moricard, Y., Moutier, R., Rimbaut, C., Buffe, D. and Juster, M. (1981) Osteopetro-rickets: a new congenital bone disorder. *Metab. Bone Dis. Rel. Res.* **3**: 91-97

Mills, B. G., Yabe, H. and Singer, F. R. (1988) Osteoclasts in human osteopetrosis contain viral-nucleocapsid-like nuclear inclusions. *J. Bone Min. Res.* **3**: 101-106

Nesbitt, T., Popoff, S., Drezner, M. K., McGuire, J. L. and Marks, S. C. Jr. (1988) Elevated renal 25 hydroxyvitamin D-1-hydroxylase in osteosclerotic (*oc*) mice and its suppression with a high calcium diet. *J. Bone Min. Res.* **3**: Suppl 1, Abstr 198

Nussey, A. (1938) Osteopetrosis. *Archs. Dis. Child.* **13**: 161-172

Osier, L. K., Popoff, S. N. and Marks, S. C. Jr. (1987) Osteopetrosis in the toothless rat - failure of osteoclast differentiation and function. *Bone and Min.* **3**: 35-45

Ozdirim, E., Altay, C. and Pienar, T. (1981) Osteopetrosis with rickets in infancy. *Turk. J. Pediat.* **23**: 211-218

Popoff, S. N., McGuire, J. L., Zerwekh, J. E. and Marks, S. C. Jr. (1989) Treatment of congenital osteopetrosis in the rabbit with high dose 1,25-dihydroxyvitamin D. *J. Bone Min. Res.* **4**: 57-67

Popoff, S. N., Koevary, S. B., Devore-Carter, D. and Schneider, G. B. (1988) Natural killer cell activity is reduced in the three osteopetrotic rat mutations and restored following normal stem cell transplantation in one. *Calc. Tissue Int.* **42**: Suppl. Abstr 46

Raisz, L. G., Simmons, H. A., Gworek, S. C. and Eilon, G. (1977) Studies on congenital osteopetrosis in microphthalmic mice using organ cultures: impairment of bone resorption in response to physiologic stimulators. *J. Exp. Med.* **145**: 857-865

Raisz, L. G., Simmons, H. A. and Hansen, C. T. (1981) Studies on congenital osteopetrosis in *tl* and *ia* rats using organ cultures. *Metab. Bone Dis. Rel. Res.* **3**: 117

Reeves, J. D., August, C. S., Humberg, J. R. and Weston, W. L. (1979) Host defense in infantile osteopetrosis. *Pediatrics* **64**: 202-206

Reeves, J., Arnaud, S., Gordon, G., Subryan, B., Block, M., Huffer, W., Arnaud, C., Mundy, G. and Haussler, M. (1981) The pathogenesis of infantile malignant osteopetrosis: bone mineral metabolism and complications in five infants. *Metab. Bone Dis. Rel. Res.* **3**: 135-142

Schneider, G. B. (1985) Cellular specificity of the cure for osteopetrosis: Isolation of and treatment with pluripotent hemopoietic stem cells. *Bone* **6**: 241-247

Schneider, G. B., Relfson, M. and Nicolas, J. (1986) Pluripotent hemopoietic stem cells give rise to osteoclasts. *Am. J. Anat.* **177**: 505

Schneider, G. B. and Relfson, M. 91987) Large granualr lymphocytes and natural killer function in *ia* osteopetrotic rats. *J. Bone Min. Res.* **2**: Suppl 1, Abstr 469

Schneider, G. B. and Relfson, M. 91988a) The effects of transplantation of granulocyte-macrophage progenitors on bone resorption in osteopetrotic rats. *J. Bone Min. Res.* **3**: 225-232

Schneider, G. B. and Relfson, M. (1988b) Natural killer cell function in *ia* osteopetrotic rats: effects of bone marrow transplantation. *J. Bone Min. Res.* **3**: Suppl 1, Abstr 260

Schneider, G. B., Relfson, M. and Ellis, T. (1988) Natural killer cell activity in (*ia*) osteopetrotic rats: effects of rIL-2. *Calc. Tiss. Int.* **42**: Suppl, Abstr 185

Seifert, M. F., Bruns, M. E. and Gray, R. W. (1986) Elevated 1,25-dihydroxyvitamin D, and calcium binding protein (CaBP) levels in two osteopetrotic mutations. *J. Bone Min. Res.* **1**: Suppl 1, Abstr 192

Seifert, M. F., Gray, R. W. and Bruns, M. E. (1988) Elevated levels of vitamin D-dependent calcium-binding protein (Calbindin-D9k) in the osteosclerotic (*oc*) mouse. *Endocrinology* **122**: 1067-1073

Seifert, M. F. and Marks, S. C. Jr. (1987) Congenitally osteosclerotic (*oc/oc*) mice are resistant to cure by transplantation of bone marrow or spleen cells from normal littermates. *Tissue and Cell* **19**: 29-37

Sieff, C., Levinsky, R., Rogers, D., Muller, K., Chessells, J., Pritchard, J., Casey, A. and Hazll, C. (1983) Allogeneic bone marrow transplantation in infantile malignant osteopetrosis. *Lancet* i: 437-441

Sly, W. S., Whyte, M. P., Sundaram, V., Tashian, R. E., Hewett-Emmett, D., Guibaud, P., Vainsel, M., Baluarte, J., Gruskin, A., Al-Mosawi, M., Sakati, N. and Ohlsson, A. (1983) Carbonic anhydrase II deficiency in 12 families with the autosomal recessive syndrome of osteopetrosis with renal tubular acidosis and cerebral calcification. *New Engl. J. Med.* **313**: 139-145

Sorell, M., Kapoor, N., Kirkpatrick, D., Rosen, J. F., Chaganti, J. S. K., Lopez, C., Dupont, B., Pollack, M. S., Terrin, B. N., Harris, M. B., Vine, D., Rose, J. S., Goossen, C., Lane, J., Good, R. A. and O'Reilly, R. J. (1981) Marrow transplantation for juvenile osteopetrosis. *Am. J. Med.* **70**: 1280-1287

Stechschulte, D., Sharma, R., Dileepan, K. N., Simpson, K. M., Aggarwal, N., Clancy, J. and Jilka, R. L. (1987) Effect of the *mi* allele on mast cells, basophils, natural killer cells and osteoclasts in C57Bl/6J mice. *J. Cell. Physiol.* **132**: 565-570

Thesingh, C. W. and Scherft, J. P. (1985) Fusion disability of embryonic osteoclast precursor cells and macrophages in the microphthalmic osteopetrotic mouse. *Bone* **6**: 43-52

Trelstad, R. L. (1983) Glycosaminoglyocans: mortar, matrix, mentor. *Lab. Invest.* **53**: 1-4

Vaananen, H. K. and Parvinen, E.-K. (1983) High active isoenzyme of carbonic anhydrase in rat calvaria osteoclasts. *Histochemistry* **78**: 481-485

Van Slyke, M. A. and Marks, S. C. Jr. (1987) Failure of normal osteoclasts to resorb calcified cartilage from osteosclerotic (*oc*) mice *in vitro*. *Bone* **8**: 39-44

Walker, D. G. (1966a) Elevated bone collagenolytic activity and hyperplasia of parafollicular light cells of the thyroid gland in parathormone-treated grey-lethal mice. *Zeit. Zellforsch.* **72**: 100-124

Walker, D. G. (1966b) Counteraction to parathyroid therapy in osteopetrotic mice as revealed in the plasma calcium level and ability to incorporate ^{3}H-proline into bone. *Endocrinology* **79**: 836-842

Walker, D. G. (1972) Congenital osteopetrosis in mice cured by parabiotic union with normal siblings. *Endocrinology* **91**: 916-920

Walker, D. G. (1973) Osteopetrosis cured by temporary parabiosis. *Science* **180**: 875

Walker, D. G. (1975a) Bone resorption restored in osteopetrotic mice by transplants of normal bone marrow and spleen cells. *Science* **190**: 784-785

Walker, D. G. (1975b) Spleen cells transmit osteopetrosis in mice. *Science* **190**: 785-787

Walker, D. G. (1975c) Control of bone resorption by hematopoietic tissue. The induction and reversal of congenital osteopetrosis in mice through use of bone marrow and splenic transplants. *J. Exp. Med.* **142**: 651-663

Whyte, M. P., Murphy, W. A., Fallon, M. D., Sly, W. S., Teitelbaum, S. L., McAlister, W. H. and Avioli, L. V. (1980) Osteopetrosis, renal tubular acidosis and basal ganglia calcification in three sisters. *Am. J. Med.* **69**: 64-74

Wittman, K. S., Krupa, P. L., Pesetsky, I. and Hamburgh, M. (1972) Electron microscopy and histochemistry of tail regression in the Brachyury mouse. *Develop. Biol.* **27**: 419-424

Zamboni, G., Cecchettin, M., Marradi, P., Foradori, M. and Zoppi, G. (1977) Association of osteopetrosis and vitamin D-resistant rickets. *Helv. Paediat. Acta* **32**: 363-368

Zerwekh, J. E., Marks, S. C. Jr. and McGuire, J. L. (1987) Elevated serum 1,25 dihydroxyvitamin D in osteopetrotic mutations in three species. *Bone and Mineral* **2**: 193-199

Index

iii

T

V

X